CULTURAL FORMULATION

CULTURAL FORMULATION

A Reader for Psychiatric Diagnosis

Edited by
Juan E. Mezzich
and Giovanni Caracci

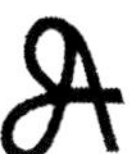

JASON ARONSON
Lanham • Boulder • New York • Toronto • Plymouth, UK

The preparation of this reader has been supported by the Veterans Administration VISN3 Mental Illness Research, Education, and Clinical Center (MIRECC)

Published in the United States of America
by Jason Aronson
An imprint of Rowman & Littlefield Publishers, Inc.

A wholly owned subsidiary of
The Rowman & Littlefield Publishing Group, Inc.
4501 Forbes Boulevard, Suite 200, Lanham, Maryland 20706
www.rowmanlittlefield.com

Estover Road
Plymouth PL6 7PY
United Kingdom

British Library Cataloguing in Publication Information Available

Library of Congress Cataloging-in-Publication Data

Cultural formulation: a reader for psychiatric diagnosis / edited by Juan E. Mezzich, Giovanni Caracci.
p. ; cm.
ISBN-13: 978-0-7657-0489-4 (cloth : alk. paper)
ISBN-10: 0-7657-0489-7 (cloth : alk. paper)
eISBN-13: 978-0-7657-0607-2
eISBN-10: 0-7657-0607-5
1. Cultural psychiatry. 2. Mental illness—Diagnosis—Social aspects. 3. Mental illness—Classification—Social aspects. 4. Diagnostic and statistical manual of mental disorders—Evaluation. I. Mezzich, Juan E. II. Caracci, Giovanni, 1952–
[DNLM: 1. Diagnostic and statistical manual of mental disorders. 2. Mental Disorders—diagnosis. 3. Mental Disorders—ethnology. 4. Cultural Diversity. 5. Mental Disorders—classification. WM 141 D8105 2008]
RC455.4.E8D76 2008
616.89′075—dc22 2007022379

Printed in the United States of America

™ The paper used in this publication meets the minimum requirements of American National Standard for Information Sciences—Permanence of Paper for Printed Library Materials, ANSI/NISO Z39.48-1992.

Contents

Acknowledgments

THE EDITORS ARE GRATEFUL to the following publications for permission to reprint materials used in this book. Some minor editorial changes were made, as deemed appropriate for an anthology of this kind.

- "Psychiatric Diagnosis: A Cultural Perspective" by H. Fabrega. From: *The Journal of Nervous and Mental Disease*, 175:383–394, 1987.
- "Cultural Context of Diagnosis and Therapy: A View From Medical Anthropology" by B. J. Good and M-J. Good. From: *Mental Health Resource & Practice in Minority Communities*, 1–27, 1986.
- "Help Seeking Pathways: A Unifying Concept in Mental Health Care" by L. H. Rogler. From: *the American Journal Psychiatry* 150:554–561, 1993.
- "On Illness Meaning and Clinical Interpretation" by A. Kleinman. From: *Culture, Medicine, and Psychiatry* 5:373–377, 1981.
- "On Culturally Enhancing The DSM-IV Multiaxial Formulation" by J. E. Mezzich and B. J. Good. From: *DSM-IV Source Book* 3:983–989, 1997
- "Cultural Comments on Multiaxial Issues" by P. Guarnaccia. From: *Culture and Psychiatric Diagnosis a DSM-IV perspective*, 335–338, 1996.
- "Cultural Formulation Development and Critical Review" by J. E. Mezzich. Original Paper.
- "Cultural Formulation of Psychiatric Diagnosis" by R. Lewis-Fernandez. From: *Culture, Medicine, and Psychiatry*, 20:133–144, 1996.
- "Cultural Formulation and Comprehensive Diagnosis" by J. E. Mezzich. From: *Cultural Psychiatry*: Psychiatry Clinics of North America 18:649–656, 1995.

- "Issues in the Assessment and Diagnosis of Culturally Diverse Individuals" by F. G. Lou. From: *The American Psychiatric Association Review of Psychiatry,* 14:447–510, 1995.
- "Framing Research on Culture in Psychiatric Diagnosis: The Case of DSM-IV" by L. H. Rogler. From: *Psychiatry,* Vol. 59, 145–154, May 1996.
- "The Place of Culture in DSM-IV" by J. E. Mezzich. From: *The Journal of Nervous and Metal Disease* 187:457–462, 1999.
- "Using the DSM-IV Cultural Formulation to Enhance Psychodynamic's Understanding" by G. Caracci. From: *Dynamic Psychiatry,* 245–256, 2000.
- "Introducing the Cultural Formulation to Mental Health Care in Stockholm, Sweden" by S. Bäärnhielm. Original Paper.
- "The Cultural Interview in Netherlands: The Cultural Formulation in Your Pocket" by H. Rohlof. Original Paper.
- "Psychosis Following Qi-Gong in a Chinese Immigrant" by R. F. Lim. From: *Culture Medicine and Psychiatry,* 20:369–378, 1996.
- "Diagnosis and Treatment of Nervios and Ataques in a Female Puerto Rican Migrant" by R. Lewis Fernandez. From: *Culture, Medicine, and Psychiatry,* 20:155–163, 1996.
- "Treatment of an Indian Woman with Major Depression by a Latino Therapist: Cultural Formulation" by M.A. Oquendo. From: *Culture, Medicine, and Psychiatry,* 21:115–126, 1997.
- "Cultural Formulation: Depression and Back Pain in a Young Male Turkish Immigrant in Basel, Switzerland" by M. G. Weiss. From: *Culture, Medicine, and Psychiatry,* 24:259–272, 2000.
- "Cultural Formulation Psychiatric Diagnosis: Sakit Jiwa Ng (Amuk) and Schizoaffective Disorder in a Japanese Woman" by K. O'Browne. From: *Culture, Medicine, and Psychiatry,* 25:411–425, 2001.

Introduction

THE PUBLICATION OF THE Cultural Formulation Outline in DSM-IV represented a significant event in the history of standard diagnostic systems. It was the first systematic attempt at placing cultural and contextual factors as an integral component of the diagnostic process. The year was 1994 and its coming was ripe since the multicultural explosion due to migration, refugees, and the impact of globalization on the ethnic composition of the U.S. population made it compelling to strive for culturally attuned psychiatric care.

Understanding the limitations of a dry symptomatological approach in helping clinicians to grasp the intricacies of the experience, presentation, and course of mental illness, the National Institute of Mental Health (NIMH) Group on Culture and Diagnosis proposed to appraise, in close collaboration with the patient, the cultural framework of patients' identity, illness experience, contextual factors, and clinician-patient relationship, and to narrate this along the lines of five major domains. By articulating the patient's experience and the standard symptomatological description of a case, the clinician may be better able to arrive at a more useful understanding of the case for clinical care purposes. Furthermore, attending to the context of the illness and the person of the patient may additionally enhance understanding of the case and enrich the database from which effective treatment can be planned.

This reader intends to assemble selected literature relevant to the Cultural Formulation originally published in the DSM-IV. Most of the selected articles appeared after the publication of DSM-IV, except the papers on background. The articles were selected for their theoretical relevance and patient care usefulness.

Structurally the reader is divided into the following sections:

I. Historical and Conceptual Background of the Cultural Formulation
II. Development and Characteristics of the Cultural Formulation
III. Reflections on and Prospects of the Cultural Formulation
IV. Clinical Case Illustrations on the Cultural Formulation

It is hoped that this reader will be a helpful component of a learning program on the DSM-IV Cultural Formulation. As such, it may contribute to enhance cultural competence for clinical care as practiced by younger and seasoned clinicians alike.

Part I

Historical and Conceptual Background of the Cultural Formulation

In this first part papers relevant to understanding the theoretical bases of the Outline for Cultural Formulation are presented. They argue for placing cultural considerations at the center of the diagnostic and therapeutic process.

Fabrega's (1987) paper on the cultural perspectives of psychiatric diagnosis is an acute analysis of the principles of categorization in medicine and psychiatry. It is clear that categorizing behavioral phenomena is far more difficult than that of most other domains. Much of the categorization of mental/behavioral problems is subject to symbolic interpretation in the context of the society and culture where these problems emerge. This seminal contribution lays a theoretical and conceptual groundwork for the cultural formulation as it posits the cultural framework as essential to understanding illness, its presentation and implications.

Good and Good's (1986) article zeroes in on the cultural context of mental illness, raising important questions about basic tenets of psychiatric diagnosis and interpretation of the meaning of symptoms. Their argument is that a meaning-centered anthropological approach can provide a critical perspective on controversial clinical issues that invariably surface in the evaluation and treatment of culturally diverse populations. Misdiagnosis and erroneous interpretation of culturally colored expressions of distress are viewed as especially prevalent in minorities and disadvantaged populations. Although anthropology and psychiatry have often been at odds over the issues of diagnostic interpretation, this paper succeeds in clarifying the importance of cultural meaning, which is at the very basis of a cultural formulation.

Rogler and Cortes's (1993) paper discusses the concept of help-seeking pathways viewed through the various phases of dealing with distress, and the engagement of social supports as well as of popular and professional healers. The process through which a mentally distressed person arrives at clinical services provides a glimpse at a culturally mediated itinerary that may be of considerable use to the clinician for adequate assessment and treatment. Centering their analysis on Puerto Rican immigrants, the authors extrapolate their observations to other ethnic groups. By broadening the scope of the discourse from the basic patient-doctor encounter to a larger multilayered interactive system, some of the bases of the cultural formulation are cogently presented.

Kleinman's (1981) paper on illness meanings and clinical interpretation makes a powerful argument for their place in effective clinical practice. Far from creating a stereotyped "rational man" for the clinician, he proposes that sensitively eliciting and interpreting complex illness meanings helps the clinician to understand and care. The author suggests that this process, which is similar to the anthropological approach of the ethnographer, has the potential to greatly humanize medical care.

Mezzich and Good (1997) offer a concise review of cultural considerations for the five axes of DSM-IV. The article attempts to make the case for understanding the cultural correlates of multiaspectual standardized diagnosis. It also highlights the limitations of applying measurement instruments that are not adequately validated in the setting where Guarnaccia's (1996) paper examines the cultural limitations of the DSM-IV axial system and proposes elements for an additional axis as a way to enhance the cultural applicability of the standard diagnostic system. In this context, he offers some helpful suggestions to increase the cultural validity and sensitivity of the multiaxial system. These include the assessment of language used, extent of acculturation, and the role of religion in the person's life.

1

Psychiatric Diagnosis

A Cultural Perspective

Horacio Fabrega, Jr.

TO A TRADITIONALIST, diagnosis involves using a body of knowledge and a system of classification based on that knowledge to appropriately name the clinical disorder that an individual shows to best initiate treatment. Each historical epoch relies on conventions and theories regarding diagnosis (King, 1963; Stevenson, 1965). In psychiatry we have come to rely on a medical biological model and currently use a multiaxial approach embodied in DSM-III. Modern psychiatrists as physicians are taught a body of biomedical knowledge and learn to use it critically and prudently. General theoretical questions implicit in diagnosis are often left aside or neglected altogether. Such questions implicate basic ontological and epistemological issues that apply to medicine; some of these have been covered in the literature (Brody, 1964; Dewhurst, 1966; Fabrega, 1976; Goodwin and Guze, 1984; King, 1963, 1970; Kraupl-Taylor, 1979, 1980; Temkin, 1973). In this study we emphasize diagnosis as classification and rely on theoretical ideas germane to the social and cultural sciences.

Any large group of individuals seeking evaluation and treatment in a mental health diagnostic clinic provides an opportunity for studying how the system of psychiatric diagnosis functions. In the study reported here, some of the analogies between psychiatric classification and diagnosis and related enterprises of classification in other fields are discussed. Theoretical aspects about illness classification in general and psychiatric illness classification in

From *The Journal of Nervous and Mental Disease* 175, no. 7 (July 1987)

particular are the central topics that anchor the discussion. In the analysis, patients are viewed not just as embodying a concrete illness or disorder that needs to be reduced to a diagnosis, but also as possessing a quantum of behavioral complexity that needs to be classified in a relatively unambiguous way. This is achieved by means of symbolic conventions tied to the knowledge base of modern psychiatry, generally, and to the current diagnostic rationale of DSM-III, more specifically. This study constitutes a theoretical account of psychiatric diagnosis viewed in a broad and comparative medical approach. In other words, the idea of illness having to be identified and treated using a culture's prevailing medical conventions is the general focus, and for this reason the study is judged as comparative. Studies that have focused on the way in which DSM-III functions empirically as a measuring system when it is applied to a large sample of individuals seeking psychiatric evaluation will be reported in subsequent publications.

Classification of Psychiatric Illnesses

Most phenomena in the world are heterogenous and not bounded naturally into groupings or classes; humans, through symbolic conventions, impose order on them. A preliminary step in classification is to delineate phenomena into classes that serve distinctive purposes and/or facilitate some sort of action. Such classes of phenomena, when viewed conceptually, may be termed "domains of interest." Objects in the domain of interest are assigned names or taxa and the latter are organized symbolically into nomenclatural and taxonomic systems. These generalizations are usually valid for classification of phenomena that are concrete, such as plants or animals, but are problematic in the case of phenomena that are abstracted from observations of the behavior of natural objects.

A taxon may be viewed as a named location in a taxonomic system. The system names and, by virtue of its organization, describes abstractly and more or less coherently a domain of interest in the real world. In thinking about a taxonomic system, then, we must keep separate the system from that of the "objects" that it references. In a taxonomy, only one taxon can occupy a particular position in the system. This is in contrast to the world of objects, where there exist many objects conforming to a particular taxa. As an example, one can consider a common type of taxonomy, one governed by the principle of class inclusion (hierarchical), which references plants in the real world. The "logic" of this type of classification allows one to say, for example, that an oak is a kind of tree, which itself is a kind of plant. In the hierarchical taxonomic system describing plants, however, there is only one taxon entitled "oak tree." At a level below this one in the system there may exist taxa designating *varieties* of oak trees (e.g., swamp, white oak, and other varieties), but at the higher level, only one oak taxon is found in the system. It should be clear that any number of concrete objects or entities in the world (i.e., in the domain of the system) provide an occasion for the application of a taxon. Thus, it is the case that many oak trees exist in a given location as well as swamp oak trees, and each one of these trees provides an occasion for the application of the taxon that names it. Looked at differently, a particular tree cannot be both an oak and a cypress. These examples allow one to claim that there is a direct link between the taxonomy and the worldly domain that it references. Thus, a one-to-one correspondence seems to exist between the taxa and the objects of the world (Berlin et al., 1973; Brown, 1986; Frake, 1961; Kay, 1973).

Some similarities to the above exist with respect to human medical illnesses as conceptualized in Western biomedicine. One can say, for example, that major depression with melancholia is a kind of major depression, which itself is a kind of affective illness in the hierarchical taxonomy of psychiatric illnesses, and psychiatric illnesses are referenced by the overarching taxonomy of human illness that include general medical and surgical illnesses. In the taxonomy of psychiatric illnesses there exists only one taxon, major depression, although varieties of major depression exist (e.g., major depression with melancholia). Moreover, the number of persons to whom can be applied the illness taxon major depression is also a large one indeed, just as there exist many oak trees to which its taxon can be applied. However, at this point, several differences emerge between the way taxonomies of natural objects are used and the ways taxonomy is used in medical care systems, generally, and Western clinical psychiatry, more specifically.

In a cross-cultural comparative or "ethnomedical" context, and also in Western medicine, a clinician-taxonomist attempts to diagnose sick people through the conventions of medical taxonomy. In a fundamental sense, the clinician deals with what we shall term "clinical conditions": he or she is attempting to diagnose ill individuals with a constellation of symptoms and distinctive histories. Given the primacy of the healer-patient relationship and the compelling exigencies of helping, there is a tendency for the clinician-taxonomist to judge that the "objects" classified through the use of his or her diagnostic system are sick individuals (whereas this is not the case, as elaborated below). However, sick individuals are not like plants or animals: objects, in other words, that are concrete, fully formed and static. Instead, the conventional taxa of a people's medical diagnostic system are applied to behaving (i.e., symptomatic) persons. Moreover, in Western biomedicine generally, and in contemporary psychiatric practice specifically, illness taxa are not like plant taxa that apply uniquely to a concrete plant; nor, for that matter, are they like names or social security numbers, *identifiers* that individuals receive or are assigned but once in their lives. Instead, one of several psychiatric illness taxa can be applied properly to a particular behaving, symptomatic person who presents with a clinical condition needing identification.

Human illness is an example par excellence of a domain of abstract "objects" set apart conceptually for important practical social reasons (Fabrega, 1974b). However, the phenomena we term human illness constitute a domain particularly difficult to classify insofar as units in the domain—actual occurrences of illness in space and time—are protean, dynamically changing, and they differ as to severity and duration. Taxonomies of illness in elementary societies appear to function much as do taxonomies of concrete objects. When brought to bear on systemically ill individuals, the taxa that comprise them generally reference one and only one individual who is judged as being ill with one and only one illness (Fabrega, 1979d). Of course, an illness has a temporal extension and, characteristically, its identity or name can change across time. However, in general, persons in elementary societies behave as though the clinical condition of the person ill has one name or identity. The contemporary biomedical taxonomy of illness is different in that individuals showing a clinical condition can be referenced by more than one of its taxa and this is taken to be an unproblematic issue.

Given the evolution of psychiatric knowledge in Western European societies, it seems clear that the taxonomy of psychiatric illnesses embodied in its diagnostic system has as its domain not a world of natural objects (i.e., clinical conditions of persons) but rather one of abstract, conceptual, and man-made objects (i.e., "ideal conditions of illness"). The interposition of a domain of ideal conditions of illness between the psychiatric diagnostic system, on one hand, and symptomatic sick persons, on the other, is what allows the psychiatric taxonomy of illness to function and operate in a manner one could term formally consistent. As a result of such an interposition, then, applying the taxonomy makes it possible for a person to embody more than one illness condition because the taxa of the diagnostic system do not strictly reference sick people (with clinical conditions) but rather (one and only one) ideal condition of illness. Between the taxonomic system and the conceptual domain of psychiatric illnesses, a one-to-one correspondence does exist, that is, one taxon, one ideal condition of psychiatric illness. However, the domain of real people stands at one stage removed from the medical psychiatric taxonomy. It is the case that between people and illnesses a *one-to-many relation* can exist in contradistinction to biological taxonomies wherein a one taxon-one natural object correspondence holds. The property of biomedicine to reference ideal conditions of illness and not persons creates problems and ambiguities, given the exigencies of medical diagnosis and treatment. The implications of the ambiguities inherent in what categories of the psychiatric system reference are discussed below.

Problems in Psychiatric Classification

Psychiatric Illnesses Are Not Manifest Concretely and Are Not "Frozen" or Static Entities

If human illnesses were like plants or animals, that is, like concrete, fully formed, and static biological entities that existed in nature as discrete and discontinuous phenomena, hence easily identified through one's sensory apparatus, then diagnosis would conform nicely to biological classification (Feinstein, 1967; Kraupl-Taylor, 1980). One might then be able to apprehend the concrete "natural object" referent of the taxonomy and merely label or point out (i.e., "identify") its properties. However, as already indicated, in a certain sense general medical and psychiatric illnesses, as construed in contemporary biomedical theory, are first and foremost conceptual and/or abstract objects that are manifest in behaving individuals. Behavior is not an object, but a set of actions that involve intentions, motives, and purposes, all of which are conditioned by social and cultural conventions. Although, as the architects of DSM-III have attempted to do, one may anchor behavioral descriptions in objective and clearly specified actions, this is often impossible.

The differences between the indicators of psychiatric and medical illnesses have been reviewed in other publications (Edgerton, 1966; Fabrega, 1972; Kendell, 1975).

Psychiatric Illness and Category Structure Models

Even if psychiatric illness were like concrete and "frozen" objects, a problem might still exist regarding its classification. This problem devolves from a consideration of what taxonomists mean when they speak of the traditional "in-or-out" model versus the prototypical model of category structure (Rosch and Lloyd, 1978). In the former, an object clearly does or does not belong in the category in question. As an example, a particular animal does or does not belong in the category "dog." The essence of "dogness" is discretely bound in nature and readily apprehended by our senses (and genetically determined). Because of this, one can relatively easily decide whether a referent animal is in or out of the category. On the other hand, in the prototypical model of category structure and definitions, one is confronted by "degrees of membership." Furniture, for example, constitutes a domain the entities of which appear structured in a prototypical way. Chairs, tables, and couches are prototypical members of this domain. Problematic candidates are certain types of stools or rectangular objects that can pass as chairs or couches. The criteria of the category and, hence, for determining membership are functional attributes involving home fashion items and living arrangements. In the prototypical model dealing with referents that more or less belong in a category, "degrees of membership" is a prevailing rule.

It is not clear whether the domain of psychiatric illness conforms to the traditional biological taxonomy model, the in-or-out model, or the prototypical model. A traditional perspective in medicine is the classical biological one and in psychiatry this rationale has been dominant in the past. It is ambiguous which category structure model underlies the formulation of DSM-III. In certain instances, criteria of illness are formulated as though the in-or-out model were the appropriate one. In other instances, however, reliance on inclusionary and exclusionary criteria suggests assumptions like those of both the prototypical and the traditional in-or-out category structure model (Cantor et al., 1980). For reasons that will be made clearer below, there are grounds for questioning which category structure model is appropriate in the case of psychiatric illnesses.

Psychiatric Illness and Cultural Conventions

Because many of the symptoms of psychiatric illness involve emotions, beliefs, intentions, or impulses, and acts or behaviors fully interpretable only in the light of symbolic conventions, it is difficult to specify criteria of illness that lead to clear boundaries. This problem is, of course, heightened significantly in the attempt to arrive at criteria that are general in nature, that is, ideally, universal. Cultural conventions about the self, reality, social rules, and patterns of emotional expression, for example, simply make universal criteria of psychiatric illness difficult to attain and the idea itself problematical (Fabrega, 1974a, 1975a, 1975b; Gillis et al., 1982; Hanck et al., 1981; Kleinman and Good, 1985; Morice, 1978; Murphy, 1976; Orley and Wing, 1979; Plog and Edgerton, 1969; Tseng and McDermott, 1981; Westermeyer, 1985). In the absence of clear boundaries between illness categories and instances of illness in individuals of differing biographical circumstances, it is difficult to develop and apply a general taxonomy of psychiatric illness regardless of its category structure mode.

A related problem involves what is normative in a social group. In a culturally pluralistic society such as that in the United States, it is difficult to establish norms, and norms appear necessary insofar as illnesses are framed in terms of indicators that entail deviations from norms (i.e., either group based or individual based; Fabrega, 1975a, 1975b; Mechanic, 1968, 1974). Even in the realm of neurovegetative behaviors (seemingly more "objective" and nonsymbolic behaviors) the problem of what is truly normal versus what constitutes a deviation still applies, creating problems for a taxonomist in search of clear category structures (Hanck, et al., 1981; Kleinman, 1982). Finally, it should be kept in mind that illness occurrences (manifest behavioral changes) are outcomes of underlying physiological, biochemical, and biophysical changes. The latter changes, which one may term *disease changes*, differ in severity and duration and manifest differently in individuals of different ages, genders, physical characteristics, and social backgrounds. A key factor influencing manifestations of illness is the individual's culture, which is "carried" in his or her mind and brain (Fabrega, 1979c). These factors all contribute to heterogeneity in the way an illness manifests, raising questions about the reliability and ease of diagnosis. Indeed, all of these factors underscore the differences between the classification of psychiatric illness versus that of concrete and relatively static and uniform natural objects that are referenced by biological category structure models (Eisenberg, 1977; Kleinman, 1980, 1982).

Psychiatric Illness and Historical Conventions

For purposes of this discussion, one can assume that psychiatric illnesses have been a component of human populations throughout recorded and unrecorded time (Haldipur, 1984; Jeste et al., 1985; Li Chiu, 1980). There are in fact reasons for entertaining the notion of phylogenetic precursors of human illnesses in general and psychiatric illnesses in particular (Fabrega, 1979a, 1979b). Be that as it may, it should be apparent that in thinking of psychiatric illness in terms of population and evolution, the issue of its genetics and biology is invoked. At this point, it is useful to introduce the idea of "theories of illness," an idea that appears to be universal in human cultures, and, more specifically, the idea of "biomedical theory of illness," which underlies the contemporary practice of medicine and psychiatry in modern nations influenced by European culture conventions (Kleinman, 1978; Kleinman et al., 1978; McEwan, 1980).

Such a theory of illness dominates psychiatric practice, and central to it is the assessment of a clinical condition as a possible illness (or of several illnesses). The latter may be related to a possible state (or states) of *disease*. A clinical condition of course may not meet criteria of illness, and many illnesses may, in turn, not yet be linked to clearly specified disease changes in the central nervous system. In line with the biomedical theory of illness, however, an assumption in psychiatry as in the rest of medicine is that a disease condition, that is, a neurological substrate having a genetic component, underlies an occurrence of illness. These disease changes are transformed into, or expressed in, altered behaviors that are maladaptive and socially dysfunctional and, in addition, psychologically as well as psychophysiologically disabling. In short, they are behaviors that constitute symptoms and that theoretically coalesce into illness pictures. A psychiatric illness, or several of them, is embodied in what we earlier termed a clinical condition of a person, which is the "object" the psychiatrist confronts and attempts to diagnose and treat. Moreover, it should be emphasized that it is clinical conditions, and not the ideal conditions of illness, that medical taxonomists and theoreticians ultimately rely on to develop category structures and that clinicians address to diagnose and treat. It is through the observation and study of "real" clinical conditions that "ideal" illness conditions are stipulated.

Western European societies have been under the influence of a variety of psychiatric taxonomists and clinicians (Jackson, 1969). We are still influenced by those eighteenth- and nineteenth-century taxonomist-clinicians who formally codified those clinical conditions of psychiatric illnesses the names of which we still use. It is important to emphasize, however, that they codified clinical conditions of persons that they equated with illnesses and that the latter, and not diseases, served as the referents of their category structures. Moreover, the illness picture (i.e., human behaviors of different types) that they used as data were influenced by the symbolic and cultural conventions of their times. For these reasons, the entities diagnosed by earlier psychiatric taxonomists can be seen as created on the basis of such conventions.

Given the above considerations, it is useful to reintroduce the idea of category structure models discussed previously. Should it not be the case that the category structure major depression, for example, is best judged as conforming to a prototypical category structure model and not to a traditional biological category structure model? Although underlying disease processes were operating, Kraepelin (1893) and then Bleuler (1911) were actually classifying clinical conditions consisting of illness pictures of different varieties. Moreover, the illness pictures at their disposal were conditioned by the prevailing symbolic rules, cultural conventions, and normative patterns of behavior. Their historically accessible depressions resembled earlier melancholia, versions that had in turn reflected prevailing conventions (Klibansky et al., 1964; Snyder, 1965). Our current attempts at category structure definition rely partly on their "prototypes," yet we appear to search for entities we judge to conform to traditional biological taxa. Perhaps we should acknowledge that clearly bound depression illness pictures conforming to the in-or-out category structure mode are not likely and that only instances that *more or less* fit a prototype model are possible. Many social symbolic rules are entailed in enculturation and brain maturation; all contribute to the formation of behavior. Hence, it seems reasonable to assume that there are many varieties of major depression continually changing over time (i.e., across historic epochs). In summary, if cultural conventions condition depressive illness manifestations, then it may be the case that, to the extent that earlier "prototypes" of depression anchor current efforts at category structure definitions, the model we should be using is not the in-or-out traditional category structure of biological taxa but the prototypical one. In the latter, illnesses more or less conform to prototypes that elude specification because of the influence of culture and changing culture and historical conventions that influence the content and form of behavior as well as its interpretation (Fabrega, 1974b, 1975a, 1977; Hanck et al., 1981; Kleinman, 1982; Lutz, 1981; Marsella and White, 1982). If and when truly biological markers, or indicators, of psychiatric *disease*-related phenomena are identified, then it may be the case that the in-or-out biological category structure model is the appropriate one for psychiatry, but even this is problematic.

Psychiatric Diagnosis as an Information Measuring Enterprise

Diagnosis in psychiatry can be conceptualized as an approach that involves codifying and measuring information. The rationale required, and the classification schema that implements it, embodies a system for organizing, through categories and ratings, a variety of clinical information about psychiatric disorders; and by extension, about individuals who potentially may manifest such disorders. In an ideal system, one would be provided with a rationale that allows one to codify clinical information such that the nature of the disorders, their treatment, and the factors bearing on overall prognosis would be specified. An ideal diagnostic system in this sense offers a "full" clinical statement about a patient and would allow one to predict the life course of the person diagnosed. In the discussion that follows, DSM-III will be used for purposes of illustration. It is handled as the discipline's current system and is assumed to be moving in the direction of an ideal system of psychiatric diagnosis. Psychiatric diagnosis and the resources of DSM-III specifically are examined as in the previous sections, from a general ethnomedical perspective.

The conceptualization that diagnosis in psychiatry can be likened to an information-measuring system will be illustrated from four separate but interrelated points of view: from that of the individual *patient*, from that of the *classification scheme* itself, from that of *illness conditions* or disorders, and from the standpoint of the *value or purpose* inherent in psychiatric diagnosis.

Viewed from the standpoint of a referred individual (i.e., a potential patient) who presents with what we have termed a clinical condition, arriving at a psychiatric diagnosis in terms of the categories and ratings of an ideal system (or as stipulated in the various axes of DSM-III) involves measuring the amount of information that is clinically relevant about that individual. In this light, the referred individual may be likened to a measure of "clinical uncertainty" that requires specification, and, ideally, measurement. The uncertainty inherent in the referred individual is, hopefully, significantly reduced by means of a full diagnosis, which is articulated in the form of entries in the various categories and ratings as illustrated in the five axes of the DSM-III system. One may assume that with an ideal system of diagnostic classification, the uncertainty posed by the referred individual would be eliminated through the assignment of a diagnosis, the specification of a treatment plan, and the stipulation of a prognostic statement, all of which are culturally and biomedically constituted by the diagnostic statement. These three types of information may be viewed as addressing the descriptive and predictive validity and the pragmatic clinical utility of any disorders that are present. Some of the problems involved in attempting to meet the requirements of an ideal system have been reviewed and are discussed further in this section.

The information-measuring aspects of psychiatric diagnosis can also be approached from the point of view of the classification schema. We have indicated that a diagnostic system is directed at a domain of nature that is more or less unlimited and has some significance to a human group. Leaving aside for the moment aspects of the domain of psychiatric illness, one can say that a classification schema can differ in a number of respects, such as the degree of comprehensiveness of coverage of the domain in question, the number of categories and their clarity of articulation, and the mutual exclusivity of these categories. Notwithstanding issues tied to general and specific criteria of illness, some of the problems that a psychiatric diagnostic system may encounter when it is handled purely as a classification system can be surmised. The system of categories designating disorders, as currently handled in axis I, may not be sufficiently exhaustive to cover all possibilities of illness; the boundary between its domain and that of nonillness may not be sharply covered by available categories. Some of the categories of illness may partially overlap with others, and still other categories may be conjoined with such regularity that they may, for this reason, be said to be redundant. Moreover, controversy may exist over how clearly some categories are articulated and distinguished from others, whether categories are omitted that should not be, and, lastly, whether certain categories may coexist together in one person as is currently the case with DSM-III.

In an ultimate sense, the information-measuring properties of a psychiatric diagnostic system, viewed purely from the standpoint of the classification schema, depend on how accurately the schema captures and allows the specification of the whole domain of psychiatric illness. For example, the rationale followed in the classification of upper body garments in terms of neck circumference and sleeve length reflects the domain of human male upper torsos reasonably well, although some individuals' shirts may be fitted better than others. However, how well this classification system fits the domain in question is ascertainable given the role that a metric system of measurement plays in it. The domain is always richer and more varied than the classification schema because the latter is an abstraction of the former. Shirts, for example, come in different colors and styles and are worn for many purposes, but the system used for classifying them need not make reference to all of this. The purposes of any classification system, especially that of human illnesses, are obviously of fundamental importance. Equally important is that the rationale of a classification cull essential features or criteria of its domain.

This leads to a third way of examining a psychiatric diagnostic system as an information system: from the standpoint of how well it handles the "objects" of its domain, namely, specific psychiatric illnesses. One must keep in mind that in some respects it is largely through a classification schema (and its underlying rationale) that one, through specification, comes to understand a domain of nature and that this is especially true with respect to man-made objects (i.e., abstract and culturally constituted objects). We have already made reference to the importance of singling out criteria of psychiatric illness, a task made especially difficult for reasons involving the nature of symbolic behavior that were covered earlier. In addition, it is important to reemphasize that a system of psychiatric diagnosis should ideally purport to offer a means of arriving at a "full" clinical statement about a patient. However, the system is itself finite and may omit many types of clinically relevant information about human adaptation.

In the rationale of DSM-III, arriving at a diagnosis is conceptualized as an initial step in a comprehensive evaluation and it is explicitly acknowledged that other types of information will be necessary. As an example, the clinician who uses DSM-III is only partially (and then only in certain instances) guided by information pertaining to family history, intellectual ability, emotional control, or cognitive-attentive clarity. All of the latter parameters play a role in the way an ill individual adapts and functions; however, they are (in most instances) conceptualized as falling outside the specific confines of the functions or purposes of DSM-III. The value of a psychiatric diagnostic system viewed as an effective measuring and pragmatic system is enhanced to the extent that it handles such factors clearly and unequivocably. When all relevant data about psychiatric disorders, as they pertain to the individual patient, are retrieved and measured through a diagnostic system one would be provided with a full clinical interpretation.

Some of the issues discussed so far can be seen as outcomes of the problem mentioned earlier involving the domain of a psychiatric diagnostic system. We have indicated that the rationale, as well as the objects, of a psychiatric diagnostic system is ambiguous. We suggest that the objects that the system references are idealized illness entities; yet these can only be realized or manifested in behaving (i.e., symptomatic) persons and what earlier were termed clinical conditions. Clinical conditions embody one or several varieties of illness, the criterial features of which can be difficult to specify precisely. Moreover, illnesses embodied in the same clinical condition are likely to influence each other and adaptation of the person in ways difficult to specify. Finally, an illness is itself the outcome, and a cultural interpretation, of a posited disease entity or process that is difficult to specify and map precisely because such undertakings require understanding disease outcomes in illness behaviors. An indeterminancy thus obtains at every level of examination of a psychiatric problem (i.e., at level of clinical condition, at level of illness, and at level of disease), and interlevel analyses are also required for full understanding. To be sure, even if a clinical condition were known to embody only one psychiatric illness and one disease, the parameters for arriving at a "full" clinical statement of the ill person require many different types of information that is complex and difficult to obtain currently. Therefore, the goal of an ideal diagnostic statement, that is, a complete clinical description of the person, is very difficult to achieve. Stated differently, the varieties of information bearing on human adaptive behavior generally, and on the effects of psychiatric illness specifically, limit the level of descriptive and especially of predictive validity that psychiatric entities can attain.

When one attempts to evaluate the informational value of a psychiatric diagnostic system from the standpoint of how well it embraces its domain of psychiatric illness, some of the limitations in our understanding of psychiatric illness become clearer. For example, earlier it was indicated that a diagnostic system is directed at a domain of human concern. However, how clearly the domain of psychiatric illness is separated from "normal" adaptive social behavior from maladaptive but nonillness behavior, from illness but not specifiable disease centered behavior, and lastly from nonpsychiatric but other medical illness behaviors is very problematic. In referring to the clarity of the domain of a psychiatric diagnostic system viewed purely as a taxonomy, the behavioral problems linked to social deviance and somatization immediately come to mind as well as the basic fact that the nature and relation of psychiatric illness to other medical conditions is imperfectly understood. How can a psychiatric diagnostic system viewed as a classification schema be expected to reflect accurately the domain of psychiatric illness if this domain is simply not yet well understood? Setting these limitations aside, one would judge highly the information-measuring value of psychiatric diagnosis to the extent that it accurately captures current understanding of its domain (psychiatric illness) and to the extent that it omits misclassifying material from other related domains (i.e., that of nonillness and/or nonpsychiatric illness).

In summary, the objects of a psychiatric diagnostic system are ideal conditions of illness. Knowledge about them is abstracted from observations of sick individuals showing clinical conditions that are affected by a number of factors logically unrelated to such illness entities. All of the problems related to an understanding of the behavior of psychiatric illnesses (i.e., involving manifestations, diagnosis, course, duration, and treatment outcome) need to be seen as a consequence of the fact that because such illnesses are ideal entities they are never observed directly. However, we think of and refer to these illnesses as though they were real and natural objects. A diagnostic system may be judged favorably to the extent that its ideal objects are easily identified in natural settings and their effects or consequences in such settings are well understood. This amounts to saying that the realizations of ideal illnesses in people (as clinical conditions) conform to expectations derived from the rationale and knowledge base embodied in the diagnostic system. A lack of perfect fit between ideal illnesses and real instances of them in the natural world of people can be expected given the complexity of the diagnostic enterprise as illustrated by a review of selected problems above (also see below).

A fourth way one may conceptualize the informational aspects of a psychiatric diagnostic system is from the standpoint of questioning the reasons for diagnostic classification. Viewed generally, diagnosis is an aspect of biomedicine, an institution with a body of scientific knowledge of Western European societies that evolved, literally, to eliminate illness problems. Illness problems are, in a fundamental sense, culturally constituted or created through diagnosis to be eliminated ultimately from nature. More specifically, physicians and researchers, as agents of the social/biomedical system of medicine, diagnose to study, treat, and thereby, hopefully, ameliorate and/or eliminate the condition of illness that was diagnosed. We earlier pointed to unique features of the "objects" referenced by psychiatric diagnosis (e.g., their dynamic and protean versus concrete and static quality). The eliminating feature of medical diagnosis also sets it apart from most other forms of classification, which do not aim to eliminate their objects. Be that as it may, this property of biomedical diagnosis of necessity requires an analyst to inquire about the efficacy of treatment because this is the fundamental purpose of medical diagnosis. In this light, the informational value of a psychiatric diagnostic system may be judged as good to the extent that instances of diagnosis, by means of its categories, ratings, and so on, lead unambiguously to clearly articulated treatment plans that are, moreover, clearly efficacious. One would judge the measurement of clinical information as low if only a small proportion of diagnosed entities (be they persons or disorders) could be linked to an identifiable treatment plan that offered the possibility of amelioration. On the other hand, it is obvious that a psychiatric diagnostic system constitutes an evolving theoretical and empirical "object" that aims to eventually provide a means for arriving at a full understanding of psychiatric illness. A diagnostic system such as DSM-III, which is in a stage of evolution, provides illustrations of this fact. DMS-III allows the clinician to specify clearly any number of conditions for which there is no effective treatment (e.g., paraphilias). Clearly, DSM-III is providing a means for conducting research aimed precisely at improving treatment plans.

That these four ways of viewing psychiatric diagnosis as an information system are interrelated and not mutually exclusive should be clear. This can be illustrated by drawing emphasis to a basic guiding assumption, namely, our level of understanding of psychiatric illness. We emphasize that known psychiatric disease conditions may be imperfectly codified because their manifestations are imperfectly known. New illness conditions may come to be discovered not only because our understanding will improve but also because new illness conditions will arise and/or be caused, given the potential changes that take place in the mixture of factors that can produce illness and the continuous modification of the ecosystem that societies bring about, although the genetically anchored stability of brain anatomy and physiology pose obvious limits to variability. For this reason, it is impossible to specify treatment plans for many illness conditions let alone specify and articulate their properties clearly. A basic purpose in the development of a psychiatric diagnostic system is to refine the description of entities so as then to be able to develop treatment-oriented research studies. Thus, on purely a priori grounds, one can stipulate that the value of a natural (i.e., not ideal) diagnostic system like DSM-III, viewed purely as an information codifying and measuring system, will show large limitations if specificity of treatment plan is used as a criterion. And, to reemphasize, insofar as the domain of a psychiatric diagnostic system is imperfectly known *and changing*, then using as a criterion of informational value elements drawn purely from the schema of classification itself (e.g., its comprehensiveness, degree of clarity, etc.) also proves problematic because it will never fully capture a domain that itself is changing and ultimately unknown other than by means of the classification system itself. More mundane issues in judging a psychiatric diagnostic system in information terms can be surmised. Thus, if persons can show more than one illness, and the clinical effect of co-occurrence (e.g., manifestations, severity, response to treatment) is not well-known, then evaluation of the information-measuring aspects of the diagnostic system from the standpoint of illness conditions and ill individuals is made difficult to the extent that illness entities can co-occur in individuals. The problems of multiple diagnoses and the related problem of changing diagnoses are additional factors that require consideration.

Problem of Multiple and Changing Psychiatric Diagnoses

An individual seeking a psychiatric evaluation is guided by one or both of two sets of considerations: (a) a perceived sense of psychological need or of troubling symptoms and/or (b) a perception followed by a recommendation on the part of another that such a need exists. In either case, it is reasonable to assume that both perceptions are grounded in the basic assumption that an individual is a whole psychological-behavioral entity and the person as a whole is coterminous with his or her problem or psychological illness. In brief, the phenomenology of self is intricately linked to the idea and experience of psychiatric illness. This fact needs to be examined in a broad cultural-medical frame of reference so as to better appreciate problems related to the idea of multiple diagnoses in psychiatry.

By definition, general systemic physical illnesses are linked to the body and disorders in it give rise to an *experiential whole.* This of course is the reason that, in simpler societies, individuals showing systemic disease changes are ordinarily seen as having one, and only one, illness (i.e., are named by one and only one illness taxon). Insofar as the body is a concrete entity with anatomically distinct parts and organs that are differentiated perceptually and hence conceptually, and given that the body has a particularized sensorimotor representation, people of simpler societies will usually think of fractures, contusions, and discretely localizable lesions and/or pains when present together as multiple ailments but not as true illnesses. Their general orientation to such discrete pains and/or ailments as opposed to an experientially and whole illness is very different (Ohnuki-Tierney, 1981). To some extent, these generalizations apply to reports of how people in earlier premodern Europe dealt with medical phenomena (Forbes, 1979; MacDonald, 1981; Thomas, 1971; Veith, 1965; Walker, 1981). When one takes into account this holistic basis for illness experiences, one can appreciate the power of biomedicine viewed purely as a system of social symbols (Eisenberg, 1977; Kleinman, 1973). Among other things, these symbols make possible the idea of an underlying physical disease that can be asymptomatic and the idea of multiple diseases underlying clinical conditions of persons that are usually experienced as whole entities.

To a modern Western European enculturated person, then, biomedically produced knowledge and beliefs about the body as an anatomical, physiological, and biochemical structure leads easily to ideas of multiple parts, segments, and/or functions. Phenomenologically, the particularized sensorimotor representation of the body provides complementary evidence, in the way of variegated sensations and awareness of body functions that can make the idea of multiple physical disorders a natural one even though the total illness experience is holistic. It is necessary to emphasize the cultural (i.e., symbolic) basis of these allegedly medical "facts." In other words, biomedical knowledge has profound implications for the ontology of a medical problem and such problems are conceptualized, experienced, and responded to differently in societies governed by different medical symbol systems (Brody, 1981; D'Andrade, 1984; Eisenberg and Kleinman, 1981; Fabrega, 1976, 1977, 1979c; Geertz, 1973; Lakoff and Johnson, 1980).

In contrast to general medicine, where the idea of multiple diseases is relatively unproblematic, in psychiatry this idea can prove awkward given quandaries devolving from the mind/body problem. We reiterate that in a formalistic sense (i.e., as stipulated by biomedical theory), multiple psychiatric diseases or disorders prove no more difficult to conceptualize than multiple physical disorders. However, given the nature of the assumptions about the self, individuality, and the mind that have evolved in Western European societies, the notion of multiple psychiatric disorders proves existentially cumbersome. An individual's reflexive powers and his or her sense of personal wholeness and identity compellingly lead to the assumption that a perceived psychological/behavioral problem or need may reflect the existence of a single disorder or illness. Psychological functions such as affect, cognition, perception, and will are not easily separable subjectively, and, of course, most behavior is felt and conceptualized as a whole. In brief, the domain of psychiatric illness incorporates the self and its social extensions in a unique way, and the latter sets apart psychiatric from general medical phenomena in spite of the fact that a similar underlying theory of illness is operative. The implications of the point have already been discussed and will not be elaborated further. Notwithstanding these special aspects of psychiatric illness, a reasonable question to raise is whether any additional problems attach to ideas of (a) multiple psychiatric diagnoses or (b) changing psychiatric diagnoses over time in an individual.

Multiple Diagnoses

An analysis of the question of multiple diagnoses brings into play fundamental epistemological and ontological questions linked to psychiatric practice already mentioned. The biomedical theory of illness embodied in DSM-III is similar to that of general medicine and in it the possibility of multiple disorders is unproblematic. Consequently, just as an individual can be ill with pneumonia and coronary heart disease, as an example, so an individual can, in theory, have more than one psychiatric illness (e.g., major depression and schizophrenia). However, with regard to psychiatric classification with DSM-III, one notes stipulations in the form of exclusionary criteria that make the coexistence of certain disorders impossible (Boyd et al., 1984). Such criteria, perhaps understandable in view of accumulated knowledge about psychiatric illness, represents a restriction on the "free play" of DSM-III as a taxonomy. In other words, the frequent coexistence of symptoms conforming to disorders such as schizophrenia and affective disorder, obsessive-compulsive disorder and major depression, and/or affective and anxiety disorders points to problems in our theory of psychiatric illness and in our assumptions underlying classification and taxonomy since restrictions are often placed on which diagnoses may coexist at one point in time. Quandaries devolving from the similarities that can exist between functional versus organic clinical pictures provide a related example. It is obvious that problems resulting from the interpretation of symbolic behavior that were discussed earlier play a large role in how clearly boundaries can be established between certain psychiatric illnesses. Finally, a number of DSM-III disorders are considered secondary, reactive, or adjunctive to other, presumably primary, disorders; for example, substance use disorders, dissociative disorders, psychological factors affecting physical illness, and even somatoform disorders can, in some instances, be conceptualized as secondary to others (e.g., depression, anxiety). Given our imperfect knowledge about traditional entities in psychiatry, it is not always clear which disorders are primary, which are secondary, and which together may reflect one larger more encompassing disorder. It is certainly the case that certain disorders frequently judged as secondary (e.g., those involving abuse of substances) can occur independent of other more traditional ones (i.e., as primary or autonomous) and that there is considerable information suggesting that either of the two need to be seen as quintessentially biological entities.

Changing Diagnoses

Logical and empirical quandaries tied to the issue of multiple diagnoses (of psychiatric illness) play a large role in one's understanding of the question of stability of psychiatric diagnoses over time. Here, as it were, the matter of theoretical and conventional versus empirical boundaries between the coexistence of psychiatric illnesses is simply spread out in time. Rather than constituting a dilemma in the *cross-sectional* analysis of psychiatric disability it becomes one in the *longitudinal* analysis and understanding of psychiatric disability. An important question, in fact, becomes whether diagnostic categories confounding an understanding of a patient's condition at one point in time play a similar role in the understanding of a patient's condition at a later point in time when presumably a "natural history" of the underlying disease processes has had an opportunity to further unfold. Do the categories that confound understanding at one point in time persist in salience, do they disappear to be replaced by others, and, lastly, do the possible roles of primary versus secondary diagnoses become untangled and more clearly bound as time elapses? Such questions have to be answered in light of the knowledge that, insofar as psychiatric illnesses are culturally constituted behavioral entities, they are of necessity influenced drastically by happenings in the social system, not only in the long run, as the earlier discussions have emphasized, but also in the short run, as research involving the course of schizophrenia has made clear (Sartorius et al., 1977).

Summary and Conclusions

In this study we have looked at the enterprise of medical and especially psychiatric diagnosis as this is conducted within biomedical theory with an emphasis on theoretical issues. Throughout the study, diagnosis as classification was the focus of analysis. Users of the biomedical theory appear to assume that the basic or fundamental happenings pertaining to human health take place at a physiological, biochemical, and/or biophysical level. When these happenings are disturbed or negatively altered, they constitute states or conditions of "disease" that humans label by means of biomedical conventions. How discrete and clearly autonomous or bound are disease changes in man is highly problematical. The next happenings of medical significance above this in the hierarchical system are termed "illness" and consist of disordered behaviors of different varieties. Not all disease changes readily manifest as illness phenomena, but an assumption in the theory of biomedicine is that a clearly specified illness has a given substrate of disease. Illnesses can occur singly or multiply in a human being, but in either instance they present as "clinical conditions," which clinician-taxonomists must classify and name according to their taxonomy. In psychiatry, this is embodied through the use of the prevailing diagnostic system. A psychiatric diagnostic system has thus been handled here as a rationale and device that a clinician-taxonomist brings to bear to a clinical condition and his or her task is to identify and name the illness entities that are accounting for the clinical condition of the person. We have emphasized that a medical and psychiatric diagnostic system is a cultural object that constitutes abstract clinical entities based on distinctive symbolic conventions.

Some of the theoretical issues involved in handling psychiatric diagnosis as a problem of classification and by means of a taxonomy have been discussed. The type of category structure model that appears to underlie psychiatric diagnosis was given attention. The similarities and differences between the use of biological versus medical and psychiatric taxonomies were also given attention. The special problems linked to psychiatric classification and diagnosis because of its reliance on behavioral indicators of illness (versus biological markers of disease) were emphasized in particular. Some of the problematical aspects devolving from the notion that psychiatric diagnoses can be applied singularly and/or multiply to persons were also discussed. The thrust of the discussion has been the variety of theoretical and empirical problems embodied in rendering accurate and valid clinical psychiatric diagnoses by means of a psychiatric diagnostic system. Moreover, throughout the study, the assumption that in certain ways psychiatric diagnosis can be conceptualized as an information-measuring enterprise was used implicitly and explicitly. This view of psychiatric diagnosis as an information-measuring system will be handled empirically in a future study.

Medical and especially psychiatric diagnosis in biomedical theory presents a scientific dilemma that is difficult to resolve and yet one that, despite its problems, researchers must endeavor to work around. The opposing issues in this dilemma, to a large extent implicit in this study, can be articulated in different ways. In this light, it is fruitful to consider the following two sets of questions. On the one hand: How "messy" is the domain of clinical conditions of persons? Recall that a "clinical condition" is a potentially complex entity comprising one or several illness occurrences. Similarly, consider the following question: How frequently do disease states appear singly versus multiply underlying a particular condition? Finally, one can pose the following: How "clean" is the domain of clinical conditions such that it can be explained by the employment of a single diagnosis? Opposed to these questions are the following: How well partitioned is the psychiatric classification system and how well-defined are its categories such that they enable the clinician-taxonomist to apply them singularly so as to fully account for the clinical uncertainty posed by the clinical condition of a person? Alternatively, how ambiguous and overlapping are the categories of a diagnostic system such that they require the clinician to use them together to explain clinical conditions?

These two sets of questions address scientific problems intrinsic to the domain of human illness and scientific questions intrinsic to illness classification, respectfully. At the same time, the two sets of questions encompass a dilemma posed by human illness diagnosis as this is made possible through the biomedical system of medicine, generally, and psychiatric diagnosis, particularly, a system that in theory allows partitioning the body into ever smaller units of function and of disease mechanisms linked to each. In other words, with the advance of biomedicine, ever more discrete disease conditions will be identified and the task of the clinician confronted with clinical conditions (which are complex wholes comprised of one or several illness occurrences) will be to identify the possible disease states that underlie the illness.

Each of the two sets of questions posed above is legitimate; heuristically valuable; and, when comprehensively explored, useful, vital, and productive for medicine and public health. However, the fact that both sets of questions are equally relevant and applicable whenever the system of biomedicine is applied, and attempts are made to refine it, presents intrinsically difficult problems to one interested in studying medical diagnosis in a naturalistic setting. This problem can be formulated by means of the following questions: How can one be totally sure that a clinical condition is made up of but a single illness occurrence as opposed to multiple illness occurrences? Alternatively, how can a researcher be certain that underlying a clinical condition is a condition of disease, and how can he or she determine that conditions of disease are truly independent occurrences and not linked to as yet undiscovered disease mechanisms? The issues devolving from the dilemma reviewed here contribute to and influence the kinds of problems tied to psychiatric classification and diagnosis. The fact that the latter enterprises are quintessentially cultural, that is, grounded in cultural meaning systems that implicate a range of symbolically constituted as well as natural phenomena, is what makes the dilemma especially acute in psychiatry.

References

Berlin, B., Breedlove, D. E., Raven, and P. H. (1973). General principles of classification and nomenclature in folk biology. *Am Anthropol* 75:214–242.

Bleuler, E. (1911). *Dementia Praecox oder Gruppe der Schizophrenien*. Leipzig, DDR: Deuticke.

Boyd, J. D., Burkee, J. D., Gruenberg, E., et al. (1984). Exclusion criteria of DSM-III. *Arch Gen Psychiatry* 41:983–989.

Brody, E. B. (1964). Some conceptual and methodological issues involved in research on society, culture, and mental illness. *J Nerv Ment Dis* 139:62–74.

Brody, E. B. (1981). The clinician as ethnographer: A psychoanalytic perspective on the epistemology of field work. *Cult Med Psychiatry* 5:273–298.
Brown, C. H. (1986). The growth of ethnobiological nomenclature. *Curr Anthropol* 27:1:1–19.
Cantor, N., Smith, E. E., Mezzich, J., et al. (1980). Psychiatric diagnosis as prototype categorization. *J Abnorm Psychol* 89:181–193.
D'Andrade, R. G. (1984). Cultural meaning systems. In R. A. Shweder, and R. A. LeVine (Eds.), *Culture theory: Essays on mind, self, and emotion*, pp. 88–119. Cambridge, UK: Cambridge University Press.
Dewhurst, K. (1966). *Dr. Thomas Sydenham (1624–1689): His life and original writings*. London: Wellcome Historical Medical Library.
Edgerton, R. B. (1966). Conceptions of psychosis in four East African societies. *Am Anthropol* 6:408–425.
Eisenberg, L. (1977). Disease and illness: Distinctions between professional and popular ideas of sickness. *Cult Med Psychiatry* 1:9–23.
Eisenberg, L., and Kleinman, A. (Eds.). (1981). *The relevance of social science for medicine*. Hingham, MA: Reidel.
Fabrega, H. (1972). The study of disease in relation to culture. *Behav Sci* 17:182–203.
Fabrega, H. (1974a). Problems implicit in the cultural and social study of depression. *Psychosom Med* 36:377–398.
Fabrega, H. (Ed.) (1974b). *Disease and social behavior: An interdisciplinary perspective.* Cambridge, MA: MIT.
Fabrega, H. (1975a). The need for an ethnomedical science. *Science* 189:969–975.
Fabrega, H. (1975b). The position of psychiatry in the understanding of human disease. *Arch Gen Psychiatry* 32:1500–1512.
Fabrega, H. (1976). Toward a theory of disease. *J Nerv Ment Dis* 162:199–312.
Fabrega, H. (1977). Culture, behavior, and the nervous system. *Annu Rev Anthropol* 6:419–455.
Fabrega, H. (1979a). Phylogenetic precursors of psychiatric illness: A theoretical inquiry. *Compr Psychiatry* 20:275–288.
Fabrega, H. (1979b). The scientific usefulness of the idea of illness. *Perspect Biol Med* 22:545–558.
Fabrega, H. (1979c). Neurobiology, culture, and behavior disturbances: An integrative review. *J Nerv Ment Dis* 167:467–474.
Fabrega, H. (1979d). Elementary systems of medicine. *Cult Med Psychiatry* 3:167–198.
Feinstein, A. R. (1967). *Clinical judgment*. Baltimore: Williams & Wilkins.
Forbes, T. R. (1979). By what disease or casualty: The changing face of death in London. In C. Webster (Ed.), *Health, medicine, and mortality in the sixteenth century*, pp. 117–140. Cambridge, UK: Cambridge University Press.
Frake, C. O. (1961). The diagnosis of disease among the subanum of Mindanao. *Am Anthropol* 63:113–132.
Geertz, C. (Ed.). (1973). *The interpretation of cultures*. New York: Basic.
Gillis, L. S., Elk, R., Ben-Arie, O., et al. (1982). The present state examination: Experiences with xhosa-speaking psychiatric patients. *Br J Psychiatry* 141:143–147.
Goodwin D., and Guze, S. B. (Eds.). (1984). *Psychiatric diagnosis*. Oxford, UK: Oxford University.

Haldipur, C. V. (1984). Madness in ancient India: Concept of insanity in charaka samhita (1st century A.D.). *Compr Psychiatry* 25:335–344.

Hanck, C., Ayuso Gutierrez, J. L., and Ramos Brieva, J. A. (1981). Clinical forms of depression in African and in Spanish cultural communities: A new comparative study. *Acta Psychiatr Belg* 81:437–443.

Jackson, S. W. (1969). Galen—On mental disorders. *J Hist Behav Sci* 5:376–384.

Jeste, D. V., del Carmen, R., Lohr, J. B., and Wyatt, R. J. (1985). Did schizophrenia exist before the eighteenth century? *Compr Psychiatry* 26:493–503.

Kay, P. (1973). A model-theoretic approach to folk taxonomy. *Soc Sci Info* 14:151–166.

Kendell, R. E. (1975). *The role of diagnosis in psychiatry.* Oxford, UK: Blackwell.

King, L. S. (1963). *The growth of medical thought.* Chicago: University of Chicago Press.

King, L. S. (1970). *The road to medical enlightenment, 1650–1695*, pp. 5–7. New York: American Elsevier.

Kleinman, A. (1973). Medicine's symbolic reality. *Inquiry* 16:203–216.

Kleinman, A. (1978). Concepts and a model for the comparison of medical systems as cultural systems. *Soc Sci Med* 12:86.

Kleinman, A. (1980). *Patients and healers in the context of culture.* Berkeley: University of California.

Kleinman, A. (1982). Neurasthenia and depression: A study of somatization and culture in China. *Cult Med Psychiatry* 6:117–190.

Kleinman, A., Eisenberg, L., and Good, B. (1978). Culture, illness, and care. *Ann Intern Med* 88:251–258.

Kleinman, A., and Good, B. (1985). *Culture and depression: Studies in the anthropology and cross-cultural psychiatry of affect and disorder.* Berkeley, CA: University of California Press.

Klibansky, R., Panofsky, E., and Saxl, F. (1964). *Saturn and melancholy: Studies in the history of natural philosophy, religion, and art.* New York: Basic.

Kraepelin, E. (1893). *Psychiatrie* (4th ed). Leipzig, DDR: Barth.

Kraupl-Taylor, F. (1979). *The concepts of illness, disease, and morbus.* Cambridge, UK: Cambridge University Press.

Kraupl-Taylor, F. (1980). The concepts of disease. *Psychol Med* 10:419–424.

Lakoff, G., and Johnson, M. (1980). *Metaphors we live by.* Chicago: University of Chicago Press.

Li Chiu, M. (1980). Insanity in imperial China: A legal case study. In A. Kleinman and T. Y. Lin (Eds.), *Normal and abnormal behavior in Chinese culture*, pp. 75–94. Hingham, MA: Reidel.

Lutz, C. (1981). Situation based emotion frames and the cultural construction of emotions. In *Proceedings of the third annual conference of the Cognitive Science Society*, pp. 84–89. Berkeley, CA.

MacDonald, M. (1981). *Mystical bedlam: Madness, anxiety, and healing in seventeenth-century England* (p. 107). Cambridge, UK: Cambridge University Press.

Marsella, A., and White, G. M. (Eds.).(1982). Culture and mental health: An overview. In *Cultural conceptions of mental health and therapy*, pp. 359–388. Hingham, MA: Reidel.

McEwan, P. J. M. (Ed.). (1980). Part B: Medical anthropology. *Soc Sci Med* 14B:8.
Mechanic, C. (1968). *Medical sociology: A selective view.* New York: Free Press.
Mechanic, D. (1974). *Politics, medicine, and social science.* New York: Wiley.
Morice R. (1978). Psychiatric diagnosis in a transcultural setting: The importance of lexical categories. *Br J Psychiatry* 132:87–95.
Murphy, J. M. (1976). Psychiatric labeling in cross-cultural perspective. *Science* 191:1019–1028.
Ohnuki-Tierney, E. (1981). *Illness and healing among the sakhalin ainu: A symbolic interpretation.* Cambridge, UK: Cambridge University Press.
Orley, J., and Wing, J. K. (1979). Psychiatric disorders in two African villages. *Arch Gen Psychiatry* 36:513–520.
Plog, S., and Edgerton, R. B. (Eds.). (1969). *Changing perspectives in mental illness.* New York: Holt, Rinehart and Winston.
Rosch, E., and Lloyd, B. B. (Eds.). (1978). *Cognition and categorization.* New York: Wiley.
Sartorius, N., Jablensky, A., and Shapiro, R. (1977). Preliminary communication: Two-year follow-up of the patients included in WHO international pilot study of schizophrenia. *Psychol Med* 7:529–541.
Snyder, S. (1965). The left hand of God: Despair in medieval and renaissance tradition. *Studies in the renaissance* 12:18–59.
Stevenson, L. G. (1965). "New diseases" in the seventeenth century. *Bull Hist Med* 39:1–21.
Temkin, O. (Ed.). (1973). *Galenism: Rise and decline of a medical philosophy.* Ithaca, NY: Cornell University Press.
Thomas, K. (Ed.). (1971). *Religion and the decline of magic.* London, UK: Penguin.
Tseng, W-S., and McDermott, J. F. (Eds.). (1981). *Culture, mind, and therapy: An introduction to cultural psychiatry.* New York: Brunner/Mazel.
Veith, I. (1965). *Hysteria: The history of a disease.* Chicago: University of Chicago Press.
Walker, D. P. (Ed.). (1981). *Unclean spirit: Possession and exorcism in France and England in the late sixteenth and early seventeenth centuries.* Philadelphia: University of Pennsylvania.
Westermeyer, J. (1985). Psychiatric diagnosis across cultural boundaries. *Am J Psychiatry* 142:798–805.

2

The Cultural Context of Diagnosis and Therapy

A View from Medical Anthropology

Byron J. Good and Mary-Jo DelVecchio Good

TRADITIONAL MEDICAL ANTHROPOLOGY dealing with ethnicity and mental health care focused almost exclusively on popular or folk beliefs, on culture specific folk-illness categories, and on native healers. This work had important strengths. It challenged the prevailing assumption that professional psychiatric clinics are *the* mental health providers in a community, focusing attention on the variety of popular care providers in a community, including families, traditional practitioners, social service agencies, religious specialists, and others who provide social support and treatment to the mentally ill. Traditional medical anthropology also drew attention to the ethnocentrism and racism embodied in the general assumption that common Anglo-American patterns of expressing distress and seeking treatment should be considered normative and that distinctive illness forms or culture-specific therapies of particular ethnic groups represent developmentally prior or inferior patterns of psychological or cultural functioning.

On the other hand, by the late 1960s, much of the work of anthropologists seemed ethnocentric in its own way. Ethnicity was often analyzed by anthropologists in "belief" terms: an ethnic group, it was held, can be identified by its distinctive set of beliefs, especially about the cause of illness and the appropriate means of its treatment. Given the great diversity of members of

From *Culture Medicine and Psychiatry* 20, no. 2 (September 1986)

any ethnic community and the rapid cultural change within communities, such accounts increasingly appeared as stereotyped characterizations, even when researchers indicated the particular subcommunity from which the data were drawn. Furthermore, anthropologists often seemed almost exclusively interested in exotic, even rare, aspects of culture—"folk illnesses" and traditional healers, in particular—rather than either the clinical or the social, political, and economic issues that play a critical role in the lives of persons seeking mental health care. Cultural issues in diagnostic work and psychotherapy, for example, were seldom the focus of anthropological research and writing.

If a rather narrow focus on folk culture has often limited the relevance of anthropologists' work for clinicians, so too have the questions put to those anthropologists who began working in clinical settings. Several years ago in a course we were teaching on culture and mental health care to third-year residents in a department of psychiatry in California, a psychiatric resident put to us a question we were to hear over and over again. "We don't want to know about social theory or about foreign cultures," he said. "Just tell us what is relevant for treating the patients we are most likely to see. What do we need to know about blacks, Mexican Americans, and Asians? What are their most important beliefs? What are the special tricks we need to know to do successful therapy with them?" Such questions place anthropologists in a kind of double bind. The immediate impulse is to respond that one cannot characterize the beliefs or patterns of interaction of any entire ethnic group, including Anglo-Americans, without maintaining and teaching stereotypes. Such a response, however, seems to imply that cultural differences are not important or cannot be conveyed in a manner relevant to the clinician. This too flies in the face of what the anthropologist believes. There is an enormous literature on the cultures represented by American immigrants and minorities, and it is our experience that a deep understanding of culture is critical to empathic and successful clinical work. So what is the response to the resident's questions?

This paper grows out of several years of experience of not only trying to teach in a manner that gives relevant answers to these questions, but also attempting to reformulate the questions that are important to ask. We spent seven years as members of a department of psychiatry in California teaching residents, clinical psychologists, and medical students. We were often called to consult in cases involving Middle-Eastern, especially Iranian, patients. We spent one year working with a Mexican American psychiatrist, Dr. Henry Herrera, in an experimental "cultural consultation clinic," seeing Hispanic patients along with spiritualist healers from the community. We are currently directing a postdoctoral research training program in clinically relevant medical anthropology. In each of these settings, several questions about the relevance of anthropology for clinical practice in multicultural contexts have been central to our work. What is different about the way someone who is "culturally competent" evaluates or diagnoses a patient and conducts psychotherapy, in contrast with someone who is not? For example, when we are called to consult with cases involving patients from a culture we know well, what are we able to do that others are not? For what aspects of diagnosis and treatment does cultural competence really make a difference? Can a clinician be taught to do those things that a good clinician from within the culture does naturally? Are years of learning about a particular culture necessary, or can we identify general skills or approaches to therapy that may make a therapist better able to function in multicultural settings? What are the critical research areas that can advance our understanding of these issues?

Several developments within psychiatry and anthropology since the 1960s have altered the context for discussing these issues. Within psychiatry, diagnosis has become a more central activity. When few effective medications were available for treatment of the mentally ill, diagnostic characterizations made relatively little difference in treatment. The emergence of medications for the affective disorders to complement anxiolytic drugs and the major tranquilizers, and the discovery that some drugs have "paradoxical" effects (for example, that antidepressants are effective in treating at least one form of anxiety—panic disorder), have focused enormous research attention on diagnostic criteria. Such work continues to provoke heated debate about the extent and consequences of misdiagnosis, especially in public care facilities (Lipton and Simon, 1985). In this context, the possibility that diagnostic criteria may be culturally relative, that criteria for a disorder such as depression may vary across cultures or ethnic groups, has far more importance than it did twenty years ago. At the same time, increasingly complex research within social psychiatry is provoking new hypotheses about the social origin and consequences of psychopathology, many of which implicate culture-specific features of social organization (kin patterns, social support, and the perception and evaluation of stressors) and require sophisticated analysis of culturally distinctive social groups. Thus psychiatric knowledge has supported a more sophisticated view of *both* biologically grounded disease phenomena, and the social production of illness phenomena.

Anthropology too has changed in the past two decades. While lively debate continues among materialist, cognitive, structuralist, and psychoanalytic theorists, "interpretive" anthropology has emerged as an important theoretical paradigm. Within medical and psychiatric anthropology, interpretive, or meaning-centered, theorizing has been wedded with new attention to clinical phenomena to produce an increasingly sophisticated literature. In general, leading figures within this paradigm reject both a "health belief" approach, which characterizes individuals or groups in terms of a distinctive set of beliefs, and a personality approach, which hypothesizes a distinctive personality type for members of a particular cultural group. Focus is rather on the "social production" and "cultural construction" of illness (e.g., Kleinman, 1980; Kleinman et al., 1977; Marsella and White, 1982), on the use of culturally distinctive meaning systems to interpret personal and social realities (e.g., Good, 1977; Good and Good, 1981, 1982; Young, 1976), on cultural idioms of distress and modes of discourse (Nichter, 1981; Csordas, 1983), and thus on processes through which forms of illness are generated, constructed as social realities, and maintained or treated. The primary object of analysis, from this perspective, is neither the typical personality of a group nor the beliefs typical of its members, but the meanings through which both are fashioned. As Geertz (1973, p. 5), one of the leading advocates of this perspective writes: "Believing, with Max Weber, that man is an animal suspended in webs of significance he himself has spun, I take culture to be those webs, and the analysis of it to be therefore not an experimental science in search of law but an interpretive one in search of meaning." This also has been the belief of interpretive medical and psychiatric anthropologists.

In this paper we will argue that an interpretive, or meaning-centered, anthropology provides a critical perspective on unresolved issues facing clinicians, teachers, and researchers working in multiethnic and cross-cultural settings. Anthropology's distinctive focus on "local" discourse and knowledge (cf. Geertz, 1983)—on individual clinical phenomena, on the complex relations among public and private meanings of symptoms and complaints, on the struggle to come to understanding and to impose authoritative interpretations on such phenomena, and on the social sciences as yet another form of interpretation—provides an important vantage for viewing clinical work and methods appropriate to its analysis. We hope to show that research from this perspective raises serious questions about the direction of much of current psychiatric research and practice. In the remainder of this paper we focus on two issues: first, the role of cultural differences in psychiatric diagnosis and the implications of such differences in psychiatric diagnosis, and second, the implications of such differences for psychotherapeutic process. Equally important issues concerning the social origins and consequences of mental illness are not addressed here.

The Cultural Context of Diagnosis

A wide variety of publications over the past two decades indicate that the diagnosis a patient receives is closely linked to his or her ethnicity and social class. Some studies provide convincing evidence that certain minority populations, owing to substantial social inequities, are at very high risk for particular disorders. For example, the prevalence of depression may be four to six times higher within select Native American communities than that observed for the U.S. population at large (see Manson et al., 1985 for an overview). Other studies indicate that misdiagnosis of minority patients is extremely high in certain clinical settings, probably because of biases implicit in the client-therapist transaction. The most classic examples of this are findings that hospitalized blacks are far more commonly diagnosed as schizophrenic and rarely diagnosed as depressed, in comparison with whites in the same institutions, and that rediagnosis using research diagnostic teams eliminates these differences (Simon et al., 1973; Raskin et al., 1975; see Adebimpe, 1981 for an excellent review). A majority of studies in the field, however, are much more difficult to interpret. Are differences in levels of psychopathology among various ethnic groups a result of *actual* differences in incidence and prevalence of psychiatric disorders, or do they result from biases in the diagnostic process or the research instruments being used?

To provoke our thinking, it may be useful to recall the findings of the famous Midtown Manhattan Study. This study did not specifically sample from strata defined in ethnic terms; however, when the small, naturally occurring Puerto Rican sample was analyzed separately, not one person was rated "well" and 52 percent were rated "impaired," a rating assigned to only 23 percent of other persons in the study (Srole et al., 1962, p. 291). These findings are particularly difficult to interpret. Are high rates of symptoms among Puerto Ricans, a finding replicated in other studies (e.g., Abad and Boyce, 1979), evidence for higher rates of psychopathology, or do they simply indicate a difference in styles of communicating distress? Do other studies that find differences in rates of symptoms or diagnoses across ethnic groups (e.g., Kuo, 1984; Vernon et al., 1982; Roberts, 1980; Quesada et al., 1978; see also reports on differences among blacks and nonblacks in the ECAC studies [Robins et al., 1984]) reflect actual differences in prevalence of mental illness or are the findings artifacts of the research instruments employed? Do these studies indicate actual differences among groups in level of distress, produced by social inequities, or do they represent differences in judgments made by clinicians representing mainstream American culture or psychometric instruments that replicate such biases in judgment? In addition, do findings such as those of the Midtown Manhattan Study that *social functioning* varies across ethnic groups reflect differences in actual levels of functioning, or are they also a result of biases in the judgments made by the raters? This latter issue takes on special significance in light of recent findings that hospital admission correlates more closely with practitioner's evaluation of level of functioning (axis V) than with diagnosis (Mezzich et al., 1985).

The problem of establishing validity of psychiatric diagnosis and assessment, and the associated problem of training clinicians to make correct diagnoses in cross-cultural and multiethnic settings, is an essential problem; it is inherent in the enterprise and is not simply a matter of bias or technique. As with many of the phenomena anthropologists study across cultures, there simply is no "gold standard" for psychiatric assessment. Recent efforts to use Research Diagnostic Criteria and the Diagnostic and Statistical Manual III (DSM-III) criteria as the "gold standard" are clearly an advance in providing grounds for overcoming bias. However, the DSM-III relies on symptoms criteria; if the content and frequency of symptoms vary across cultural groups, diagnosis using these criteria will be strongly affected. What evidence do we have? Do symptoms vary systematically across cultural groups? Are differences significant enough to produce systematic bias in diagnosis? How does this source of bias relate to that resulting from clinicians' attitudes toward, or ways of communicating with, clients from particular ethnic groups or social classes?

In the following two sections we will examine the question of diagnostic bias and raise the issue of the indeterminacy of diagnostic criteria. We will conclude by arguing for a cultural or interpretive understanding of the relation of symptoms to psychiatric illness and outline issues for research and training that follow.

Culture, Race, and Bias

Considerable evidence indicates bias on the part of the clinician influences diagnostic judgments that are made. Before reviewing this issue, a few words are in order about its significance. Whether in matters of research or teaching, why should we be so concerned about psychiatric diagnosis?

As we described in the introduction to this paper, the past fifteen years have seen dramatic changes in methods of assessment and diagnosis of mental illness. Whereas diagnosis was once primarily the domain of theoreticians rather than practitioners, the discovery of psychoactive drugs that have differential effects upon particular psychiatric conditions lent urgency to efforts to establish valid and reliable criteria for psychiatric diagnosis that would be an important part of routine clinical work. Such efforts resulted in the DSM-III and in associated epidemiological instruments (see Weissman and Klerman, 1978; and Murphy, 1982 for excellent reviews of changes in epidemiological research). The widespread use of these medications and the discovery that the diagnoses upon which their prescription is based varies enormously from country to country—in particular that American psychiatrists vastly overdiagnose schizophrenia (Cooper et al., 1972)—led to major efforts not only to establish validity of diagnosis but also to increase adherence to these criteria in actual practice. Such efforts were spurred on by awareness of the enormous iatrogenic effects of psychiatric medications, in particular the major tranquilizers.

Recent research indicates that in many clinical settings, diagnostic style has not changed nearly as much as this history would lead one to believe. For example, a recent study in part of the same hospital system in which the study by Cooper and his colleagues (1972) was conducted, the Manhattan Psychiatric Center, found that as many as 75 percent of all patients may be misdiagnosed (Lipton and Simon, 1985; cf. Goleman, 1985). Whereas hospital diagnoses showed 68 percent of patients with schizophrenia and 12 percent with affective disorders, the research team found that only 12 percent met criteria for schizophrenia. Thus, failure to use new criteria for psychiatric diagnosis and prescription of medication appears to be widespread, even to this day, at least in public institutions.

Why should social scientists interested in mental health practice and research in minority communities take special note of such a finding? First, it should be remembered that minority persons are disproportionately represented in public clinics and the public hospital system, and that members of various ethnic groups have quite different hospitalization rates. Any negative effects of misdiagnosis will thus bear most heavily on those overrepresented groups. Second, differential diagnosis is closely linked to medication practices. The diagnosis of schizophrenia is routinely followed by treatment with neuroleptics, prescribed, as Lipton and Simon (1985, p. 371) point out, "in doses sufficient to 'quiet' the 'disturbing' symptoms." Tardive dyskinesia, a significant complication of neuroleptics, may be found in as many as 30 percent of persons using antipsychotic drugs. In addition to increasing social dysfunction and representing the clearest evidence to the patients that they are "crazy," tardive dyskinesia seems to increase risk for disease and suicide (Lipton and Simon, 1985, p. 371). Thus, not only are persons suffering from depression or manic depressive disorders prevented from receiving effective treatment, they are also treated with drugs having very significant iatrogenic effects. Third, mislabeling individuals "schizophrenic" is likely to have profound effects on their life course. Hospitalization is likely to be vastly lengthened, medications are likely to mask symptoms of manic or depressive episodes, as well as of organic disorders, and the risks of chronic institutionalization and social breakdown syndrome are dramatically increased. While much of the debate of the late 1980s around social labeling was probably misplaced, given its focus on deviance and its questioning the existence of mental illness as disease, clearly misdiagnosis has many of the deleterious effects associated in that literature with labeling. Because these issues so profoundly affect members of minority groups, it is worth giving special reconsideration to the issue of misdiagnosis.

While misdiagnosis seems very high among all ethnic groups in some clinical settings, there is what Adebimpe (1981) in an interesting review describes as "a modest body of circumstantial evidence" that members of minority subcultures are at a particularly high risk for error in diagnosis and assessment. Several explanations run through the literature. First, cultural differences associated with language, modes of expressing symptoms, meanings associated with experiences such as altered states of consciousness, typical idioms of distress, sociolinguistic patterns, and differences in explanatory models and value systems are often reported to lead to unintended but systematic bias in assessment and diagnosis of persons from very different life worlds from that of the clinician. Second, both institutionalized racism (Hankins-McNary, 1979) and cultural stereotypes translated into psychiatric language and maintained by clinicians have been found to influence assessment. Stereotyped images of blacks as "jovial" may in part account for the widespread impression of low levels of depression (Adebimpe, 1981, p. 281); images of Puerto Ricans or blacks as lacking impulse control or having primitive character structure translates cultural differences into normative psychiatric language and can only lead to more severe diagnostic ratings (Sabshin et al., 1976; Abad and Boyce, 1979); and views of somatization as a primitive defense system, rather than a cultural idiom, has led to readiness to assume many are inappropriate for psychotherapy. Third, related to this problem, are reports of culturally based forms of transference and countertransference that strongly influence the nature of clinical presentation, especially during initial stages of evaluation and therapy, and that influence the judgments made by therapists (e.g., Ticho, 1971). For example, the clinical expression of hostility and other affects is influenced not only by cultural patterns of expressing emotion, as greatly as these vary across cultures, but by implicit rules for cross-ethnic communications. Carter (1974), for example, cites the "masking" of self and affect as a historically grounded survival mechanism: and notes the special fears associated with black patients' expression of hostile or aggressive feelings to white therapists. On the other hand, clinicians often have relatively little experience dealing with patients of other ethnic groups (Jones and Gray, 1985), and, because of their own discomfort, often engage unknowingly in ways of relating that play out stereotypical images and expectations (see Maduro, 1975 for perhaps the best case report and analysis of this phenomenon in the literature). Individual clinicians may respond in various ways. Beiser (1985) reports that young psychiatrists stationed in the Native American health services tend to respond in two ways. Some become rigidly and authoritatively "medical," dismissing beliefs and values of patients and concentrating on disease. Others become enamored with native culture and rationalize symptoms rather than recognizing them as signs of illness. This results from a process similar to that reported by McDermott (1967), who found that physicians underdiagnose organic brain conditions in children from lower social classes because they believe the symptoms to be the result of cultural deprivation that the children will "grow out of."

From an anthropological perspective, these biases in the diagnostic process are not simply aberrations or biases based in attitudes of practitioners; they are examples of a more general process that is often hidden from view when clinician and patient are from a similar culture and social class. All diagnostic and therapeutic encounters are transactions across distinctive subcultures and are embedded in local systems of power relations. Not only do clinicians as individuals belong to particular subcultures, their theoretical position itself is a cultural form and one that incorporates a set of values, explanatory models, "structures of relevance," and ways of interpreting the discourse of patients. A psychoanalyst, biomedical psychiatrist, and family therapist will interpret a particular symptom from a radically different vantage. In addition, individual background and culture influence the assessments made, even when explicit diagnostic paradigms are used. Gaines (1979), for example, shows to what extent the implicit paradigms or models of psychiatric residents influence their decisions in emergency rooms. Thus not only do clinical algorithms and explanatory models frame diagnostic judgments, but the personal meanings associated with these models and with the issues raised by the patient's distress influence those assessments as well. What psychiatric theory analyzes as transference and countertransference are particularly important subtypes of more general cultural phenomena that have been the focus of interpretive anthropological studies (e.g., see Good et al., 1982, 1985).

Several important training issues emerge from a view of clinical practice as transactions across distinctive cultures. First, clinicians in training should be encouraged to develop explicit awareness not only of their own psychological responses, which is a goal of most programs, but of unexamined aspects of their working clinical knowledge, its relation to their own subculture, and the personal meanings with which they invest their clinical paradigms. Second, clinicians should be taught to elicit and identify critical aspects of the patient's culture—the explanatory models of patients and their families, the popular illness categories used to identify aspects of their condition, and the meanings associated with particular affects or symptoms. Third, the role of culture and acculturation in transference and countertransference phenomena should be addressed explicitly in clinical training. Individuals establish personal identity in relation to society; for members of immigrant groups or distinctive subcultures, identity in relation to the dominant culture is often problematic. Individuals may identify themselves as traditional, as bicultural, as adherents of a distinctive ethnic identity, or as fully acculturated members of the dominant culture, or may have different identity strategies in various domains of their lives. A clinician can never be neutral in relation to the client's stance toward the dominant culture; the therapist will always represent, to some extent, a particular aspect of that culture. Self-presentation of the client during assessment and therapy will thus reflect a particular stance toward mainstream culture, and the data upon which assessment is based will thus be grounded in a particular subjective stance toward what the clinician represents.

The anthropological perspective on diagnosis raises even more fundamental questions, however. If diagnosis is always an evaluative transaction across systems of meaning or culture, how can we be certain that such cross-cultural interpretations (i.e., diagnoses) are valid? How can we be certain we are not committing a "category fallacy"? In a cross-cultural context, a category fallacy is the reification of a nonsological category developed for a particular cultural population and the application of that category to members of another culture without establishing its validity for that culture. Having dispensed with indigenous categories because they are culture specific, psychiatrists and researchers often go on to impose their own "scientific" categories on some sample of behavior in another culture as if their own disease categories were culture free (Kleinman, 1977; cf. Good and Kleinman, 1985b). Does this fundamental problem in cross-cultural psychiatry also plague diagnostic work and epidemiological research with American minority groups?

The Indeterminacy of Diagnostic Criteria

As we argued earlier in this paper, we believe the establishment of explicit diagnostic criteria, such as those found in DSM-II, provides an important advance over previous approaches to diagnosis and, if applied in a reliable manner, should reduce bias in cross-ethnic situations. On the other hand, DSM-III and the associated diagnostic instruments, such as the Diagnostic Interview Schedule (DIS) of the National Institute of Mental Health, are currently being translated into various languages to serve as the basis for making comparable diagnostic and treatment decisions. For example, the DIS has been translated for use among Mexican Americans (Hough et al., 1983) and several Native American groups (Manson et al., 1985). Such an approach to translation must assume not only that psychiatric disease categories are universal, but that symptoms that serve as diagnostic criteria are also, with minor variations, universal. Current work in medical and psychiatric anthropology suggests several problems inherent in the translation of symptom criteria for use in another culture, whether in clinical practice or in research. We will briefly review five.

The Problem of Normative Uncertainty

"Cultural anthropology, if properly understood, has the healthiest of all skepticisms about the validity of the concept 'normal behavior,'" wrote Edward Sapir (1970, p. 150) in 1932. "It cannot deny the useful tyranny of the normal in a given society, but it believes the external form of normal adjustment to be an exceedingly elastic thing." We now know that many mental health problems are more diseaselike than Sapir and his psychoanalyst friends believed in the 1930s, that certain forms of disordered experience appear quite similar across cultures and universally cause suffering. At the same time, however, one of the major difficulties facing any clinician working with a patient whose culture is different is to determine whether particular behaviors or forms of experience are abnormal and therefore a symptom of illness or simply different but normal within the patient's own cultural context. Is there a cultural basis for explaining why the mother of a hospitalized Iranian patient is spending fifteen hours a day in the waiting room outside the psychiatric unit, we were asked, or is this a sign of a pathologically enmeshed family relationship? (See Good and Good, 1981, for analysis of this case.) Is the complaint of a Puerto Rican woman that she has suffered an *ataque*, which included momentary loss of consciousness, a symptom of a neurological disorder, a culturally labeled panic attack, or simply a culturally normal—though troubling—response to an acutely stressful situation? Given great differences among the ways members of various cultures experience and communicate emotion, how should the clinician determine whether a Vietnamese or American Indian patient meets the criterion of "dysphoria"? May the presence of altered states of consciousness, even when intrusive and unwanted, be normal rather than pathological in some societies? For example, Liss and his associates (1973) found that delusions and hallucinations were associated with a definitive diagnosis of schizophrenia among white but not black patients, indicating these symptoms do not have the same diagnostic import in the latter (Adebimpe, 1981, p. 282).

If the problem of determining whether a particular behavior or a particular level of distress should be considered normal or symptomatic is difficult for clinicians, it has been a plague for cross-cultural psychological studies. Studies using psychological scales, such as the State-Trait Anxiety Inventory (see Spielberger and Diaz-Guerrero, 1976), have been remarkably ambiguous as to whether differences in scale scores across cultures should be interpreted as differences in what is normal for a group (i.e., the norm, a characteristic response pattern of a normal population) or represent actual differences in levels of distress or pathology in the groups studied (for a review of cross-cultural psychological studies of anxiety, see Good and Kleinman, 1985b, pp. 300–303). Similar problems exist for symptom checklists used to identify psychopathology across cultures. Researchers have found higher levels of psychological symptoms among Puerto Ricans than other North American populations for over twenty years (e.g., Srole et al., 1962; Dohrenwend and Dohrenwend, 1969); however, the issue is still unresolved whether levels of psychiatric illness are higher among Puerto Ricans or whether this represents culturally prescribed differences in ways of communicating symptoms. Haberman (1976), for example, found that symptom scores on the twenty-two-item screening instrument used in the Midtown Manhattan Study were higher for Puerto Ricans living on the island than for those living for a long period in New York, indicating these rates represent "culturally patterned differences in modes of expressing distress" rather than level of psychopathology. In addition, symptom levels seem to have quite different relationships to impairment levels across cultures. For example, in the Sterling County and Yoruba studies, the Yoruba were found to have far higher levels of symptoms (particularly of somatic symptoms) than Canadians but far lower rates of significant social impairment (see Murphy, 1982, p. 53, for a discussion).

Diagnostic instruments such as the DIS were designed in part to overcome difficulties in determining norms and cutoff points. However, the problem of the indeterminacy of norms is embedded in the instrument as it is in diagnostic work. How serious should heart palpitations or loss of energy be before a person is considered to have met criteria for these symptoms? Given enormous cultural differences in care-seeking patterns (e.g., Lin et al., 1978), can the fact that an individual has or has not sought help for a particular symptom be used to determine whether the individual has met a particular symptom criterion [as is the case for both the DIS and the Schedule for Affective Disorders and Schizophrenia (SADS)]?

Cleary, one of the identifying features of culturally competent clinicians is that they are able to make a reasonable determination of whether a particular behavior or experience is culturally normal or is a symptom of pathology. However, cultural judgments about normalcy often masquerade in diagnostic manuals and epidemiological instruments as scientific objectivity.

The Problem of Centricultural Bias

Wober (1969) has labeled those research strategies that begin with a research instrument developed exclusively in one culture and directly translate them into languages for use in other cultures as "centricultural." Difficulties associated with the centricultural approach are common to diagnostic work and research.

Anthropological and cross-cultural psychiatric research has found great variation in the content of symptoms across cultures. For example, the Yoruba literature (Murphy, 1982) indicates that anxiety disorders are associated with three primary clusters of symptoms: worries about fertility, dreams of being bewitched, and bodily complaints (Collis, 1966; Jegede, 1978). Research by an Ibo psychologist indicates that a rich somatic vocabulary is typical of Nigerian psychiatric patients (Ebigbo, 1982). For example, patients commonly complain that "things like ants keep on creeping in various parts of my brain," or "it seems as if pepper were put into my head," in a fashion that would be interpreted in nearly any American patient as delusional. Chinese patients commonly present with a variety of somatic and somatopsychic complaints, including such culture-specific symptoms as heaviness or pressure depressing into the head or chest, fear of excessive loss of semen with diminished vital energy, excess of hot inner energy, and fear of cold in the body (Kleinman, 1982). Iranians often complain that their hearts are upset (Good, 1977).

In addition to these clinical and anthropological reports, factor analytic studies have found distinct variations in symptom clusters associated with particular psychiatric disorders. For example, Binitie (1975) found that while depressed patients in England exhibited most of the typical symptoms that serve as DSM-III criteria for affective disorder, many of the symptoms were absent or rare in depressed Nigerians. They rarely contemplate suicide, and they are more apt to complain of somatic symptoms and delusions of persecution or neglect self-care. English patients more commonly express guilt, self-reproach, and suicidal thoughts.

Culture-specific idioms of distress and symptom vocabularies are not merely typical of exotic or non-Western cultures; they are the language in which members of any culture express distress. Complaints of feeling stress or pressure, of feeling sinful and deserving God's punishment, are cultural idioms. Complaints of *nervios* and *ataques* seem common among some Hispanic cultures (e.g., Abad and Boyce, 1979; Low, 1981). Somatic idioms are certainly more prevalent among Puerto Ricans and blacks than among Anglos (Abad and Boyce, 1979; Carter, 1974) and may have quite different diagnostic implications among different groups.

Two very clear difficulties arise from the centricultural approach to translating diagnostic criteria and epidemiological instruments. First, a wide range of symptoms typical of a particular culture may simply be omitted from consideration because they are not present for the development of the criteria. Morbid concerns about fertility or dreams of being bewitched simply do not appear as criteria in the DSM-III and thus would not appear in a Nigerian manual, despite their importance (see Orley and Wing, 1979, for such an example). Imagine reversing the process: if Ebigbo's Psychiatric Screening Form were translated from Ibo into American English, how would those somatic symptoms mentioned above be translated? What typical American symptoms with significance for differential diagnosis would simply be eliminated from consideration?

Second, it seems likely that there are differences in content and duration of symptoms of diagnostic significance across cultures. Simple translation of those symptoms found to result in valid diagnosis among particular American populations does not ensure the validity of these symptoms as criteria among other cultures.

The extent to which these difficulties raise problems for diagnosis among various American ethnic groups is not yet clear. There are certainly indications that the centricultural bias raises problems of validity not only for cross-cultural work but for diagnosis among some American populations as well. Manson et al. (1985) indicate that the thirty-day duration criterion for major affective disorder is inappropriate for the Hopi.

The Problem of Indeterminacy of Meaning

The major method of translation of psychiatric criteria is designed to find "semantic equivalents." Items are translated, back translated, and administered to bilingual subjects. Such a method assumes the existence of objective and universal referents, which may be represented by different symbolic forms in different cultures. For a term like "headache," this may be true. In general, however, the referents of symbols—i.e., their meanings—are aspects of a culture or a life world, not objects outside of language through which language obtains meaning (see Good, 1977; Good and Good, 1982, for elaboration). "Heart discomfort" for Iranians is not the equivalent of "heart palpitations" for Americans; it does not *mean* the same thing (Good, 1977). It is a symbol that condenses a distinctive set of meanings, a culture-specific "semantic network," for Iranians. Complaints of feeling impure in India refer to a semantic domain of profound cultural significance, one that regulates caste, sexuality, and social hierarchy; there simply is no equivalent among Americans. Feelings of guilt and sinfulness are rooted in Christian culture. When Orley and Wing (1979) translated the PSE question for "pathological guilt" into Luganda (in research in Uganda), they used the question "Do you sometimes blame yourself for something that was a mistake?" Is it any wonder they found unexpectedly high levels of guilt associated with depression, or that there has been such debate over whether guilt is associated with depression for Africans?

We do not question that translation of criteria should include those domains that appear to have biological significance, for example the vegetative signs associated with neuroendocrine functioning for the depressed. However, anthropological techniques are available for identifying the *semantic domains* associated with a particular illness in the discourse of patients. (See Kinzie et al., 1982, for an example of development of a Vietnamese depression scale beginning with such an approach.) For example, such domains for depressed Iranians include "grief and sadness" (*gam o gosseh*), "anger" (*asabani*), "sensitivity" (*hassasiyat*), and "mistrust" (see Good et al., 1985). These refer to culture-specific forms of social life and personal distress for Iranians. No only are they of diagnostic significance, they are complaints that open onto a culture-specific world of suffering for the culturally competent clinician.

The Problem of Narrative Context

Put simply, people of any culture express symptoms differently in different contexts. This may have unrecognized significance for the determination of diagnostic criteria. Chinese have long been believed to "somatize" depression (Tseng, 1975; Kleinman, 1977). Cheung (1982, 1984), in research in Hong Kong, found that outside of medical settings Chinese report experiencing a high level of psychological symptoms. However, they prefer to discuss these with friends and to discuss somatic symptoms with physicians. It seems likely that an important part of what has been seen as the Chinese tendency to somatize is a characteristic of the communicative context in which research was undertaken, rather than primarily on the range of feelings or experiences typical of Chinese.

Our review of the work on misdiagnosis among American minority groups made it clear that important aspects of clinical presentation of ethnic patients with Anglo clinicians result from norms for communication within the clinical context; a sampling of the same patient's complaints in other contexts—at home, with primary care practitioners, with native healers, in a church healing ritual—might well give a very different picture of the patient's symptoms. Symptom criteria for diagnosis might thus vary by narrative context.

The Problem of Category Validity

We have been arguing that cultural meanings and norms for expressing distress significantly alter the relationship between symptoms and diagnostic entity, posing serious problems for translation of diagnostic criteria and symptom-based epidemiological instruments. Ultimately, however, one must ask whether psychiatric diagnostic entities are universal categories—whether diagnostic categories primarily reflect medical culture (and therefore change with changes in medical theories), whether they characterize certain American and European populations (and therefore are only valid within those populations), or whether they are universal psychobiological and/or psychological entities. We have little doubt that schizophrenia and some forms of depression and anxiety can be found in all populations. However, whether depressive illnesses experienced primarily in psychological terms and associated with strong feelings of remorse and guilt should be equated with that experienced primarily in sociosomatic terms is open to question (see Kleinman and Good, 1985, for extended discussion of this issue; cf. Marsella, 1979). It may be that those affective disorders defined by DSM-III are cultural variants of an underlying depressive disorder, expressed in significantly different ways in some cultures. The same is certainly true for anxiety disorders (see Good and Kleinman, 1985b) and for even more vaguely defined "somatoform disorders." Thus the problem may lie at a deeper level than simply mapping the correct symptoms for each culture onto universal categories. Only research that is open to this issue can tell us whether particular categories are universal or whether seeming universality is produced as an artifact of research and clinical method.

Anthropology, Diagnosis, and Ethnicity

A meaning-centered or interpretive anthropology challenges psychiatric researchers and clinicians on two grounds. First, it challenges the assumption that symptoms are reflections of psychobiological phenomena and that their primary meaning resides in those biological phenomena to which they stand as signs. Instead, it argues for a recognition that "symptoms" are medical abstractions from culture-specific forms of discourse, that is from persons' narrative accounts of their own suffering or that of someone in their primary social network. Their meanings reside not only in disordered biology, though biology certainly constrains and in some cases actively constructs experience; the meanings of symptoms are also grounded in and open onto life worlds that are as distinctive as the cultures of our universe. Second, anthropology thus challenges the centriculturalist view of interpretation of diagnostic criteria. It suggests that interpretation should follow after inductive studies of psychopathology within cultures provide grounds for real comparisons of quite distinctive discourses of distress, rather than simply beginning with criteria found valid within particular American populations and assuming that finding "semantic equivalents" of diagnostic criteria will define a population suffering from the same universal disease.

We recognize that we are here defining ethnic groups as distinctive cultures or subcultures and that there are difficulties with this definition. However, while analysis of social factors producing psychopathology and inequities in access to services requires a primarily social view of ethnicity, we believe that issues of cultural meanings come to the fore in discussing competence for diagnosis and psychotherapy.

The anthropological perspective developed here provides an approach to analyzing culturally competent diagnosis—in terms of various dimensions of translation between diagnostic criteria and culture and context-specific discourses of patients—and points to a similar analysis of culture and psychotherapy.

The Cultural Context of Psychotherapy

We will simply outline several issues for understanding cultural competency in psychotherapy that follow from the kind of analysis developed in the preceding sections. Our work in a "cultural consultation clinic" in a university department of psychiatry in California (see Good et al., 1982, 1985) suggested to us that symbolic and interpretive processes play a central role in (1) the establishment of intimate therapeutic relations; (2) the control of "affective distance" in therapy; (3) the development of metaphors critical to healing; and (4) issues of reflexivity and countertransference that emerge in therapy. These provide grounds for defining culturally competent psychotherapy.

First, the definition and establishment of intimate relations varies enormously across cultures. We find that members of one culture often complain that those from another are "shallow," that their family relations, their rituals, their friendships lack depth and feeling. They complain that it is difficult to feel close to persons from another society, that persons from that society are distant or intrusive. These qualities are often seen as characteristic of that culture rather than as problems in intercultural interpretation and communication. A central quality of a therapist is that he or she is able to establish intimate relations with patients and manage levels of intimacy as the therapeutic relationship develops. We believe that culturally based difficulties in establishing intimacy lie at the root of common claims that members of particular cultural groups are not appropriate candidates for psychotherapy.

Second, a critical feature of competent psychotherapy is the ability to manage "affective distance." Scheff (1977) argues that individuals may be emotionally "underdistanced" or "overdistanced"; for example, a person may be totally and hopelessly overcome with grief or, on the other hand, unable to experience a grief that still has power for that person. A person may be in a violent rage or completely out of touch with anger. A central function of both ritual and psychotherapy is management of emotional distance so that the affect can be safely experienced and discharged or integrated (see Kapferer, 1979, for an example). Again, management of affective distance is a culturally fraught process. Particular symbols have not only unique personal significance but affective meanings that are as much a feature of the cultural landscape as family relations and cultural values. Manipulation of these symbols in psychotherapy thus has quite different effects depending on the "semantic networks" (Good, 1977) in which they are embedded. We found in our cultural consultation clinic that the spiritualist healers with whom we worked could very quickly recognize issues having emotional potency for the patient, use ritual means for inducing relaxation, then help the patient to experience with directness overdistanced emotions. We believe the ability to manage emotional distance therapeutically is a central feature of cultural competence.

Third, much of the work of healing is done through the development of culturally powerful metaphors. Lakoff and Johnson (1980) argue that much of our phenomenal world is metaphorically constructed, and that the central metaphors vary greatly by society. Traditional healing systems draw on metaphors resonant within the culture to construct the illness reality and then symbolically manipulate it to effect healing. A central image, such as a spirit, will be constructed in a ritual setting; the sick person will be encouraged to identify the image as the source of the illness, thereby associating personal meanings with a public ritual symbol; and therapy will be directed at removing or transforming the illness reality constituted in this ritual (clinical) process. (See Lienhardt, 1961, for a classic account in anthropology.)

Much psychotherapy proceeds along a similar course—sometimes consciously, as the therapist likens the patient's condition to a culturally syntonic image, sometimes without explicit awareness, as patient and therapist share metaphors as part of their assumptive world. Therapy may also fail because the patient's metaphoric understanding of the illness condition is hidden from or rejected by the therapist, or because the therapist is unable to construct a metaphor with adequate power to provide the patient leverage to transform the grounds of suffering. One of the hallmarks of the culturally competent psychotherapist is the ability to recognize the metaphors that have power within the patient's discourse or to construct powerful metaphors, then to work through the patient's problems through the symbolic transformation of the metaphor.

Finally, as we have discussed above, the transferential relationship always has an "ethnic" component when therapeutic encounters take place across cultures or subcultures. The culturally competent psychotherapist should be able to recognize and manage this dimension for the good of the patient.

Conclusion: Two Proposals for Training and Research Relevant to Cultural Competence in Diagnosis and Therapy

In conclusion, we offer two suggestions we believe may contribute both to research and programs of training relevant to the issues we have been discussing. We believe it is critical that training for cultural competence be combined with research. As indicated by the body of this paper, we simply do not have the data to indicate precisely how psychopathology and appropriate techniques for psychotherapy vary across American subcultures; even if we did, so important is relationship and context to the work of assessment and therapy that such knowledge could not be learned simply as a set of criteria or techniques. Our suggestions thus deal with approaches to assessment and psychotherapy processes, rather than simply content.

First, we propose the development of "cultural consultation clinics" as sites for research and training relevant to cultural issues in assessment and therapy. In our previous experience (Good et al., 1982, 1985), a cultural consultation clinic was developed as part of a behavioral medicine clinic associated with a psychiatric consultation-liaison program. In our current experience at Harvard, one of our postdoctoral training fellows (in a program in clinically relevant medical anthropology) is working with hospital clinicians to develop a clinic to specialize in assessment and treatment of Hispanics. In other contexts, such a clinic might be multiethnic, that is, a clinic with a variety of cultural specialists available to make culturally relevant assessments and therapy recommendations or to provide specialized treatment.

A cultural consultation clinic should have integrated clinical, teaching, and research functions. As a clinical facility, it can provide assessments (either within its own setting or in another hospital or clinic setting) of the cultural issues involved in diagnosis and treatment of patients, where these have come to be a problem. Diagnostic issues (e.g., Is a particular behavior normal within the patient's culture? What are the meanings associated with a particular complaint?) and treatment questions (e.g., How can a more intimate therapeutic relationship be negotiated? What are the critical affective issues that need to be addressed?) such as those discussed in the body of this paper are appropriate issues for consultation. Such a clinic might also provide culturally appropriate therapies in some cases.

As a teaching site, such a clinic can serve to clarify the role of cultural issues for trainees. Trainees can work alongside cultural specialists, either clinicians or community persons, to learn awareness of their own cultural countertransference, to learn to deal openly and explicitly with the culture-specific meanings associated with symptoms and therapies (for example, to learn to elicit explanatory models and patients' metaphors), and to try approaches to therapy not taught as regular modalities.

A cultural consultation clinic can serve as a site for research into the kinds of issues raised in this paper. We focused here on diagnostic issues because we believe they are particularly urgent. While it is encouraging that the DIS is being adapted for use with great care, we believe this approach should be combined with research into central issues, such as investigation of culture-specific symptoms and illness idioms, research into semantic networks and semantic domains to which symptoms and elements in patients' discourse belong, the effect of clinical context on presentation of symptoms, and culture-specific cognitive schemata associated with particular illnesses.

Our second recommendation points to one specific mode of combining research and assessment. We propose that a cultural axis be developed as a research axis to be added to the psychiatric diagnostic and statistical manual, and that social and cross-cultural psychiatrists, anthropologists, psychologists, and other social science researchers be challenged to demonstrate the utility of such an approach in their research (cf. Good and Kleinman, 1985a). The axial structure of DSM-III represents a compromise among competing and complementary views of psychiatric disorder. It construes psychopathology as a heterogenous psychiatric disease entity (axis I), as a pathology embedded in a particular personality (axis II), as a response to stressful social precursors (axis IV), and as a level of social dysfunction (axis V). These represent current ways in which clinicians evaluate the nature and extent of psychopathology, each from the perspective of the clinician. However, none of these axes represent evaluation of the patient's condition from the patient's own perspective or that of the patient's family or primary social group. The cultural axis we propose would represent this perspective, what anthropologists have called the "emic" perspective or that from "the native point of view" (Geertz, 1983, pp. 55–70).

There is a strong evidence to suggest that the cultural meaning of a disorder, the idiom in which the disorder is experienced and communicated, and the social evaluation of the disorder by members of the sufferer's primary social network have an important influence on the illness as a social reality and thereby on the course of the disorder and its effect on the social functioning of the sufferer. In some cases such evaluation may have more significance than the axis I diagnosis. Researchers should specify the sources of data, the categories of data to be gathered, and the means of recording the data (categorical, descriptive, or linear). We suggest that researchers and clinicians should record the culture-specific illness category, the explanatory model, the illness idiom, the predominant care-seeking pattern, and the perceived level of disability. For example, an axis VI assessment might record that a juvenile Puerto Rican patient's family interprets the disorder as an *ataque de nervios*, that they believe began with the patient's learning suddenly of the death of a friend, that they believe the disorder seriously affects the patient's ability to function in public and work settings, but that they believe the disorder is acute and likely to pass as the patient resolves his grief and matures as an adult. Such information would add significantly to a diagnostic assessment that recorded generalized anxiety disorder, dysthymic disorder, and undiagnosed epileptiform seizures. Perhaps more to the point, an axis VI assessment that a major depression is interpreted by one patient and his or her family in somatic terms (as neurasthenia, as undiagnosed medical illness) and by another in a religious idiom (as punishment of God for sins) *may* turn out to have greater implications for prognosis and treatment than the diagnosis major depression alone. Establishment of a cultural axis would promote systematic investigation of the nature of culture-specific evaluations of psychiatric disorders and of their effects on phenomenology, prognosis, and appropriate treatment. Employed in training, it would encourage clinicians to systematically review cultural aspects of patient care often neglected. We believe it would both promote cultural competence and serve to focus research on what constitutes culturally competent assessment and therapy.

References

Abad, V., and Boyce, E. (1979). Issues in psychiatric evaluations of Puerto Ricans: A socio-cultural perspective. *Journal of Operational Psychiatry* 10:28–39.

Adebimpe, V. (1981). Overview: White norms and psychiatric diagnosis of black patients. *American Journal of Psychiatry* 138:279–285.

Beiser, M. (1985). The grieving witch: A framework for applying principles of cultural psychiatry to clinical practice. *Canadian Journal of Psychiatry* 30:130–141.

Binitie, A. (1975). A factor analytic study of depression across cultures—African and European. *British Journal of Psychiatry* 127:559–563.

Carter, J. (1974). Recognizing psychiatric symptoms in Black Americans. *Geriatrics* 29:95–99.

Cheung, F. M. (1982). Psychological symptoms among Chinese in urban Hong Kong. *Social Science and Medicine* 16:1339–1344.

Cheung, F. M. (1984). Preferences in help-seeking among Chinese students. *Culture, Medicine, and Psychiatry* 8:371–380.

Collis, R. (1966). Physical health and psychiatric disorder in Nigeria. *Transactions of the American Philosophical Society* 56(4):1–45.

Cooper, J., et al. (1972). *Psychiatric diagnosis in New York and London.* Oxford: Oxford University Press.

Csordas, T. (1983). The rhetoric of transformation in ritual healing. *Culture, Medicine, and Psychiatry* 7:333–376.

Dohrenwend, Bruce, and Dowhrenwend, Barbara. (1969). *Social status and psychological disorder: A causal inquiry.* New York: Wiley Interscience.

Ebigbo, P. O. (1982). Development of a culture-specific (Nigeria) screening scale of somatic complaints indicating disturbance. *Culture, Medicine, and Psychiatry* 6:29–43.

Gaines, A. (1979). Definitions and diagnoses: Cultural implications of psychiatric help-seeking and psychiatrists' definitions of the situation in psychiatric emergencies. *Culture, Medicine, and Psychiatry* 3:381–418.

Geertz, C. (1973). *The interpretation of cultures.* New York: Basic Books.

Geertz, C. (1983). *Local knowledge.* New York: Basic Books.

Goleman, D. (1985, April 23). State hospital accused of wrong diagnoses: Fueling debate over nation's mental care. *New York Times*, pp. C1, C8.

Good, B. (1977). The heart of what's the matter. *Culture, Medicine, and Psychiatry* 1:25–58.

Good, B., and Good, M. (1981). The semantics of medical discourse. In E. Mendelsohn and Y. Elkana (Eds.), *Sciences and cultures: Sociology of the sciences.* Vol. V. Dordrecht: Reidel.

Good, B., and Good, M. (1982). Toward a meaning-centered analysis of popular illness categories: "Fright illness" and "heart distress." In Iran. In A. J. Marsella, and G. M. White (Eds.) *Cultural conceptions of mental health and therapy.* Dordrecht: Reidel.

Good, B., Good, M., and Moradi, R. (1985). The interpretation of Iranian depressive illness and dysphoric affect. In A. Kleinman and B. Good (Eds.), *Culture and depression.* Los Angeles: University of California Press.

Good, B., and Kleinman, A. (1985a). Epilogue. In A. Kleinman and B. Good (Eds.), *Culture and depression.* Los Angeles: University of California Press.

Good, B., and Kleinman, A. (1985b). Culture and anxiety: Cross-cultural evidence for the patterning of anxiety disorders. In H. Tuma and J. Maser (Eds.), *Anxiety and the anxiety disorders.* Mahwah, NJ: Lawrence Erlbaum Publishers.

Good, B., et al. (1982). Reflexivity and countertransference in a psychiatric cultural consultation clinic. *Culture, Medicine, and Psychiatry* 6:281–303.

Good, B., et al. (1985). Reflexivity, countertransference, and clinical ethnography: A case from a psychiatric consultation clinic. In A. Gaines and R. Hahn (Eds.), *Physicians of Western medicine.* Dordrecht: Reidel.

Haberman, P. W. (1976). Psychiatric symptoms among Puerto Ricans in Puerto Rico and New York City. *Ethnicity* 3:133–144.

Hankins-McNary, L. (1979). The effect of institutional racism on the therapeutic relationship. *Perspectives in Psychiatric Care* 17:25–31, 58.

Hough, R., Kamo, M., Burnham, A., Escobar, J., and Timbers, D. (1983). The Los Angeles Epidemiologic Catchment Area Research Program and the epidemiology of psychiatric disorders among Mexican Americans. *Journal of Operational Psychiatry* 14:42–51.

Jegede, R. O. (1985). Outpatient psychiatry in an urban clinic in a developing country. *Social Psychiatry* 13:93–98.

Jones, B., and Gray, B. (1985). Black and white psychiatrists: Therapy with blacks. *Journal of the National Medical Association* 77:19–25.

Kapferer, B. (19792). Emotion and feeling in Sinhalese healing rites. *Social Analysis* 1:108–152.

Kinzie, J. D., et al. (1982). Development and validation of a Vietnamese-language depression rating scale. *American Journal of Psychiatry* 139:1276–1281.

Kleinman, A. (1977). Depression, somatization, and the new cross-cultural psychiatry. *Social Science and Medicine* 11:3–10.

Kleinman, A. (1980). *Patients and healers in the context of culture.* Berkeley: University of California Press.

Kleinman, A. (1982). Neurasthenia and depression. *Culture, Medicine, and Psychiatry* 6:117–190.

Kleinman, A., Eisenberg, L., and good, B. (1977). Culture, illness, and care. *Annals of Internal Medicine* 88:251–258.

Kleinman, A., and Good, B., eds. (1985). *Culture and depression: Anthropological, cross-cultural psychiatric, and psychological studies of illness and affect.* Berkeley: University of California Press.

Kuo, W. H. (1984). Prevalence of depression among Asian-Americans. *Journal of Nervous and Mental Disorders* 172:449–457.

Lakoff, G., and Johnson, M. (1980). *Metaphors we live by.* Chicago: University of Chicago Press.

Lienhardt, G. (1961). *Divinity and experience.* Oxford: Clarendon Press.

Lin, T., et al. (1978). Ethnicity and patterns of help-seeking. *Culture, Medicine, and Psychiatry* 2:3–14.

Lipton, A., and Simon, F. (1985). Psychiatric diagnosis in a state hospital: Manhattan State revisited. *Hospital and Community Psychiatry* 36:368–373.

Liss, J. L., et al. (1973). Psychiatric symptoms in white and black inpatients. I: Record study. *Comparative Psychiatry* 14:475–481.

Low, S. (1981). The meaning of *nervios:* A sociocultural analysis of symptom presentation in San Jose, Costa Rica. *Culture, Medicine, and Psychiatry* 5:25–48.

Maduro, R. (1975). Hoodoo possession in San Francisco: Notes on therapeutic aspects of regression. *Ethos* 3:425–447.

Manson, S., Shore, J., and Bloom, J. (1985). The depressive experience in American Indian communities: A challenge for psychiatric theory and diagnosis. In A. Kleinman and B. Good (Eds.), *Culture and depression.* Berkeley: University of California Press.

Marsella, A. (1979). Depressive experience and disorder across cultures. In H. Triandis and J. Draguns (Eds.), *Handbook of cross-cultural psychology.* Vol. 6, Psychopathology. Boston: Allyn and Bacon.

Marsella, A., and White, G., eds. (1982). *Cultural conceptions of mental health and therapy.* Dordrecht: Riedel.

McDermott, F. (1967). Social class and mental illness in children: The diagnosis of organicity and mental retardation. *Journal of the American Academy of Child Psychiatry* 6:309–320.

Mezzich, J. E., et al. (1985). Admission decisions and multiaxial diagnosis. *Archives of General Psychiatry* 41:1001–1004.

Murphy, H. B. M. (1982). *Comparative psychiatry: The international and intercultural distribution of mental illness.* New York: Springer-Verlag.

Nichter, M. (1981). Idioms of distress. Alternatives in the expression of psychosocial distress: A case study from south India. *Culture, Medicine, and Psychiatry* 5:379–408.

Orley, J., and Wing, J. K. (1979). Psychiatric disorders in two African villages. *Archives of General Psychiatry* 36:513–520.

Quesada, G. M., Spears, W., and Ramos, P. (1978). Interracial depressive epidemiology in the Southwest. *Journal of Health and Social Behavior* 19:77–85.

Raskin, A., et al. (1975). Psychiatric history and symptom differences in black and white depressed inpatients. *Journal of Consultation and Clinical Psychology* 43:73–80.

Roberts, R. (1980). Prevalence of psychological distress among Mexican Americans. *Journal of Health and Behavior* 21:134–145.

Robins, et al. (1984). National Institute of Mental Health Diagnostic Interview Schedule. *Archives of General Psychiatry* 38:381–389.

Sabshin, M., Disenhaus, M., and Wilkerson, R. (1976). Dimensions of institutional racism in psychiatry. *American Journal of Psychiatry* 127:787–793.

Sapir, E. (1970). *Culture, language, and personality: Selected essays.* Berkeley: University of California Press.

Scheff, T. (1977). The distancing of emotion in ritual. *Current Anthropology* 18:483–505.

Simon, R. J., Fleis, J. L., Garland, B. J., Stiller, P. R., and Sharp, L. (1973). Depression and schizophrenia in hospitalized black and white mental patients. *Archives of General Psychiatry* 28:509–512.

Spielberger, C. D., and Diaz-Guerrero, R., eds. (1976). Cross-cultural anxiety. New York: John Wiley & Sons.

Srole, L., et al. (1962). *Mental health in the metropolis: The Midtown Manhattan Study.* New York: McGraw-Hill.

Ticho, G. (1971). Cultural aspects of transference and countertrans-transference. *Bulletin of the Menninger Clinic* 35:313–334.

Tseng, Y. (1975). The nature of somatic complaints among psychiatric patients: The Chinese case. *Comparative Psychiatry* 16:237–245.

Vernon, S., Roberts, R., and Lee, E. S. (1982). Response tendencies, ethnicity, and depression scores. *American Journal of Epidemiology* 116:482–495.

Weissman, M., and Klerman, G. (1978). Epidemiology of Mental Disorders. *Archives of General Psychiatry* 35:705–712.

Wober, M. (1969). Distinguishing multi-cultural from cross-cultural tests and research. *Perceptual and Motor Skills* 28:488.

Young, A. (1976). Some implications of medical beliefs and practices for social anthropology. *American Anthropologist* 78:5–24.

3

Help-Seeking Pathways

A Unifying Concept in Mental Health Care

Lloyd H. Rogler and Dharma E. Cortes

In the now voluminous and ever-increasing body of research seeking to explain why some persons, but not others, turn to professional mental health care, the concept of help-seeking pathways occasionally appears. Sometimes it is used to structure the research and organize the findings. Other times it is alluded to, as if it hovered in the background of the research, penumbra-like, a shadow outlined by detectable boundaries. In either case, the idea of help-seeking pathways remains undeveloped both conceptually and methodologically. It has not attracted the explicit and sustained programmatic attention it deserves. Our purpose here is to invite such attention by showing that, if the concept is formulated in generic terms and oriented toward institutional structures, it can help integrate much of what we know about the use of mental health care facilities. We propose that help-seeking pathways provide the critical link between the onset of psychiatric problems and the provision of mental health care.

The proposal stems from our efforts to understand the relation between epidemiologic findings regarding the distribution of mental health problems in the social structure and the interpersonal coping efforts of psychologically distressed persons. The findings repeatedly demonstrate that those at the very bottom of the social stratificational system experience mental health problems disproportionately (1, 2). They have such problems more often and are less likely to receive professional mental health care (3). These findings, and

From *American Journal of Psychiatry* 150, no. 4 (April 1993)

many others as well (4, 5), should be seen in the context of the following statement of Ware et al. (6), based on findings in a sample of 4,444 individuals in families randomly assigned to diverse health insurance plans: "The great majority of those who are most psychologically distressed receive no mental health treatment even when care is free" (p. 1090).

This conclusion poses questions: Did some individuals in this "great majority" undertake help-seeking efforts? If so, who were they and under what circumstances did they undertake such efforts? Did they make use of the nonprofessional help-giving institutional structures of society? How? Finally, with respect to the persons most often studied—those who received professional care—what were the interpersonal circumstances directing them toward such care? If we are to answer these and other questions as to how the help-seeking effort deploys individuals throughout the help-giving institutional structure of society and what happens to them as a result of such deployment, the pathway concept needs to be developed. To contribute to this end, we will first examine and illustrate the concept of pathway, and then we will show how it is relevant to current issues and research findings pertaining to the onset of psychological distress, the contacting of mental health care facilities, and treatment in such facilities. In the final discussion we will argue that the pathway concept promises a unifying perspective if it is brought to the forefront of attention in the expanding research on mental health care.

To focus our discussion, we will refer to the situation of Hispanics, a population that in recent years has experienced considerable deterioration in its access to health care (7). Hispanics in general and Puerto Ricans in particular have been characterized as being at high risk for mental health problems (8). In fact, Puerto Ricans have been found to fulfill epidemiologic models of populations at high risk; at the same time, however, they tend to underutilize mental health facilities (9). Thus, they confront the paradox of being at high risk but infrequently using mental health facilities. They also confront serious socioeconomic problems (10) and problems stemming from migration-induced acculturative changes affecting mental health (11, 12). When the pathway concept is projected on the lives of Puerto Ricans, its significance is amplified, thus making it, to use Merton's phrase, a "strategic research event" (13). Since many of the ideas presented here originated in the earlier work on Hispanics of one of us (L.H.R.), we will provide illustrations taken from this work, but the general points apply to cultural groups other than Hispanics.

The Concept of Help-Seeking Pathways

By "pathways," we mean the sequence of contacts with individuals and organizations prompted by the distressed person's efforts, and those of his or her significant others, to seek help as well as the help that is supplied in response to such efforts. In mental health research, psychological distress encompasses a broad range of experiences, from those that are situationally induced to those associated with axis I and II disorders of DSM-II-R.

Research on factors influencing contacts with mental health care facilities focuses its definitions of help-seeking primarily on the initial recognition of the distress as a health problem and the subsequent decision to secure professional care (5). We begin with a more comprehensive view by looking on the pathway comprising the interpersonal help-seeking and help-receiving efforts as including cultural interpretations of the evolving distress, attempted therapeutic and social interventions by laypersons and professionals, and referral to help-giving primary and secondary groups. The pathway has direction, which is the sequential ordering of individuals and organizations contacted during the effort. The pathway also has duration, which is the time lapse between the initiation of the help-seeking effort and the formation of contacts. Psychosocial and cultural factors impinge upon direction and duration to shape the pathway's historical course. Thus, the metaphor invoked by the pathway concept is appropriate because the sequence of interpersonal contacts prompted by the distress is neither bizarre nor random. Pathways are structured.

Since the preponderance of research on this topic deals with treated patients, the customary pathway considered culminates in involvement in a mental health care facility (14, 15). This creates a gap in our knowledge because of the finding that the pathways of a majority of distressed persons do not lead to such involvement (6). A generic definition of *pathway*, oriented toward the distressed person's sequence of contacts with formal and informal institutional sources of help and the functions such sources perform as they intersect the pathway, invites the study of emergency rooms, nonpsychiatric specialized clinics, general practitioners, spiritualist sessions, the meetings of Pentecostal or charismatic religious denominations, civic groups and organizations, or repeated visits to the local pharmacist for advice. Broadly conceived, the pathway concept serves as an incessant reminder that coping with mental health distress in a culturally pluralistic, highly differentiated, and bureaucratized society such as that of the United States involves a vast range of help-giving institutional structures in addition to professionally developed mental health services.

Clinicians and their patients, of course, are aware of pathways and talk about them with varying degrees of explicitness. The story surrounding the distress brought to the clinician has been constructed in the patient's memory and forms an essential part of the presenting problem. The story is revelatory of the patient, including as it does a biography of "the events and pressures surrounding the particular problem" (16, p. 194). As the problem is being revealed, so is the pathway bringing the patient to the clinician.

We propose that what occurs routinely in clinical interviews can and should be developed extensively in field studies focusing on the pathways of clinical and nonclinical populations. *Trapped: Puerto Rican Families and Schizophrenia* by Rogler and Hollingshead (17), a study of schizophrenic individuals in the slums and public housing developments of San Juan, Puerto Rico, provides an illustration based on the experience of Mrs. Badillo. A married thirty-seven-year-old woman, Mrs. Badillo began suddenly to have violent seizures in which she collapsed on the floor, her limbs trembling, as she gasped for breath and moaned sorrowfully. A psychiatrist diagnosed her problem as a hysterical hyperkinetic seizure, but in Puerto Rican culture it was an *ataque*. Mrs. Badillo did not take her problem to a mental health professional. First she turned to her husband and then she turned to her neighbors, all of whom advised her that the problem had a spiritual cause. Third, she went to a spiritualist for consultation:

> The medium told me that there was a young man who was in love with me. The mother-in-law of this young man bewitched me through an evil spirit. The evil spirit takes me over in a violent way. When I see the mother-in-law of the young man I get an attack. This proves that the medium is right. (17, p. 248)

Mrs. Badillo's story about her *ataques* illustrates the definition of pathways: the sequence of contacts with individuals and organizations prompted by the effort to alleviate psychological distress and the help that is supplied through such contacts. The pathway's direction brought Mrs. Badillo into contact with the spiritualist medium, but its duration from the initial experience of the *ataques* to this contact remains unknown because it was not probed in the research. However, her experience shows how "cultural context affects not only the perception of potential problems; it also conditions ways of dealing with the problems" (14, p. 53). Spiritualist culture provided her with a socially verifiable interpretation of her bewildering *ataques*. The problem, having been rendered cognitively and emotionally meaningful through the succession of contacts with primary groups, was contained, at least until that time. Among Puerto Ricans living in the United States spiritualism retains its cultural vitality (18) as a form of folk psychiatry imbedded in their pathways.

The treatment of the pathway concept in research ranges from studies dealing with it as a hypothetical construct to studies that explicitly focus data collection on it. At the hypothetical construct end of this range, data directly relevant to the pathway are not collected, and the construct is used in the study only to interpret the empirical relationships found between actual utilization and the variables affecting utilization. So used, the construct signifies a process that remained unstudied in the research but is considered valuable in interpreting the relationship among variables such as age, sex, and education on the one hand and variables relevant to the type of professional service contacted and the degree to which the service is used on the other. To explain the relationship between the two sets of variables, the process may have been assumed to have involved specific types of interpersonal settings where decisions were made to secure professional services (19) or to have involved a more complex set of intervening phases—recognition of the problem, lay consultation, medical consultation, and referral to professional mental health care (20, 21). The implied argument, which we believe is correct, is that the psychosocial and cultural variables influencing utilization attain their relevance largely by affecting the intervening processes—the pathways. However, Gross and McMullen's review of the literature (14) quite correctly referred to pathway phases as "postulated" because, at this end of the continuum, they are used heuristically and not studied directly as observable processes.

Toward the other end of the continuum are efforts to deal with pathways as amenable to direct study. Here, data are used to document the proportion of individuals arrayed throughout the phases that evolve toward mental health care (22) or grid instruments are used to record data from patient interviews about the occurrence of psychiatric symptoms, the character of interventions, and the perceived effect of such interventions in the pathway (23). However, the preponderance of utilization research in mental health clearly falls away from this end of the continuum (5, 14, 24–26). Comparatively little is known objectively about the interpersonal dynamics of the help-seeking process because when the process is postulated it is not operationally assessed; thus, it is bypassed in the collection of data and then inserted heuristically in the interpretation of findings. Pathways need to be studied directly, as they evolve in one institutional direction or another, at whatever pace, whether or not they culminate in professional mental health care.

Thus, important specific issues remained unresolved in the illustration of Mrs. Badillo's *ataques*. It could well be that her problem remained intact, because the cessation of the pathway need not, empirically, coincide with the termination of the problem. How coterminous the two are depends on the interactions between the clinical manifestations of the distress and the impinging psychosocial and cultural environment. The beginning of the pathway—the initial organization of the help-seeking effort—is itself a process.

The Onset of the Distress Commencing the Pathway

The psychological problem initiating the help-seeking effort is important to study not only because it commences the pathway, if it commences at all, but also because the problem itself becomes the object of evolving interpersonal concerns and elaborations once the pathway starts. From the beginning, psychosocial and cultural factors impinge upon the severity and type of mental health problem; these factors interactively shape the pathway's direction and duration. Considerable attention has been given to this initial experience (27–29) and the underlying components that serve to define it (29, 30). Angel and Thoits (29), documenting the complexity of how cognitions structure the expression of illness, postulated a temporal sequence beginning with the proclivity of persons to monitor their own physiological and affective changes, continuing to the interpretation of such changes, then the actions taken based on the symptoms, and ending with the reevaluation of the symptoms produced by interaction with experts. Their formulations converge on the point that the initial subjective experiences of change revealed through self-monitoring are suffused with the person's cognitions and meanings. The clinical facts of the disease are only imperfectly related to the subjective experience of the illness (29), in part, at least, because of the immediate interventions of culture: "The experience of illness (or distress) is always a culturally shaped phenomenon" (28, p. 7). Errors result when culture is not taken into account. For example, the failure to consider how Mexican culture shapes the self-reports of physiological symptoms of Mexican Americans, according to Angel and Thoits (29), has produced serious errors in the findings of epidemiologic studies, which "reduce reports of illness for individuals at greater risk of poor health" (p. 470). In epidemiologic research in psychiatry this is an issue of measurement error, of how cultural components viewed as conceptually extraneous to psychological distress intrude into the observed assessments of psychological distress (31).

What is a measurement problem in epidemiologic research, however, becomes a substantive issue about culture in the development of the pathway concept. The issue is the identification of cultural factors that intervene between the self-monitored experience of change and the initiation of the help-seeking effort. For example, among Hispanics, in particular those in the first generation low in socioeconomic status, a *Weltanschauung* of fatalism is of likely importance. Fatalism views events as preordained by an overarching, metaphysically governed destiny in which the actions of human beings are largely ineffective in influencing their future lives (32). Socially, immigration selects individuals who are less fatalistic, but research indicates, nonetheless, that second-generation Puerto Ricans are substantially less fatalistic than their first-generation parents (32). Belief in fatalism diminishes an activist orientation toward life (33) and, when it encompasses orientation toward the self, suppresses the organization of distress into the help-seeking instrumental actions of the pathway.

Cultural norms can also keep distress from progressing toward help-seeking actions. More than two decades ago, Dohrenwend (34) argued that ethnically based cultural norms could well shape perceptions of the social undesirability of psychiatric symptoms. Since then, other researchers have noted that the disproportionately high expression of symptomatic distress among Puerto Ricans could be due to cultural norms not defining such symptoms as strongly undesirable (35). Puerto Rican respondents may be more willing than those in other ethnic groups to admit to mental health symptoms listed in the psychiatric inventories of epidemiologic studies; however, if the symptoms are not viewed as strongly undesirable, they are not as likely to prompt the help-seeking pathway. At onset and throughout the pathway, culture affects the proclivity to self-monitor as well as the normative content of the monitoring process (27).

Expressions of distress inevitably arise in the social interactions surrounding the distressed person (28, p. 7) and generate help-seeking efforts, usually in the context of the family, the pathway's customary starting point (36). As the quintessential primary group, the family mediates the decision to seek help by employing cultural interpretations such as those previously discussed. Culturally relevant here is one persistent epidemiologic finding: not only do women experience more psychological distress than men, but they are more likely than men with similar symptoms to seek help (37). Men are more likely than women to deny their problems and often have to submit involuntarily to the imposition of help from others (24). A considerable literature has emerged to explain these findings (38, 39), but it is still difficult to see in what way such gender-linked reactions to distress actually function in the family to prompt the pathway. We propose that such reactions are imbedded in the degree of sex-role segregation in the family. In cultural groups with strong sex-role segregation in the making of decisions, performing tasks, and leisure activities, women are cast in the role of socioemotional leadership and are absorbed in attending to matters of illness to prevent the disruption of affectional bonds in the family (17). More sensitive to the nuances and imperatives of psychological distress, they are more likely than men to mobilize the family's help-giving resources. As sex-role segregation diminishes, for example, in upwardly mobile cultural groups (32), the spouses more equally share leadership in organizing and directing the pathway.

Such leadership, however, is exercised in the context of the family's broader social organization, which varies considerably in a socially heterogeneous and culturally pluralistic society. The extremes that define the family's social organization range from the rapidly emerging pattern of single-parent households (40) to the nuclear unit of spouses and children living in one household and then to the extended family composed of collateral and intergenerationally linked kin living in the same household (41). Social organization defines the effective scope of the norm of reciprocal familial help, which, sustained by the double edge of guilt and gratitude, is implemented through the structure of kinship roles. The family's social organization reveals the character of the social unit that first mobilizes to circumscribe and treat the problem of psychological distress or to project the pathway outward toward other social networks.

Pathways to Contacts with Professional Mental Health Care

Social networks, a concept that has emerged in research on the utilization of professional mental health care (24, 25, 36, 42–45), designates "a specific set of linkages among a defined set of persons, with the additional property that the characteristics of the linkages as a whole may be used to interpret the social behavior of the persons involved" (46, p. 2). However, it is commonly recognized (21, 25, 26, 43, 44) that social networks, as is evident in the family, are suffused with cultural beliefs and serve as vehicles for transmitting them. Pathways function in the context of social networks. Let us explain what this means.

Freidson's influential theoretical formulations (43) hold to the assumption that "the whole process of seeking help involves a network of potential consultants, from the intimate and informal confines of the nuclear family through successively more select, distant, and authoritative laymen, until the professional is reached" (p. 377). The assumption points to the interaction between the lay and professional systems in explaining contacts with medical facilities. The professional system is built on medical culture and institutions; the lay system is built on lay culture and a network of personal contacts along which the client travels on the way to secure services. When the two systems are combined into a typology, substantial differences are predicted by the two extreme types in contacting medical services. The first, predicting isolation from our prolonged delays in forming such contacts, occurs when the lay referral system is large and extended and has an indigenous culture different from medical culture. The second type predicts quick contacts with the medical system when there is a loose and truncated lay referral system with beliefs congenial to medical culture. The in-between types predict a somewhat attenuated delay in contacting medical care.

Research based on the typology has sought to distinguish between kin and friendship groups as part of the lay referral system and has relied heavily on Elizabeth Bott's anthropologically developed concept of close-knit and open-knit networks (47). Close-knit networks signify strong interconnectedness among individuals; open-knit networks signify weak interconnectedness. Bott believed that social support derived from strong interconnectedness of closed networks (48). Correlatively, since social support has long been thought to be relevant to how people cope with problems, her ideas on interconnectedness were incorporated into research on the utilization of mental health facilities. Thus, to explain contacts with service providers, researchers have assessed the degree of interconnectedness among kin and in friendship groups (25) and also the interconnectedness between the two groups (42). Their findings have been promising: the stronger the interconnectedness, the longer the pathway's delay in contacting health facilities (42).

Explanations for this relationship remains speculative, but the following, advanced by Birkel and Repucci (42), reflect the ideas of other researchers, and are certainly plausible:

1. When networks are open, and the individuals are not too involved with each other, they are more exposed to information about the environment, including where to go for professional treatment. Pathways, then, are directed toward such treatment.
2. In close-knit networks, persons are pressured toward the acceptance of normative beliefs. When the beliefs do not coincide with the culture of the service facilities, pathways are restrained from reaching such facilities.
3. In close-knit networks, social support renders professional service less necessary, thus bending the pathway away from such services.

The explanations can be compressed into one general hypothesis: the degree of interconnectedness of social networks influences the social and cognitive functions of pathways—access to new help-seeking information, conformance with norms, and social support—intervening between the onset of the illness and the act of contacting mental health facilities. Such contacts are accelerated by the presence of a friend or associate knowledgable about mental health practice and removed from the distressed person's inner circle of social networks (36, 43–45). These are the "authoritative laymen" in the earlier quotation from Freidson. By using the pathway concept to unify the explanations into one general hypothesis, we can begin to see how such social and cognitive functions, are arrayed throughout the help-seeking effort and the corresponding roles persons perform in response to variations in network interconnectedness.

Minimally, this task involves the study of institutional settings where such functions intersect pathways, but even here we confront a problem of ignorance, and it affects Hispanic mental health research. In this research, it is customary to identify a priori the family, friends, neighbors, the co-parent/godfather-based relationship (49), and therapeutic folk institutions, such as spiritualism (18), but other institutional patterns that are emergent rather than traditional remain to be identified. They arise when there is a deep structural gulf separating the linguistic and cultural minority from the bureaucratic system of service delivery. Crescive networks emerge to bridge this gulf, nurtured by the efforts of the bicultural minority leaders—who have the requisite linguistic skills, knowledge, and interest—to connect the needs of compatriots to the resources of the system (50). When the attempts succeed, the emergent networks are institutionalized to channel pathways.

For example, in an anthropological study of a small Puerto Rican community in a middle-sized city on the Eastern seaboard (33), the grassroots leaders of two organizations were identified as having a virtual monopoly in orienting the newly arrived and intervening with agencies on behalf of their Puerto Rican compatriots. The constituency of a political boss consisted of the least assimilated immigrants, and a powerful civic leader represented their somewhat more assimilated compatriots. While intervening, these leaders also served as acculturative agents, transmitting to their constituents the professional ideologies of the service system. This type of leader is unpaid; his or her services on behalf of compatriots are exchanged for increments of prestige and power in the ethnic community. Since the roles they perform are crescive rather than planned or enacted, they do not appear in tables of organization, the Yellow Pages, or compendiums of community institutions. Their relevance can be uncovered only through ethnographic studies of pathways.

The studies are also likely to show that among cultural minorities, as well as broad segments of the general population, the pathway's first contact with the health delivery system is not with a mental health professional. People afflicted with a mental health problem often seek treatment in the general medical sector (51, 52). Procedurally, the identification of the presenting problem as psychiatric is often a residual diagnosis arrived at after an array of clinical and laboratory tests have proven negative. This procedure links congenially to the tendency among Hispanics and other cultural minorities to somatize distress (28, 31, 53, 54), thus serving to contain the pathway in the nonpsychiatric medical sector (51).

Pathways to Treatment in Mental Health Facilities

There are compelling reasons for continuing the development and use of the pathway concept after treatment in a mental health facility has been sought and is being provided on an inpatient or outpatient basis. The mental health practitioners and their associated personnel now become part of the pathway's network, but their insertion into the network is, at least at first, likely to be tenuous and uncertain. An abundance of research demonstrates substantial discontinuity between first contact and incorporation into a reliable treatment program. Mitchell (45) estimated that between 20 percent and 57 percent of patients in psychotherapy drop out after the first therapy session; Sue and Zane (55) reported that among cultural minorities there is 50 percent attrition after the first appointment. The discontinuity disproportionately affects cultural minorities (21, 23, 53, 56). Attrition quickly sets in, thus eliminating from professional treatment many distressed individuals whose pathway has brought them to the doorstep of the mental health facility. However, attrition may signify a change in pathway direction toward other sources of help.

Among Hispanics, cultural incongruities between patient and treatment setting play a role in such attrition (57). The inability to communicate because of language differences between the patient and the clinician is sufficient to deflect the pathway away from the treatment setting. To avoid such deflection, Hispanics often bring compatriots to serve as translators or translators are provided by the treatment facility, but these solutions are not free of problems (58). Moreover, linguistic difficulties may still continue to affect the pathway even when the patient knows some English but is Spanish dominant and must talk to an English-speaking clinician: diagnostic errors are likely to occur (59, 60) that might deleteriously affect the choice and use of a treatment modality.

To the first-generation Hispanic immigrant with limited socioeconomic resources and accustomed largely to traditional forms of primary group interaction, contact with a professional therapist means incorporation into a new and different network of relationships. For the relationships to be successful, both patient and therapist must become meaningfully involved in the help-seeking pathway that already has been shaped by a history of primary group network interventions before the patient entered a setting with bureaucratic regulations. That setting has waiting rooms, offices, charts and interview schedules, testing protocols, and all the other accoutrements and paraphernalia of daily bureaucratic life. However, unlike the usual contacts with service bureaucracies, the expectation is for repeated appointments and prolonged treatment with no predictable end in sight. Appointments must be kept on time and end after so many minutes. Patients are seen serially, and therapists can be changed. The relationship is premised on an implied contract: the patient is to fulfill the organization's expectations and the therapist is obligated to bring expertise to bear on the psychological problem presented without assuming responsibility for the client's total welfare. In this impersonal and segmented environment, the patient is invoked to reveal the inner turmoil of his or her private life to a virtual stranger—usually representing a higher status and often a different culture as well as speaking a different language—through potentially compromising confessions. During initial contacts, the patient's bewilderment and anxiety are exacerbated by the experience of altered, disjunctive relationships. Mitchell (45) found that when individuals in treatment received positive feedback for being in therapy from members of their personal network, they continued to attend therapy sessions. Without shedding primary group involvements, the pathway encounters a troublesome threshold as it is incorporated into a network of secondary, professional contacts.

The concentrated attention given by so much research to explanation of the use of professional services may inadvertently create the view that, when used, such services monopolize the patient's help-seeking efforts. The point is our need to know how professional interventions intertwine with the patient's retention of primary group bonds and what happens when the intervention ceases. We are reminded of an illustration in the previously cited study by Rogler and Hollingshead (17): a man prone to violent eruptions was taken to a psychiatrist by relatives so that he could be tranquilized and then taken to a "genuine" therapist, a spiritualist medium. As long as the help-seeking effort continues, the pathway concept has relevance.

Discussion

Pathways begin at some identifiable point in the social structure, prompted by the culturally mediated help-seeking interactions between the distressed person and his or her significant others. The quality and seriousness of the distress provide the impetus to the pathway (25, 30), but its duration and direction are shaped by the convergence of psychosocial and cultural factors (3, 23, 24, 30, 56). Some factors affect the pathways directly, and some affect it indirectly through the social networks that bind the distressed person to his or her significant others. Thus, the concept of pathways emerges in this analysis as having sufficient integrity to be considered scientifically as a distinct and identifiable process. If brought to the forefront of programmatically organized research, it can help to integrate much of our understanding about the use of mental health care.

Reliable procedures for the prospective and retrospective assessment of pathways need to be developed in studies incorporating clinical and nonclinical samples. Clinical samples are convenient, and their study fits the ethos of a highly bureaucratized society oriented toward the flow of needy clients into the service sector. Pathways, however, have many directions. Even though recent years have witnessed notable efforts to study nonclinical samples through the National Institute of Mental Health's Epidemiologic Catchment Area program (52), the purpose has been to document primarily the magnitude and type of mental health problems. The development of procedures to assess pathways will make a complementary but essential contribution by showing how countless numbers of people, prompted by such problems, are being distributed throughout the informal and formal help-giving institutions of our society.

The use of such procedures must be accompanied by the recognition that help-giving institutions are not equally capable of rendering help, either quantitatively or qualitatively (61, 62). Paraphrased, Litwak's formulations (62) assert that kinship structures, resting on permanent relationships, can deal with long-term commitments; friendship ties, resting on free choice and affectivity, can deal with the provision of new information; neighbors, because of geographical proximity, can deal with emergencies; and bureaucracies, resting on trained expertise and concentrated resources, can provide specialized segmented services. These formulations define the outlying limits of help-giving structures and serve also to remind us of the social selection that occurs in successive contacts with such structures. We believe that social selection, filtering individuals into pathways bending in one direction or another, functions across the entire spectrum of help-seeking efforts, affecting people who do not reach psychiatric care or, having reached it, stabilize their involvement or drop out. What appear to be dropouts falling by the wayside, victims of attribution, may have in fact been selectively channeled toward other organizations or selectively encapsulated within the confines of their primary groups. Or they may have been selectively projected toward the street culture of the homeless. The identification of the help such structures actually give and how the help is arrayed sequentially to selectively filter individuals from one structure to the next awaits the development and implementation of the pathway concept (22, 23).

Even though the pathway concept remains methodologically undeveloped, its clinical unity is evident. It renders understandable the underlying processes of recent innovative efforts to provide Hispanics and other cultural minorities with culturally sensitive mental health care: the attraction of indigenous help-seeking pathways to mental health care facilities (63), allaying the uncomfortable discontinuity of incorporating the distressed person's pathway into new sets of professional relationships (55), and stabilizing the pathways' linkages to the therapeutic setting (63). Appropriately developed, the pathway concept promises to integrate much of our understanding of mental health care while increasing our vision of how to make such care more accessible and effective.

References

1. Dohrenwend, B. P., Dohrenwend, B. S., Gould, M. S., Link, B., Neugebauer, R., and Wunsch-Hitzig, R. (eds). (1980). *Mental illness in the United States: Epidemiological estimates.* New York: Praeger.

2. Kressler, R. C., and Cleary, P. D. (1980). Social class and psychological distress. *Am Sociol Rev* 45:463–478.

3. Link, B., and Dohrenwend, B. P. (1980). Formulation of hypotheses about the ratio of untreated and treated cases in the true prevalence studies of functional disorders in adults in the United States. In B. P. Dohrenwend et al., eds. *Mental illness in the United States: Epidemiological estimates.* New York: Praeger, 1980.

4. Regier, D. A., Goldberg, I., and Taube, C. (1978). The de facto U.S. mental health services system. *Arch Gen Psychiatry* 35:685–693.

5. Horwitz, A. V. (1987). Help-seeking processes and mental health sciences. In D. Mechanic (Ed.), *Improving mental health services.* San Francisco: Jossey-Bass, 1987.

6. Ware, J. E., Manning, W. G., Duan, N., Wells, K. B., and Newhouse, J. P. (1984). Health status and the use of outpatient mental health services. *Am Psychol* 39:1090–1100.

7. Access to Health Care in the United States (1987). Results of a 1986 Survey, vol 2. Princeton, NJ: Robert Wood Johnson Foundation.

8. Moscicki, E. K., Locke, B. Z., Rae, D. S., and Boyd, J. H. (1989). Depressive symptoms among Mexican Americans: the Hispanic Health and Nutrition Examination Survey. *Am J Epidemiol* 130:348–360.

9. Rodriguez, O. (1987). *Hispanics and human services: Help-seeking in the inner city*: Monograph 14. New York: Hispanic Research Center, Fordham University.

10. Bean, F. D., and Tienda, M. (1987). *The Hispanic population of the United States.* New York: Russell Sage Foundation.

11. Rogler, L. H., Gurak, D. T., and Cooney, R. S. (1987). The migration experience and mental health: Formulations relevant to Hispanics and other immigrants. In M. Gaviria and J. D. Arana (Eds.), *Health and behavior: Research agenda for Hispanics*: Monograph 1. Champaign: University of Illinois Press.

12. Rogler, L. H., Cortes, D. E., and Malgady, R. G. (1991). Acculturation and mental health status among Hispanics: Convergence and new directions for research. *Am Psychol* 46:585–597.

13. Merton, R. K (1987). Three fragments from a sociologist's notebook: Estab-

lishing the phenomenon, specified ignorance, and strategic research materials. *Annual Rev Sociology* 13:1–28.

14. Gross, A. E., and McMullen, P.A. (1983). Models of help-seeking process. In B. M., DePaulo, A. Nadler, and J. D. Fisher (Eds.), *New directions in helping*, vol. 2. New York: Academic Press.

15. Williams, P., Wilkinson, G., and Rawnsley, K. (Eds.). (1991). *The scope of epidemiological psychiatry.* New York: Routledge.

16. Howard, C. S. (1991). Culture tales: A narrative approach to thinking cross-cultural psychology and psychotherapy. *Am Psychol* 46:187–197.

17. Rogler, L. H, and Hollingshead, A. B. (1985). *Trapped Puerto Rican families and schizophrenia*, 3rd ed. Maplewood, NJ: Waterfront Press.

18. Harwood, A. (1977). *Rx: Spiritist as needed: A study of a Puerto Rican community mental health resource.* New York: John Wiley & Sons.

19. Briones, D. F., Hellet, P. L., Chalfant, H. P., Roberts, A. E., Aguirre-Hauchbaum, S. F., and Farr, W. F. Jr. (1990). Socioeconomic status, ethnicity, psychological distress, and readiness to utilize a mental health facility. *Am J Psychiatry* 147:1333–1340.

20. Kadushin, C. (1958). Individual decisions to undertake psychotherapy. *Administrative Science Quarterly* 3:379–411.

21. Lin, K. M., Inui, T. S., Kleinman, A. M., and Womack, W. M. (1982). Sociocultural determinants of the help-seeking behavior of patients with mental illness. *J Nerv Ment Dis* 170:78–85.

22. Goldberg D., and Huxley, P. (1980). *Mental illness in the community: The pathway to psychiatric care.* London: Tavistock Publications.

23. Lin, T. Y., Tardiff, K., Donetz, G., and Goresky, W. (1972). Ethnicity and patterns of help-seeking. *Cult Med Psychiatry* 2:3–14.

24. Horwitz, A. V. (1977). The pathways into psychiatric treatment: Some differences between men and women. *J Health Soc Behav* 18:169–178.

25. Horwitz, A. V. (1987). Social networks and pathways to psychiatric treatment. *Social Forces* 56:86–105.

26. McKinlay, J. B. (1973). Social networks, lay consultation, and help-seeking behavior. *Social Forces* 51:275–292.

27. Mechanic, D. (1968). *Medical sociology: A selective view.* New York: Free Press.

28. Kleinman, A. (1988). *Rethinking psychiatry: From cultural category to personal experience.* New York: Free Press.

29. Angel, R., and Thoits, P. (1987). The impact of culture on the cognitive structure of illness. *Cult Med Psychiatry* 11:465–494.

30. Greenley, J. R., and Mechanic, D. (1976). Social selection in seeking help for psychological problems. *J Health Soc Behav* 17:249–262.

31. Rogler, L. H. (1989). The meaning of culturally sensitive research in mental health. *Am J Psychiatry* 146:296–303.

32. Rogler, L. H., and Cooney, R. S. (1984). *Puerto Rican families in New York City: Intergenerational processes*: Monograph 11. New York: Hispanic Research Center, Fordham University.

33. Rogler, L. H. (1984). *Migrant in the city*, 2nd ed. Maplewood, NJ: Waterfront Press.

34. Dohrenwend, B. P. (1966). Social status and psychological disorder: An issue of substance and an issue of method. *Am Sociol Rev* 31:14–34.

35. Haberman, P. (1976). Psychiatric symptoms among Puerto Ricans in Puerto Rico and New York City. *Ethnicity* 3:133–144.

36. Horwitz, A. V. (1978). Family, kin, and friend networks on psychiatric help-seeking. *Soc Sci Med* 12:297–304.

37. Kessler, R. C., Brown, R. L., and Broman, C. L. (1981). Sex differences in psychiatric help-seeking: Evidence from four large scale surveys. *J Health Soc Behav* 22:49–64.

38. Leaf, P. J., and Bruce, M. L. (1987). Gender differences in the use of mental health-related services: A re-examination. *J Health Soc Behav* 28:171–183.

39. Veroff, J. B. (1981). The dynamics of help-seeking in men and women: A national survey study. *Psychiatry* 45:189–200.

40. Sweet, J. A., and Bumpass, L. L. (1987). *American families and households.* New York: Russell Sage Foundation.

41. Hill, R. (1970). *Family development in three generations.* Cambridge, MA: Schenkman.

42. Birkel, R. C., and Repucci, N. D. (1983). Social networks, information-seeking, and utilization of services. *Am J Community Psychol* 11:185–205.

43. Freidson, E. (1960). Client control and medical practice. *Am J Sociol* 65:374–382.

44. Freidson, E. (1970). *Profession of medicine: A study of the sociology of applied knowledge.* New York: Russell Sage Foundation.

45. Mitchell, M. E. (1987). The relationship between social network variables and the utilization of mental health services. *Am J Community Psychol* 1989; 17:258–266.

46. Mitchell, J. C. (1969). Social networks in urban situations. Manchester: Manchester University Press.

47. Bott, E. (1957). *Family and social networks.* New York: Free Press.

48. Rogler, L. H., and Procidano, M. E. (1986). The effect of social networks on marital roles: A test of the Bott hypothesis in an intergenerational context. *J Marriage and the Family* 48:693–701.

49. Rogler, L. H., Malgady, R. G., and Rodriguez, O. (1989). *Hispanics and mental health: A framework for research.* Malabar, FL: Robert F Krieger.

50. Rogler, L. H. (1974). The changing role of a political boss in a Puerto Rican migrant community. *Am Sociol Rev* 39:57–67.

51. Alegria, M., Robles, R., Freeman, D. H., Vera, M., Jimenez, A. L., Rios, C., and Rios, R. (1991). Patterns of mental health utilization among island Puerto Rican poor. *Am J Public Health* 81:875–879.

52. Wells, K. B., Golding, J. M., Hough, R. L., Burnam, M. A., Karno, M. (1988). Factors affecting the probability of use of general and medical health and social/community services for Mexican Americans and non-Hispanic whites. *Med Care* 26:441–452.

53. Angel, R., and Guarnaccia, P. J. (1989). Mind, body, and culture: Somatization among Hispanics. *Soc Sci Med* 28:1229–1238.

54. Ruiz P (1985). Clinical care update: The minority patient. *Community Ment Health J* 21:208–216.

55. Sue S., and Zane, N. (1987). The role of culture and cultural techniques in psychotherapy: A critique and reformulation. *Am Psychol* 42:37–45.

56. Sue, S. (1977). Community mental health services to minority groups: Some optimism, some pessimism. *Am Psychol* 32:616–624.

57. Miranda, M. R. (1976). *Psychotherapy with the Spanish-speaking: Issues in research and service delivery*: Monograph 3. Los Angeles: Spanish-Speaking Mental Health Research Center.

58. Acosta, F., and Cristo, M. (1981). Development of a bilingual interpreter program: An alternative model for Spanish-speaking services. *Professional Psychol* 12:474–482.

59. Marcos, L. R., Alpert, M., Urcuyo, L., and Kesselman, M. (1973). The effect of interview language on the evaluation of psychopathology in Spanish-American schizophrenic patients. *Am J Psychiatry* 130:549–553.

60. Marcos, L. R., Urcuyo, L., Kesselman, M., and Alpert, M. (1973). The language barrier in evaluating Spanish-American patients. *Arch Gen Psychiatry* 29:655–659.

61. Litwak, E., and Szelenyi, I. (1969). Primary group structures and their functions: kin, neighbors, and friends. *Am Sociol Rev* 34:465–481.

62. Litwak, E. (1968). Technological innovation and theoretical functions of primary groups and bureaucratic structures. *Am J Sociol* 73:468–481.

63. Rogler, L. H., Malgady, R. G., Constantino, G., and Blumenthal, R. (1987). What do culturally sensitive mental health services mean? The case of Hispanics. *Am Psychol* 42:565–570.

4

On Illness Meanings and Clinical Interpretation

Not "Rational Man," but a Rational Approach to Man the Sufferer/Man the Healer

Arthur Kleinman

ILLNESS IS INSEPARABLE from the networks of meanings within which it is experienced and treated. These meanings—often changing, usually ambiguous, frequently tacit—sometimes are determined principally by the nature of the illness itself and its consequences for the sick person and family. But more often illness absorbs and is saturated by the web of beliefs, norms, and interests that constitute the day-to-day world of the sick person in his particular social situation. Illness, thereby, becomes a polysemic symbol, one whose referents are affect and motivation as much as cognition and social relations; it is part of an idiosyncratic meaning system that belongs to a broader, more visible cultural meaning system, which, because it is shared, is also easier (though rarely easy) to interpret. Illness meanings may or may not be understood by the sick person and his network. Probably they are appreciated more often than clinicians and social science researchers allow, but owing to their powers to manipulate social relations as well as to illness's legitimated social cachet, these meanings cannot be readily acknowledged and their function commented upon openly by social actors themselves. This would be tantamount to stripping away the fixation on content that obscures the structure of social reality, and converting social actors into sociologists

From *Culture, Medicine, and Psychiatry* 5, no. 4, 373–77 (December 1981) with kind permission from Springer Science and Business Media

and their discourse into a theoretical metalanguage. It would undermine the very fabric of social life and alienate and paralyze action. No! Illness meanings remain dense, vague, obscure, and partially interpreted or misinterpreted as a basic requirement of social life. Nonetheless, it is important to recognize that they are only partially out of awareness, that their web of significance is sensed and may be creatively manipulated in interpersonal transaction.

The very complexity of these meaning systems, their necessarily disguised condition, their polysemy—all of this makes for fundamental uncertainty in interpretation. Moreover, since each more or less overt expression of illness meaning is socially constructed for certain purposes—to obtain help, sanction failure, elicit love and attention, distance a bothersome researcher, deny a fearsome reality to the sick person, and so on—meaning is actively constituted in the very act of interpretation, so that different contexts of interpretation may generate different significances for the "same" illness. It is not just that the psychiatrist and medical anthropologist are more skilled at interpreting illness meanings or that they have more time to make sense of an obscure and obscuring reality than the family doctor, but that the meanings they "uncover," like those the family doctor confronts, are in fact created by them and for them in their transaction with patients. Each socially constructed understanding of an illness is precisely "an" understanding: partial, one-sided, tendentious, replicating a particular relationship and "interest." Perhaps only an extraordinarily sensitive novelist can resurrect a network of illness meanings in its entirety. To do that he must expose for us a complete world of signification—subtle, dense, uncertain—and this tour de force is possible for him to do precisely because he is writing fiction.

The *explanatory models* framework provides the clinician with an expeditious practical method to assess the more accessible meanings that hold clear-cut importance for care. The picture so constructed is doubtless crude, incomplete, biased. But it is usually "good enough" for the purpose at hand: namely, to alert the clinician to the psychosocial setting of the sickness and to make available to him an appreciation of at least some of the dominant meanings expressed and reproduced by the illness experience. So informed, the clinician may select to undertake a more extensive ethnography of his patient's illness, ask a liaison psychiatrist or clinical social scientist to undertake this task for him, or make do with what he has learned. The very act of inquiring into illness meanings, whatever in fact is learned, breaks the tunnel vision of biomedicine and its veterinary tendency. The explanatory models approach, however inadequate it may be for ethnographer or novelist, brings meaning, person, family, and feeling into the process of clinical judgment, and this opening to the humanness of suffering, in my experience, is often all that is needed to reaffirm for the physician the critical importance of psychological and social issues in a particular case and thereby make him less tolerant of delivering simply a technical "fix." Since the primary care physician is engaged in an ongoing conversation over the years with the families for whom he provides care, a conversation that contributes to the social construction of their shared clinical reality, it is likely that the explanatory models elicitation framework will build on and contribute to a fairly deep appreciation of particular illness meanings and, if the physician is open to the opportunity, will sensitize him to an understanding of how his professional culture's categories and relationships socially construct sickness as ideal-typical diseases. In this sense, explanatory models can lead the clinician to a multiperspective pluralistic view of sickness that liberates him from a naïve and severely limiting single-sided professional perspective.

Interpretation of illness meanings is essential for effective clinical work and it is the very essence of liaison psychiatry and clinically applied medical anthropology. The patient with chronic pain may be expressing a distressing relationship, the pain of failure, the pain of loneliness, or eliciting love and support, seeking compensation, warding off depressive thoughts and feelings that threaten to overwhelm him, or several of these meanings simultaneously. Whether he suffers from cancer, arthritis, or depression, effective care involves taking into account and dealing with these meanings as much as treating him with drugs and surgery. The explanatory models approach does not create a stereotyped rational man for clinician or researcher. It situates them in the patient's personal and social world, and makes unavoidable the human antecedents and consequences of illness, thereby humanizing medicine by anthropologizing it. Like the ethnographer who objectivizes conventional wisdom so that he can detect generative culture rules behind surface utterances, the clinician who employs the explanatory models method objectivizes his patients' and his own understandings not to construct a false dialogue between "rational men" but to take a rational approach to the social world, one hopefully that is as systematic, rigorous, and intelligently informed by social science as his assessment of physiology is by biomedicine.

Explanatory models are not ways of thinking or systems of thought but practical statements about particular illness experiences. They are expressed guides to help seeking and clinical decision making. Since by definition the elicitation process makes them public, negotiated understandings, their private sources (personal fears, family troubles, paradigmatic exemplars of moral behavior) must be inferred. The explanatory model, then, is Janus-faced: pointing outward to public metaphors, inward to private ones that are as much affect and motivation as cognition. Explanatory models disclose the interpersonal processes of denial and dissimulation, retrospective narratization and rationalization, dependence and domination, reality construction and manipulation, that are as basic to communication as are exchange of resources and transmission of information.

Hence the explanatory models framework is a useful and richly evocative technique to teach clinicians about the psychological, social, and cultural contexts and functions of clinical communication. And the same technique can be turned on its head, so to speak, and employed by the clinician or health educator to engage patients and families more fully and knowledgeably in the workings of medical care. Indeed, to my mind, systematic elicitation and negotiation of explanatory models make unavoidable to the clinical and health services researcher the mediating symbolic bridge of meanings and relationships that connects environment with physiology forming the basis for biopsychosocial integration in illness and healing. Perhaps this is why this orientation to clinical teaching and practices offends discipline-bound thinkers who want their physiology, their psychology, their philosophy straight and undiluted. It is a window on the messy, complicated human world that, for all its "quick and dirty" limitations and attempts to be quantitatively scientific, provides a view determinedly interdisciplinary, inherently ethnographic. One begins with superficial utterances and ends up with deeply troubling questions of *interpretation* that are the very essence of illness experience and clinical work.

If anthropology, as Raymond Firth contends, can be usefully thought of as "the uncomfortable science," then the explanatory models heuristic of medical anthropology can be regarded as a fairly effective means of making clinicians, and clinical teachers and researchers too, uncomfortable about the flat, dehumanized, statistical reductionism intrinsic to biomedical rationality and behavior or for that matter, uncomfortable with the distorting effect of any single analytic lens (e.g., behavioral, psychoanalytic, survey research, Marxist) applied to the complex, rapidly changing, many-sided, negotiated human world that is socially constructed by clinical categories and clinically constructed by social ones. The study of applied clinical rationality (of patients as well as practitioners) goes away when it isolates rationality from its normative context of therapeutic action and freezes it as a "thing" apart from the dynamic process of practical interpretation in which it is psychoculturally expressed and constituted.

5

On Culturally Enhancing the DSM-IV Multiaxial Formulation

Juan E. Mezzich and Byron J. Good

THE NEED FOR A CULTURALLY SENSITIVE and cross-culturally valid DSM-IV, including its multiaxial schema, is primarily based on the multicultural reality of the United States. The substantial and growing presence of African Americans, Asian Americans, Native Americans, and Latinos is impressive and presents special problems for diagnosis. So too the flow of migrant refugees to the United States and the growth of special populations such as the homeless create particular difficulties for making valid and reliable diagnoses using uniform criteria. The international visibility expected of DSM-IV, predicated on the worldwide impact of the DSM-III (American Psychiatric Association, 1980), noted by Mezzich (1987), provides an added impetus for making cultural considerations explicit within the structure of the manual.

The emerging comprehensive concepts of health status, which encompass physical health, mental condition, functioning levels, and quality of life, are also important here. As Patrick et al. (1985) pointed out, each of these aspects is influenced by cultural factors. Consequently, assessment in multicultural settings requires particular clinician sensitivity, and both reliability and validity of assessments depend on a systematic recognition of difficulties in using diagnostic categories and rating scales across cultures.

Cultural considerations offered for the multiaxial system of DSM-IV are discussed here axis by axis and then with regard to a complementary cultural formulation.

Axes I and II: Mental Disorders

The impact of cultural factors on the various aspects of psychopathology and its professional appraisal and diagnostic categorization has been a focal point of sustained anthropological and cross-cultural psychiatric research, as summarized by Fabrega (1987), Hopper (1991), Kleinman (1988), and Mezzich et al. (1996). Specific recommendations for according a measure of cultural sensitivity to the judgments and ratings corresponding to Axes I and II are for the most part contained in proposals to be inserted in the pertinent sections of the main body of DSM-IV. We also recommend that specific attention be drawn to relevant cultural issues in the section of the manual that discusses the multiaxial structure.

Axis III: General Medical Disorders

The differential distribution of certain medical diseases across ethnic groups, reflected in epidemiological findings and literature on illness behavior (for a summary, see Harwood 1981), is one consideration for sensitive diagnoses on this axis. Such variations may reflect genetic factors (as in the case of sickle-cell anemias and African ethnicity), social and environmental factors (as in the distribution of a wide variety of infectious diseases), and risk behaviors.

Of special importance to psychiatric diagnosis is the fact that general medical diseases interact with psychiatric illness in complex ways. For example, Kleinman (1988) pointed out that several of the primary criteria for major depressive disorder (weakness, tiredness, and appetite disturbance) are common symptoms of many parasitic and infectious diseases, making diagnosis of depression more difficult in populations in which such conditions are endemic. Weiss (1985) has shown that culture strongly influences both normal and pathological responses to such highly stigmatizing illnesses as leprosy, presenting significant difficulties for assessment. Similar considerations may be applicable to AIDS.

Cultural factors also powerfully influence the emergence, meaning, and ramifications of those health problems that are ill defined and difficult to diagnose, such as those often seen in primary care. Culturally distinctive somatic idioms for expressing distress and illness add to the difficulty of making valid and reliable diagnoses across cultures.

Axis IV: Psychosocial Stressors and Supports

The importance of this area has been widely recognized since the proposals of Rutter et al. (1975), despite the modest success reported with the specific procedures developed for assessment of this axis. The importance of this domain appears to be significant not only for psychiatric conditions but also for general health, as documented by House et al. (1988). Options are being formulated for shifting the focus of Axis IV from overall severity of psychosocial stressors to a list of specific stressors and/or a procedure focused on the appraisal of support factors. Because the scaling of stressors and supports assumes an implicit cultural norm, and because any list of stressors and supports will be culturally specific, it will be a challenge to make Axis IV assessments valid across social and cultural subgroups in our society or cross-culturally.

Nonetheless, the need to consider general environmental factors, specific precipitating events, and levels of support as well as the cultural factors influencing them is widely recognized. For example, Tseng (1985) emphasized the need to understand the anthropology of the family to effectively assess pertinent stressors and coping patterns. Pierloot and Ngoma (1988) documented that psychosocial stressors tend to originate in large group interactions in the case of African patients as compared with more restricted family interactions in patients with a European background. Vargas-Willis and Cervantes (1987) discussed the loss of family relations and cultural change faced by Latino immigrants to the United States.

The meaning of the stressors for the affected individuals may have a decisive etiopathogenic role. Furthermore, cultural factors may influence both the structure of social supports and the evaluation of the effectiveness of such support (Guarnaccia, 1996).

To furnish information on feasibility and fit, diagnostic proposals on psychosocial factors should be empirically validated through field trials in the major American ethnic groups and minority populations.

Axis V: Functioning

The structure and content of Axis V are subject to a number of competing perspectives. One of them refers to focusing this aspect on adaptive functioning only, without considering symptomatology. This is based on the argument that symptomatology is most relevant to the clinical syndromic axes and the inclusion of symptoms in the functioning axis heavily shifts the clinician's attention to them to the detriment of the role of social performance. Furthermore, the severity of symptoms may be best handled by severity guidelines furnished for psychopathological (Axes I and II) diagnoses.

Another proposal involves separate assessment of key functioning areas such as occupational and interpersonal performance. It has been widely demonstrated that cultural factors can have crucial effects on the design and application of measurement instruments in this area, as indicated by Alarcon (1983), particularly for personality disorders. To illustrate further, Kunce and Vales (1984) discussed the need for sensitivity in the assessment of the functioning of Mexican Americans, taking into consideration differences in behavioral expectations, values, and styles. Good and Good (1986) and Good and Kleinman (1985) summarized the difficulties in adapting psychometric instruments for cross-cultural use.

As in the case of Axis IV, it seems clear that the cultural relevance of measurement instruments or of clinician ratings must be empirically examined and that sensitivity to cultural diversity is required in their administration. In addition to assessing functioning in terms of the norms of the broader society, it should be useful to base it on the evaluation of significant others close to the patient (Guarnaccia, 1996).

Complementary Cultural Formulation

The need for dedicated attention to the cultural dimensions of diagnoses has been argued by Hughes (1985) and others. Empirical proposals for culture-relevant axes are exemplified by the octaxial schema conceptualized and implemented in the Puerto Rican mental health care system by H. Ramirez (personal communication, April 2, 1989). Critical perspectives and elements for organizing a cultural axis have been articulated by Good and Good (1986).

Key informants for a cultural formulation would be the patient and his or her primary social group (Good and Good, 1986). This represents an emic perspective or "the native point of view" (Geertz, 1983).

A major instrumental issue involves language abilities and preferences (Irvine, 1985; Marcos and Alpert, 1976). A new critical perspective in this regard is multilingualism, prompted by recent observations of Latin American immigrants (Guarnaccia, 1996). These considerations are connected to the importance of acculturation and biculturalism. Work in this area has tended to portray an individual's affiliation on a continuum from totally involved in the culture of origin to totally assimilated into the host culture (Cuellar and Roberts, 1984). Alternative perspectives have focused on the parallel appraisal of involvement in both the culture of origin and the host culture (Santisteban and Szapocznik, 1982). There is a growing literature on the contribution of acculturation stress to the emergence of psychopathology and on the adaptive value of biculturalism (Guarnaccia, 1996).

The constitutive elements of a prospective cultural formulation, as initially proposed by Good and Good (1986), would include the meaning of and explanatory models for the diagnoses made, the recognition of culture-specific syndromes and illness idioms, perceived levels of adaptive functioning, care-seeking patterns, and expectations of illness outcome and quality of life.

The proposed cultural formulation could be presented within the framework of a comprehensive psychiatric evaluation, in line with the tradition of familial-genetic and psychodynamic formulations. Further research may lead to the standardization, at least in part, of this formulation, the establishment of more solid connections with other elements of psychiatric assessment, and its effective use for treatment and prognosis.

At the 1991 Conference on Culture and Diagnosis in Pittsburgh, Pennsylvania, sponsored by the National Institute of Mental Health, there was clearly wide interest in some form of cultural statement to complement the standard diagnostic ratings in DSM-IV. The conceptual and consultation work carried out in the following years led to the development of a Cultural Formulation Guideline, growing out of wide empirical research and clinical experience (Mezzich et al., 1993). The guideline consists of the following five components.

Cultural Identity of the Individual

The clinician should specify the individual's cultural reference groups. Attend particularly to language abilities, use, and preferences (including multilingualism). For immigrants and ethnic minorities, note separately the degree of involvement with both the culture of origin and the host or majority culture.

Cultural Explanations of the Individual's Illness

Identify the following:

1. The predominant idioms of distress through which symptoms are communicated (e.g., "nerves," possessing spirits, somatic complaints, inexplicable misfortune).
2. The meaning and perceived severity of the individual's symptoms in relation to norms of the cultural reference group.
3. Any local illness category used by the individual's family and community to identify the condition.
4. The perceived causes or explanatory models that the individual and the reference group employ to explain the illness.

5. Current preferences for and past experience with professional and popular sources of care.

Cultural Factors Related to Psychosocial Environment and Functioning

Note culturally relevant interpretations of social stressors, available social supports, and levels of functioning and disability. Special attention should be given to stresses in the local social environment and to the role of religion and kin networks in providing emotional, instrumental, and informational support.

Cultural Elements of the Relationship between the Individual and the Clinician

Indicate differences in culture and social status between the individual and the clinician and problems that these differences may cause in diagnosis and treatment (e.g., difficulty in communicating in the individual's first language, in eliciting symptoms or understanding their cultural significance, in negotiating an appropriate relationship or level of intimacy, in determining whether a behavior is normative or pathological).

Overall Cultural Assessment for Diagnosis and Care

The formulation should conclude with a discussion of how these cultural considerations specifically influence comprehensive diagnosis and care.

Field trials were conducted on clinical cases corresponding to prominent ethnically identified minorities in the United States, supporting the feasibility and usefulness of the cultural formulation. We would urge researchers and clinicians, especially those in minority clinics and minority mental health research centers, to develop this cultural formulation further and systematically investigate its utility for clinical description and care.

A properly framed and annotated multiaxial schema, supplemented by an idiographic cultural formulation, would represent a qualitatively enhanced comprehensive diagnostic formulation, one that is not only culturally valid but aimed at appraising the totality of the patient's clinical condition, including the uniqueness of his or her personal experience.

References

Alarcon, R. D. (1983). Latin American perspectives on DSM-III. *Am J Psychiatry* 140:102–105.

American Psychiatric Association (1980). *Diagnostic and statistical manual of mental disorders*, 3rd Edition. Washington, DC: American Psychiatric Association.

Cuellar, I., and Roberts, R. E. (1984). Psychological disorders among Chicanos. In J. L. Martinez and R. H. Mendoza (Eds.), *Chicano psychology*. Orlando, FL: Academic Press.

Fabrega, H. (1987). Psychiatric diagnosis: A cultural perspective. *J Nerv Ment Dis* 175:383–394.

Geertz, C. (1983). *Local knowledge*. New York: Basic Books.

Good, B. J., and Good, M-J. D. (1986). The cultural context of diagnosis and therapy: A view from medical anthropology. In M. R. Miranda and H. H. L. Kitano (Eds.), *Mental health research and practice in minority communities* (DHHS Publ No ADM-86–1466). Washington, DC: U.S. Government Printing Office.

Good, B. J., and Kleinman, A. (1985). Culture and anxiety: Cross-cultural evidence for the patterning of anxiety disorders. In A. H. Tuma and J. Maser (Eds.), *Anxiety and the anxiety disorders*, pp. 297–323. Hillsdale, NJ: Lawrence Erlbaum Associates.

Guarnaccia, P. (1996). Cultural comments on multiaxial issues. In J. E. Mezzich, A. Kleinman, H. Fabrega, et al. (Eds.), *Culture and psychiatric diagnosis*. Washington, DC: American Psychiatric Press.

Harwood, A. (1981). Ethnicity and medical care. Cambridge, MA: Harvard University Press.

Hopper, K. (1991). Some old questions for the new cross-cultural psychiatry. *Medical Anthropology Quarterly* 5:299–330.

House, J. S., Landis, K. R., and Umberson, D. (1988). Social relationships and health. *Science* 241:540–545.

Hughes, C. C. (1985). Culture-bound or construct-bound? In R. C. Simons and C. C. Hughes (Eds.), *The Culture-bound syndromes*, pp. 3–24. Dordrecht, Netherlands: D. Reidel.

Irvine, J. (1985). Status and style in language. *Annual Review of Anthropology* 14:557–581.

Kleinman, A. (1988). *Rethinking psychiatry: From cultural category to personal experience*. New York: Free Press.

Kunce, J. T., and Vales, L. F. (1984). The Mexican American: Implications for cross-cultural rehabilitation counseling. *Rehabilitation Counseling Bulletin* 28:97–108.

Marcos, L. R., and Alpert, M. (1983). Strategies and risks in psychotherapy with bilingual patients. *Am J Psychiatry* 133:1275–1281.

Mezzich, J. E. (1987). International use and impact of DSM-III. In A. E. Skodol and R. L. Spitzer (Eds.), *An annotated bibliography of DSM-III*, pp. 37–46. Washington, DC: American Psychiatric Press.

Mezzich, J. E., Good, B. J., Lewis-Fernandez, R., et al. (1993). Cultural formulation guidelines. In J. E. Mezzich, A. Kleinman, H. Fabrega, et al. (Eds.) *Revised cultural proposals for DSM-IV: Technical report submitted to the DSM-IV Task Force by the steering committee, Group on Culture and Diagnosis*, pp. 163–168. Pittsburgh, PA: National Institute of Mental Health.

Mezzich, J. E., Kleinman, A., Fabrega, H., et al. (1996). *Culture and psychiatric diagnosis*. Washington, DC: American Psychiatric Press.

Patrick, D. L., Sittampalam, Y., Somerville, S. M., et al. (1985). A cross-cultural comparison of health status values. *Am J Public Health* 75:1402–1407.

Pierloot, T. A., and Ngoma, M. (1988). Hysterical manifestations in Africa and Europe: A comparative study. *Br J Psychiatry* 152:112–115.

Rutter, M., Shaffer, D., and Shepherd, M. (1975). *A multiaxial classification of child psychiatric disorders.* Geneva, Switzerland: World Health Organization.

Santisteban, D., and Szapocznik, J. (1982). Substance use disorders among Hispanics. In R. M. Becerra, M. Karno, and J. I. Escobar (Eds.), *Mental health and Hispanic Americans.* New York: Grune & Stratton.

Tseng, W-S. (1985). Cultural aspects of family assessment. *Intl J Fam Psychiatry* 6:19–31.

Vargas-Willis, G., and Cervantes, R. C. (1987). Consideration of psychosocial stress in the treatment of the Latina immigrant. Special issue: Mexican immigrant women. *Hispanic J Behav Sci* 9:315–329.

Weiss, M. (1985). The interrelationship of tropical disease and mental disorder. *Cult Med Psychiatry* 9:121–200.

6

Cultural Comments on Multiaxial Issues

Peter J. Guarnaccia

THE MULTIAXIAL SYSTEM provides considerable opportunities for incorporating social and cultural information into patient evaluation. However, the limited utilization of Axes IV and V as they are defined in recent versions of the DSM makes one pause before being either too enthusiastic or too comprehensive in selecting new axes. Well-developed systems can have several axes, which are used to enhance the utility and cultural sensitivity of diagnostic systems. Such an expanded system could be used to codify a more complete assessment of patients and provide an improved framework for clinicians and researchers.

Some of the lack of use of the current Axes IV and V may come from their attempt to summarize multiple and complex issues in too brief a form. "Unpacking" these axes and providing additional ones might make them more useful. One possibility, suggested by Mezzich (1996) and Frances and colleagues (1991) among others, would be to develop multiple axes to accompany the three diagnostic axes and to allow more flexible use of these axes depending on the needs of the clinician or researcher.

From a cultural point of view, a major problem in the conceptualization of Axis IV is that the instructions were suggesting that rating the severity of the stressor should be based on the assessment of "an 'average' person in similar circumstances and with similar sociocultural values" (American Psychiatric Association, 1987). This instruction required the clinician to make a generalization about the "average" person from a sociocultural value system that may be quite different from that of the clinician. At the same time, it led the clinician to ignore the assessment of the patient. Unless the patient's culture is well-known by the clinician, such a generalization is quite difficult and runs the risk of being stereotypic. The force of psychosocial stressors results from the meaning of those events to the person who experiences them. Thus, identifying the specific stressors (as now indicated in DSM-IV) and their meaning for the person seems more appropriate, both clinically and for research purposes. In the area of specific stressors, particular attention needs to be paid to the migration experience for individuals recently arrived from other countries or moving from rural to urban areas within countries. The reasons for migration, the migration process itself, and the situation in the new country are all potent sources of social stressors. Particularly stressful migration experiences may play either exacerbating or etiological roles in different psychiatric disorders.

Rather than confounding stressors and social supports as the present system does, construction of a separate axis on social supports would be very useful. The level of social support has been shown to be both a vulnerability factor in the onset of disorder (Brown and Harris, 1978) and a key issue in treatment planning. Cultural factors influence both the structure of social supports and the evaluation of the effectiveness of support. Clinically, the nature of social ties is critical both to therapy and to treatment planning. Assessing the degree of social support is also a key area in social research on mental health (Barrera, 1980).

Axis V also combines two issues that are not easily subsumed into one score: symptomatology and social functioning. The severity of symptomatology is best handled with the severity criteria already provided for Axis I diagnoses. Thus, Axis V could focus on social functioning. Alarcon's (1983) commentary on DSM-III highlights the problems of assessing social functioning cross-culturally, specifically in the case of antisocial personality disorder. For example, in sectors of American society where unemployment is widespread, an assessment of occupational functioning may be quite difficult. In this axis, two assessments—one based on the broader norms of society and the other based on the evaluation of significant others close to the patient—might be useful.

The proposal for a cultural axis (Good and Good, 1986) has considerable merit. Research in medical anthropology and cross-cultural psychiatry (much of it summarized in Kleinman, 1988) has strongly demonstrated the role of culture in shaping psychiatric disorder and the importance of examining popular illness categories in comparison with psychiatric diagnoses. I recommend using the cultural axis both for popular illness categories and for recording the patient's understanding of his or her disorder. The presence of a separate axis is preferable to adding cultural syndromes to Axis I. This allows for simultaneous exploration of cultural categories in relation to psychiatric diagnoses and for developing appropriate clinical interventions for culturally defined syndromes.

At least three additional areas for a cultural axis seem central to the issue of diagnosis, particularly given the multicultural dynamism of U.S. society. One important area is the assessment of language use and multilingualism. Considerable evidence has been presented on the influence of the language of assessment on the outcome of the diagnosis; particularly notable is the work of Marcos et al. (1973). An area or subaxis is needed that can assess the language abilities and preferences of multilingual individuals. A detailed assessment of language abilities and preferences is central to accurate diagnosis, to treatment, and to research on the cultural and cognitive processes in psychiatric disorder.

The area of acculturation, or preferably biculturalism, is another important sphere for axis development. Early work on acculturation focused on developing a unidimensional scale assessing an individual's affiliation on a continuum from totally involved in their culture of origin to totally assimilated to the host culture (Cuellar et al., 1980). More recent conceptualizations (Szapocznik et al., 1980) have focused on biculturalism and the parallel assessment of involvement in both the culture of origin and the host culture (see Rogler et al., 1991 for an excellent review of the acculturation literature). To assess the impact of culture on expressions of distress and recovery from psychiatric disorder, clinicians and researchers need an accurate assessment of the cultural background of the patient. Labels that focus only on national origin miss the complexities of cultural affiliation. There also is a sizable literature on the contribution of acculturative stresses to the emergence of mental disorder. There is a growing literature on the adaptive value of biculturalism. Evaluation of these propositions, both from clinical and research perspectives, requires a more rigorous and more uniform assessment of biculturalism than currently exists. Also, the bulk of the literature has focused on Latin Americans, and more work must be done to develop similar assessments for other ethnic groups in the United States.

The third axis I propose addresses issues of religious belief and practice. Religious beliefs provide one framework for structuring an individual's relationship to the world. When an individual's world becomes disordered, religious belief and practice can provide a sense of coherence that in itself may be therapeutic (Antonovsky, 1979). At the same time, religious ideas may also provide the content for hallucinations and delusions. Sorting out those ideas that are culturally consonant and those that are indicative of disorder requires an assessment by the clinician and significant others of the role of religion in the person's life and the degree to which a person's ideas are culturally appropriate. Mezzich (1989) noted that Ramirez in Puerto Rico has already developed a schema for such an axis that could serve as the basis for broader developments in this area.

Given the current focus on and reality of the multicultural nature of U.S. society, it is incumbent on us to develop diagnostic systems that are responsive to the realities already faced by clinicians and mental health researchers working in the United States and cross-culturally. DSM-IV, like its predecessors, will be used internationally and should be responsive to multicultural issues in assessment and diagnosis. A major way to expand the cultural scope of DSM-IV is through the creative enhancement of the multiaxial system.

References

Alarcon, R. (1983). A Latin American perspective on DSM-III. *Am J Psychiatry* 140:102–105.

American Psychiatric Association. (1987). *Diagnostic and statistical manual of mental disorders*, 3rd Edition, Revised. Washington, DC: American Psychiatric Association.

American Psychiatric Association. (1994). *Diagnostic and statistical manual of mental disorders*, 4th Edition, Washington, DC: American Psychiatric Association.

Antonovsky, A. (1979). *Health, stress, and coping*. San Francisco: Jossey-Bass.

Barrera, M. (1980). A method to assess social support networks in community research. *Connections* 3:8–13.

Brown, G. W., and Harris, T. (1978). *Social origins of depression*. New York: Free Press.

Cuellar, I., Harris, L. C., and Jasso, R. (1980). An acculturation scale for Mexican American normal and clinical populations. *Hispanic J BehavSci* 2:199–217.

Frances, A., Pincus, H. A., Widiger, T. A., et al. (1991). DSM-IV: Work in progress. *Am J Psychiatry* 147:1439–1448.

Good, B., and Good, M-J. D. (1986). The cultural context of diagnosis and therapy. In M. Miranda and H. H. L. Kitano (Eds.), *Mental health research and practice in minority communities* (U.S. Department of Health and Human Services Publ No (ADM) 86–1466). Washington, DC: U.S. Government Printing Office.

Kleinman A. (1988). *Rethinking psychiatry*. New York: Free Press.

Marcos, L. R., Urcuyo, L., Kesselman, M., et al. (1973). The language barrier in evaluating Spanish-American patients. *Arch Gen Psychiatry* 29:655–659.

Mezzich J. E. (1996). Culture and multiaxial diagnosis. In J. E. Mezzich, A. Kleinman, H. Fadrega, and D. L Parron (eds.), *Culture and Psychiatric Diagnosis*. Washington, DC: American Psychiatric Press.

Mezzich J. E. (1989). International diagnostic systems and Latin-American contributions and issues. *Br J Psychiatry* 154:84–90.

Rogler, L., Cortes, D. E., and Malgady, R. G. (1991). Acculturation and mental health status among Hispanics. *Am Psychol* 46:585–597.

Szapocznik, J., Kurtines, W. M., and Fernandez, T. (1980). Bicultural involvement in Hispanic American youths. *Intl J Intercultural Relations* 4:353–365.

Part II

Development and Characteristics of the Cultural Formulation

THE FOLLOWING ARTICLES were selected to illustrate both the laborious process that led to the development of the DSM-IV Cultural Formulation Outline and the wide scope of the formulation, both for clinical care as well as investigative domains. Although some overlap can be noted among the articles, each brings a unique perspective.

Mezzich's paper on the development of the DSM-IV Cultural Formulation starts by summarizing its conceptual bases. It then presents its organizing principles and various domains. It ends with a critical review of the effort involved in producing this contribution to diagnosis and care.

Lewis-Fernandez's (1996) paper provides an enlightening comment on the historical background and origins of the Cultural Formulation Outline within the U.S. diagnostic manual. It systematically addresses each component and subcomponent of the outline with helpful conceptual introductions, specific examples, and concrete suggestions.

Mezzich's (1995) paper on Cultural Formulation and comprehensive diagnosis places narrative and idiographic formulations within the context of current diagnostic systems. It points out that one of the main strengths of the Cultural Formulation is to allow subjective experience to come to the foreground of diagnostic evaluations. Admittedly the numerous clinical and therapeutic advantages facilitated by the Cultural Formulation could be even greater with further conceptual refinement, evidence-based research, and clear guidelines on how to use it. Within this scenario, the author indicates some strategic paths toward improving the Cultural Formulation, discussing potential applications as well as still unanswered questions.

Lu et al.'s (1995) paper discusses the basic principles of the Cultural Formulation within the context of case formulations. Each domain is examined and then practical examples and questions are presented to explore each subcomponent. Asian populations in particular are highlighted in the examples. The authors also elaborate on the complex process of immigration and acculturation, the use of interpreters, and developments in cultural competence in general. This article sows the seeds for practical Cultural Formulation guidelines.

7

Cultural Formulation

Development and Critical Review

Juan E. Mezzich

WITHIN THE EFFORT TO ADDRESS the cultural framework of psychiatric diagnosis for DSM-IV (American Psychiatric Association, 1994), one of the contributions that attracted high interest was the Cultural Formulation. This was probably related to the fact that the Cultural Formulation brought up the consideration of culture systematically to the majority of clinical cases rather than to isolated ones or narrow areas of psychopathology, and to its place within a broadly conceptualized diagnostic statement.

The cultural formulation is discussed first with regard to its conceptual, clinical, and anthropological background. Discussed next is its actual construction, followed by the outline published in DSM-IV. Finally, a critical assessment of the Cultural Formulation and its implications is presented.

Conceptual Bases

Over the past decade, the professional literature (Fabrega, 1987; Good and Good, 1986; Hughes, 1985; Kleinman, 1988a; Mezzich and Berganza, 1984) has offered general recommendations toward a cultural statement to upgrade or potentiate standard psychiatric diagnosis. Additionally, concentration on the personal experience of the patient is becoming a focus of convergence between anthropological considerations on the cultural matrix of psychopathology and a movement within clinical and social psychiatry. For example, Strauss (1992) has pointedly argued that psychiatrists, more than treating mental disorders, care for people who happen to experience such disorders. This coincides with the anthropologic emphasis of Geertz (1983) on the "native point of view."

Table 7.1 displays the results of a review of the literature relevant to the identification of the key elements of a cultural formulation. It reveals that a focus on the *patient's personal perspectives* is, in fact, recognized as fundamental (Good and Good, 1986; Hughes, 1993; Jones and Thorne, 1987; Kleinman, 1988b).

Four of the six papers offering specific recommendations spoke of several facets of the *cultural identity of the individual*, that is, behavioral or ideologic ethnicity (Kleinman, 1988b) and spiritual or religious involvement (Guarnaccia, 1996; Hughes, 1993; Ramírez, 1991). Another major theme was *cultural factors pertinent to the patient's illness*, recommended by both Good and Good (1986) in terms of idioms for experiencing and communicating illness, culture-specific illness categories, explanatory models, and predominant care-seeking patterns; and by Kleinman (1988b), who considered the cultural significance of symptoms, culturally salient illnesses, and explanatory models of illness. A third major theme corresponds to *cultural factors on social environment and functioning*, articulated by Good and Good (1986) with regard to perceived level of disability, as well as by Ramírez (1991) in terms of three elements in his Puerto Rican Octagonal Assessment Schema (i.e., perceived social stress, connectedness to sociocultural supports, and acquired maturity). A fourth theme involves *intercultural elements of the clinician-patient*

TABLE 7.1.
Literature Review on Elements for a Cultural Formulation

Cultural Themes	Good & Good (1986)	Jones & Thorne (1987)	Kleinman (1988b)	Ramírez (1991)	Hughes (1993)	Guarnaccia (1996)
Personal Perspective	X	X	X		X	X
Individual's Identity			X	X	X	X
Illness Explanations	X			X		
Social Environment & Functioning	X			X		
Clinician-Patient Relationship			X			

relationship, represented by negotiation between patient/family and professionals and the consideration of the clinician's biases (Kleinman, 1988b).

Developmental Process on the Cultural Formulation Guidelines

The project to develop proposals for enhancing the cultural validity and suitability of DSM-IV offered the framework for the development of specific guidelines for a cultural formulation. A National Institute of Mental Health (NIMH) Conference, held in Pittsburgh in April 1991 for a meeting of minds between a group of cultural experts and representatives of the American Psychiatric Association's DSM-IV Task Force and Work Groups, identified a number of structural elements in the new manual as foci for a cultural development program. These included a cultural statement for the introduction to the manual, cultural considerations sections for the text of the various diagnostic categories, a glossary of culture-bound syndromes, annotations on the multiaxial evaluation, and guidelines for a cultural formulation.

The initiative for conceiving a cultural formulation emerged when the possibility of a "cultural axis" was considered. Diagnostic axes, as incorporated in official diagnostic systems such as ICD-10 and DSM-IV, are contextualizing schemas that involve domains assessed with standardized instruments (typologies or dimensional scales). Diagnostic axes, therefore, were not considered appropriate for articulating a cultural statement, which, given the complexity of the cultural matrix, requires organizational flexibility and the use of all the resources of natural language.

The NIMH Group on Culture and Diagnosis undertook the preparation of the various cultural proposals for DSM-IV agreed to at the 1991 Pittsburgh conference, including a cultural formulation guideline. The process of conceptualizing a cultural formulation was informed by the literature review summarized in the preceding section. To the first four elements supported by the literature review (cultural identity of the patient, cultural factors in the patient's illness, cultural factors pertinent to social environment and functioning, and intercultural elements in the clinician-patient relationship) was added a summary, that is, an overall cultural statement for diagnosis and care.

The first presentation of a draft of the Cultural Formulation Guideline took place in January 1992 to the DSM-IV Task Force, which received it with interest and recommended its experimental piloting. This pilot project, aimed at appraising the feasibility and suitability of the Guideline, was carried out by a subgroup of the NIMH Culture and Diagnosis Group. The project included the application of the draft of the Guideline to sets of cases from the four main ethnically identified minorities in the United States, that is, African Americans, American Indians, Asian Americans, and Latinos or Hispanic Americans. For each case, a succinct clinical history, a multiaxial diagnosis, and a cultural formulation were prepared. The results of the pilot project led to the revision of the Cultural Formulation proposal (Mezzich, Good, and Lewis-Fernández, 1993), which included three parts: an introduction, the key five elements of the formulation, and four illustrative cases. This proposal was well received by the overall DSM-IV Task Force

The DSM-IV Cultural Formulation Outline

After an extensive editing and summarizing process, the first two of the three sections of the proposal were actually published in DSM-IV (pp. 843–844). They were printed without the illustrative cases in Appendix I of the DSM-IV, along with the Glossary of Cultural Bound Syndromes. The DSM-IV Cultural Formulation Outline reads as follows:

> The following outline for cultural formulation is meant to supplement the multiaxial diagnostic assessment and to address difficulties that may be encountered in applying DSM-IV criteria in a multicultural environment. The cultural formulation provides a systematic review of the individual's cultural background, the role of the cultural context in the expression and evaluation of symptoms and dysfunction, and the effect that cultural differences may have on the relationship between the individual and the clinician.
>
> As indicated in the introduction to the manual, it is important that the clinician take into account the individual's ethnic and cultural context in the evaluation of each of the DSM-IV axes. In addition, the cultural formulation suggested below provides an opportunity to describe systematically the individual's cultural and social reference group and ways in which cultural context is relevant to clinical care. The clinician may provide a narrative summary for each of the following categories:
>
> A. Cultural identity of the individual. Note the individual's ethnic or cultural reference groups. For immigrants and ethnic minorities, note separately the degree of involvement with both the culture of origin and the host culture (where applicable). Also note language abilities, use, and preferences (including multilingualism).
>
> B. Cultural explanations of the individual's illness. The following may be identified: the predominant idioms of distress through which symptoms or the need for social support are communicated (e.g., "nerves," possessing spirits, somatic complaints, inexplicable misfortune), the meaning and perceived severity of the individual's symptoms in relation to norms

of the cultural reference group, any local illness category used by the individual's family and community to identify the condition (see Glossary of Culture Bound Syndromes), the perceived causes or explanatory models that the individual and the reference group use to explain the illness, and current preferences for and past experience with professional and popular sources of care.

C. Cultural factors related to psychosocial environment and levels of functioning. Note culturally relevant interpretations of social stressors, available social supports, and levels of functioning and disability. This would include stresses in the local social environment and the role of religion and kin networks in providing emotional, instrumental, and informational support.

D. Cultural elements of the relationship between the individual and the clinician. Indicate differences in culture and social status between the individual and the clinician and problems that these differences may cause in diagnosis and treatment (e.g., difficulty in communicating in the individual's first language, eliciting symptoms or understanding their cultural significance, in negotiating an appropriate relationship or level of intimacy, in determining whether a behavior is normative or pathologic).

E. Overall cultural assessment for diagnosis and care. The formulation concludes with a discussion of how cultural considerations specifically influence comprehensive diagnosis and care.

Critical Assessment

The Cultural Formulation emerged late as a target of cultural contributions for DSM-IV and also late in the laborious process of preparing DSM-IV. This was probably due to its innovativeness and the intensive and time-consuming work, both conceptual and empirical, that it required to be crystallized in an understandable and practical way.

Its initial presentation to the DSM-IV Task Force was well received despite the advanced stage in the preparation of the Manual. This led to a busy and hectic period of empirical trials and preparation of illustrative cases, which accompanied the final proposal submitted to the DSM-IV Task Force.

While the introduction and the core elements of the Cultural Formulation were accepted for publication, this did not happen for the illustrative cases. Evidently, considerations of space predominated over those on clarity and need for guidance on how to prepare a Cultural Formulation.

In any case, work remains to be done on developing more detailed instructions and illustrations on the application of this Formulation to regular clinical care. Its empirically assessed impact on clinical effectiveness is a pressing challenge as well.

References

American Psychiatric Association. (1994). *Diagnostic and statistical manual of mental disorders,* 4th Edition. Washington, DC: American Psychiatric Association.

Fabrega, H. (1987). Psychiatric diagnosis: A cultural perspective. *J Nerv Ment Dis* 175:383–394.

Geertz, C. (1983). *Local knowledge.* New York: Basic Books.

Good, B. J., and Good, M-J. D. (1986). The cultural context of diagnosis and therapy: A view from medical anthropology. In M. R. Miranda and H. H. L. Kitano (Eds.), *Mental health research and practice in minority communities,* pp. 165–198. U.S. Department of Health and Human Services Publication No. (ADM) 86–1466. Washington, DC: US Government Printing Office.

Guarnaccia, P. J. (1996). Comments on culture and multiaxial diagnosis. In J. E. Mezzich, A. Kleinman, H. Fabrega et al. (Eds.), *Culture and psychiatric diagnosis.* Washington, DC: American Psychiatric Press.

Hughes, C. C. (1993). Culture in clinical psychiatry. In A. Gaw (Ed.), *Culture, ethnicity, and mental illness,* pp. 3–41. Washington, DC: American Psychiatric Press.

Hughes, C. C. (1985). Culture-bound or construct-bound? In R. C. Simons, and C. C. Hughes (Eds.), *The culture-bound syndromes,* pp. 3–24. Dordrecht, The Netherlands: Reidel.

Jones, E. E., and Thorne, A. (1987). Rediscovery of the subject: Intercultural approaches to clinical assessment. *J Consult Clin Psychol* 55:488–495.

Kleinman, A. (1988a). *Rethinking psychiatry: From cultural category to personal experience.* New York: Free Press.

Kleinman, A. (1988b). *The illness narratives: Suffering, healing, and the human condition.* New York: Basic Books.

Mezzich, J. E., and Berganza, C. E. (1984). Culture and psychopathology. New York: Columbia University Press.

Mezzich, J. E., Good, B. J., Lewis-Fernández, R., et al. (1993). Cultural formulation guidelines. In J. E. Mezzich, A. Kleinman, H. Fabrega, et al. (Eds.), *Revised cultural proposals for DSM-IV,* pp. 161–168. Technical Report, NIMH Group on Culture and Diagnosis, Pittsburgh, PA.

Ramírez, E. (1991) *Octagonal assessment schema.* San Juan: Technical Report, Department of Mental Health of Puerto Rico.

Strauss, J. S. (1992). The person—key to understanding mental illness: Towards a new dynamic psychiatry, III. *Br J Psychiatry* 161 (Suppl. 18): 19–26.

8

Cultural Formulation of Psychiatric Diagnosis

Roberto Lewis-Fernández

THIS ISSUE OF *Culture, Medicine, and Psychiatry* introduces a new regular feature to the Journal: a Section of Clinical Cases exemplifying the Cultural Formulation outlined in DSM-IV. The Cultural Formulation is an operationalization for clinicians of the process of cultural analysis as it relates to the clinical encounter that can be performed as part of the evaluation of every patient (Mezzich and Good, 1996 [chapter 5 of this volume]; Mezzich, 1995a). Its immediate origins lie in the process of revision of psychiatric nosology that resulted in DSM-IV. Responding to criticisms of prior insensitivity to cultural issues in past editions of the manual, the National Institute of Mental Health (NIMH) supported formation of a Group on Culture and Diagnosis in 1991 composed mainly of anthropologists and cross-cultural psychiatrists (cf. Alarcón, 1995; Mezzich, 1995b, for a history of these events). The general goal of this Group was to advise the DSM-IV Task Force on how to make culture more central to DSM-IV. From the beginning, one of its specific aims was to devise a mechanism that would facilitate the application of a cultural perspective to the process of clinical interviewing and diagnostic formulation in psychiatry.

Early notions favored supplementing the five existing axes of the manual—those that organize diagnostic formulations into separate domains for pathological syndromes, personality disorders, medical conditions affecting the psychiatric picture, relevant stressors, and resulting levels of function-

From *Culture, Medicine, and Psychiatry* 20, no. 3, 133–44 (September 1996) with kind permission from Springer Science and Business Media

ing—with a sixth, or "Cultural Axis." Investigators had previously laid out some of the conceptual components that should be included in such a proposal, indicating that a cultural axis would only be viable if it represented illness from an "emic" perspective, that is, from the perspective of the sufferer and his or her primary reference group (Good and Good, 1986). The Group realized, however, that in order to fit the existing multiaxial format, a Cultural Axis would almost certainly be reduced to a standardized typology of brief cultural characterizations, a menu of key descriptors listed in the manual for use as part of the clinical evaluation (Mezzich, 1996). These descriptors would most likely be used to hone but not fundamentally alter the basic diagnoses, following the model of other diagnostic modifiers, such as the specifier "with rapid cycling" used to characterize a subtype of bipolar disorder. Items in an Axis VI typology would include general specifiers for use in any cultural setting (such as "with prominent somatization") and indigenous labels for the presenting syndrome (such as "*nervios* illness" that describe patients' and family members' views of causation and pathophysiology). Some investigators proposed dealing with the constraints of the multiaxial schema by expanding Axis VI into a series of subaxes, covering topics such as language preference, levels of acculturation and biculturality, and religious belief and practice (Guarnaccia, 1996; Ramírez, in Mezzich 1996). In general, the Cultural Axis proposal had the obvious advantage of fitting within the existing DSM structure, thus apparently facilitating its widespread acceptance by clinicians already familiar with the multiaxial format.

The Cultural Axis concept, however, soon came under criticism as unworkable and insufficient. From the beginning, a Cultural Axis faced what appeared to be significant technical objections. Doubts arose as to whether this format could ever yield any real clinical usefulness. How might one assemble a series of brief comments on culture that are universally applicable and nonstereotyping? How would the items forming the necessarily limited typology be selected? Would the typology simply make official clinical commonsense (any clinician knows when there is an "excess" of somatic symptoms) without adding any useful information? Would this format not contribute instead to the essentializing, or stereotyping, tendency of psychiatric assessments? Is there any difference between pulling indigenous illness labels out of context, without any processual analysis of how they emerge in particular settings, and the cultural essentializing involved in the psychiatric diagnoses themselves? Consider the inadequacy of the likely Cultural Axis evaluation of the rich contextual dynamics involved in a presentation of *taijin kyofusho*. The particular Japanese exigencies of self-definition within different social circles evincing distinct relational obligations, especially problematic during adolescence, patterned by gender roles and cultural rules of social trust and reciprocity (*amae*), and showing historical changes with the loosening of social bonds as a result of the growth of corporate capitalism in Japan (Russell 1989) would all be reduced to an Axis I diagnosis of social phobia and a Cultural Axis VI evaluation of "with other-directed shame features" or a similarly worded modifier. Using the axial format, cultural contextualization came to seem practically impossible. Initial technical objections gave way to more fundamental criticisms of the Cultural Axis proposal, and then led, by contrast, to alternative views regarding how to put together a clinically useful cultural analysis that could complement DSM-IV.

In order to be truly useful, a cultural assessment of a patient should alter the diagnostic process itself, affecting the way clinicians view all five axes, not just add a sixth list of essentializing descriptors. Such an assessment should contextualize the multiaxial data within a processual view of social relations and institutions. The fundamental challenge that cultural analysis brings to diagnostic thinking is its capacity to render visible the socially constructed context that mediates key features of a patient's presentation and subsequent course. To fulfill this function, a cultural assessment must take into account intracultural as well as cross-cultural elements, paying special attention, for instance, to the complicated interactions of gender, class, race, and other intracultural factors affecting the clinical presentation (Lewis-Fernández and Kleinman, 1993). It must go beyond explanations of cross cultural differences in symptomatology to describe the cultural constituents of all clinical phenomenologies, as well as courses and outcomes; patterns of help-seeking and etiological attributions by patients and their social circles; and diagnostic practices, institutional pressures, and modes of research by clinicians.

Instead of facilitating these tasks, a Cultural Axis format would almost certainly contribute to the decontextualizing tendency of the DSM system by limiting the role of cultural analysis in clinical evaluation simply to its phenomenological component and even then to a secondary role, serving as an explanation of cross-cultural difference. At worst, a "cultural axis" so conceived might further the view that a cultural assessment of the patient is a last-minute phenomenological refinement, an ancillary and thus dispensable procedure, while leaving the rest of the diagnostic process unaffected. Given the pressures impinging on working clinicians, who already often bypass Axes IV and V and might ignore a sixth axis (Guarnaccia, 1996), a cultural axis as it would likely be accepted into the DSM-IV might paradoxically lessen the cultural contextualization of diagnostic practice. The Group saw that what was needed instead was a framework that helped clinicians realize how culture affects every aspect of the clinical encounter.

As the proposal for a Cultural Axis waned, in its place emerged a consensus in favor of outlining an approach that would complement and broaden the standard diagnostic work, leading clinicians to focus systematically on how culture influences psychiatric evaluation, which would be recorded in narrative rather than categorical terms. In place of the potential straightjacket of a nomothetic typology, this framework would permit an idiographic portrayal of the person and his/her relevant sociocultural environment (Mezzich, 1995a). The use of narrative description came to be favored by the Group first because it obviously allows much greater operational flexibility than the fixed DSM format. More important, however, is that narratives make a different kind of truth claim than diagnostic typologies. Narrative creates a humanized account of suffering fundamentally embedded in a particular setting through the assembling of telling contextual details as the signs of truth (Kleinman, 1988; Herschbach, 1995; Good, 1994). Rather than focusing on patients as the "embodied signs of pathology," emphasis falls on "the horrible variety of suffering" experienced by particular human beings and those involved with them (Weir Mitchell, in Herschbach, 1995, p. 189). The use of narrative also permits an accounting of the role of health institutions and practitioners in the evolution of the person's illness career and self-experience (Saris 1995). Turning the gaze of the profession back on itself is a major achievement of contemporary medical anthropology, as it clarifies the fluid and interactive process whereby diagnosis (and to a large extent, outcome) is reached in psychiatric practice (Good, 1994). A humanized and ethnographic narrative of illness that includes a reflexive stance on the clinician-patient interaction would truly constitute a significant contribution to patient care.

Searching for a precedent for this kind of narrative analysis within clinical practice, the Group found one in the Psychodynamic Formulation, a complementary narrative to multiaxial diagnostics that follows a prescribed structure and is often included as part of the patient's chart next to other assessment procedures. It is employed by many psychotherapists and training centers instructing young clinicians in order to assess a patient's key psychological patterns of conflicts and defenses as rooted in the details of his/her life experience (Friedman and Lister, 1987; Perry, 1989). The Psychodynamic Formulation is then used to inform the choice and progression of psychological therapies. Because of its individual specificity, it is often considered superior for these purposes to the generic descriptions of the axial diagnoses (Perry et al., 1987). The Group came to see the Psychodynamic Formulation as a good model for complementing the standard diagnostic evaluation because it is a well-known format for clinicians, it is thought to convey useful information not already included in the axis system, and it is narrative and personalized. As a result, the resulting proposal for the mini-ethnographic narrative assessment came to be known as the "Cultural Formulation."

An outline of this proposal was prepared (Mezzich, et al. 1993) and submitted to the DSM-IV Task Force. In addition, clinicians associated with the Group on Culture and Diagnosis undertook a "field trial," testing the applicability of the Cultural Formulation on actual patients. This process involved developing case analyses from the four main ethnic minorities in the United States (African Americans, American Indians, Asian Americans, and Latinos) and revealed that the Cultural Formulation could be used very successfully as currently proposed (Mezzich, 1995a). Short and long versions of the Cultural Formulation were envisioned to meet the needs of different clinical professionals. Social workers and psychotherapists, for example, might require the completeness and detail of the full Formulation, whereas psychopharmacologists could make use of an abbreviated version. The final draft of the Outline included the short versions of four cases from the field trial for inclusion in DSM-IV as models of completed formulations. The Group recommended that the Outline be prominently placed at the front of the manual, immediately following the section on Multiaxial Assessment.

The editors of the DSM-IV agreed to publish an edited and shortened version of the proposed text (see chapter 7), but only as an appendix rather than in the central text. Furthermore, rather than highlighting it in a space of its own, as recommended by the Group on Culture and Diagnosis, they combined it with what they titled the "Glossary of Culture-Bound Syndromes," a glossary that had been prepared by the Group as a separate submission under the title "Glossary of Cultural Syndromes and Idioms of Distress." The effect of joining these two disparate proposals is to exoticize the Cultural Formulation, which now seems relevant only to "culture-bound" presentations among non-Western ethnic groups, rather than as an evaluation process applicable to every patient in every cultural setting. Moreover, the illustrative cases were removed, thereby decreasing the persuasiveness and the pedagogic effect of the Outline. These alterations to the Cultural Formulation proposal were not unique; they formed part of an admittedly conservative editorial policy (Frances et al., 1990) of simplifying or rejecting many of the Group's cultural proposals in order to maintain the universalistic position of DSM-IV (Lewis-Fernández and Kleinman, 1995).

Despite its efforts, therefore, the Group on Culture and Diagnosis was only able to exert a slight influence on DSM-IV. Nevertheless, the need for the cultural expansion of DSM categories remains and can be illustrated with great force. To this end, two strategic fronts may acquire greater relevance in the future. The first is the intensification of research on the epidemiology of indigenously defined syndromes, heralded by Rubel's work on *susto* in Mexico (1964) and Carstairs and Kapur's investigation of possession and other forms of psychopathology in India (1976), and developed by Manson on models of depression among the Hopi (1985), by Guarnaccia and Canino on *ataques de nervios* among Puerto Ricans (Guarnaccia et al., 1993), and by Kleinman (1986) and later by Lin and Weiss on neurasthenia in Chinese communities (Lin, 1995), among others. Documenting alternate nosologies affecting whole nations and ethnic groups that account for much of the variance in validity assessments of standard epidemiologic surveys by indigenous clinicians is a powerful way of problematizing the universality of the established Western nosologies used in those surveys (Guarnaccia et al., 1990).

The second front in the struggle to make culture more central to the process of clinical evaluation and treatment consists of the systematic development of case-based clinical ethnography as operationalized by the Cultural Formulation (cf. Kleinman's [1988] recommendations for the place of "mini-ethnographies" in clinical work). Marshalling the empirical evidence of many case analyses will reveal the contextual embeddedness of illness, and thus the limited usefulness of purely descriptive diagnostics and the fallacy of universalistic course predictions and outcome measures (Canino et al., 1997). It will also establish the impact of cultural factors on clinical phenomenology by revealing the poor fit between existing nosologies and many non-Western presentations of psychopathology.

The new Clinical Cases section initiated here in the pages of *Culture, Medicine, and Psychiatry* constitutes part of the vanguard of this second front. This section will be a testing ground for the Cultural Formulation, where the current proposal will be honed in practice and improved by critique and elaboration. These developments should help inform the subsequent work of the Group on Culture and Diagnosis. The Group has already begun to push forward the Formulation proposal by preparing a booklet that describes the Formulation guidelines and contains two illustrative cases. Entitled *Introduction to the Cultural Formulation*, it will be distributed to most medical schools and training programs for mental health professionals. Following the booklet, planning is underway for a Cultural Casebook of hundreds of cases canvassing the application of different Cultural Formulation formats to diverse psychopathology categories and cultural populations. The *CMP*'s Clinical Cases section will continue in the tradition of the booklet and pave the way for the *Casebook*, so that Formulation refinements obtained through the section will inform the Casebook, and cases published first in *CMP* will be available for subsequent republication.

The Clinical Cases editorial policy will give priority to psychiatric cases in which cultural elements make a difference to illness phenomenology, to diagnostic assessment, to patients' outcome, to health services utilization, or to a combination of these factors. The first two cases published in the journal illustrate these tendencies. The Puerto Rican case highlights some of the diagnostic difficulties involved in assessing the phenomenology of *nervios* and *ataques*. It also discusses the impact on illness outcome of different cultural conceptualizations of the patient's presentation. A shorter version of this case was one of the four illustrations of the Cultural Formulation Outline submitted to DSM-IV that were not included in the published manual. The American Indian case disentangles the complicated effects of ethnicity and of different explanatory models of illness on the health-seeking behavior and the clinician-patient interactions of a young woman suffering from depression, alcoholism, and the sequelae of sexual abuse.

The Clinical Cases section will publish case discussions of patients from any cultural or ethnic group, including those that highlight the cultural aspects of clinical presentations by Euro-Americans or majority European populations. Since child and adolescent cases are generally underrepresented in cross-cultural work, their submission is encouraged. We are also interested in cases where clinical variables are significantly affected by intracultural differences, for instance, class, gender, or sexual orientation. In general, we find that the best cases are those that aim to expand the boundaries of the established nosology or that show how cultural information clarifies a complex phenomenological treatment or health services picture.

Table 8.1 lists the features that each case submitted to the Clinical Cases section must contain. A submission should start with a standard brief psychiatric description of the patient that includes a full multiaxial assessment. Authors should present a level of detail necessary to establish the diagnoses and to anticipate any obvious questions regarding relevant rule-outs. The latter is obviously especially important when standard categories are challenged by the case data: nosologists will want to know that all the established categories have been explored before entertaining NOS or mixed-category diagnoses. Both DSM-TV and ICD-10 categories may be applied, but the DSM-IV multiaxial structure must be utilized throughout, including the standard format for Axes IV and V and the use of diagnostic codes. If comparison between the two nosologies is pertinent, it could become a very interesting aspect of the case. Attention to help-seeking strategies and explanatory models is requested, particularly when these affect outcome. Information on long-term treatment and follow-up is especially desirable, as these validate initial diagnoses: readers may suspect that presentations appearing culturally particular at first will be revealed over time to conform to established nosologies. In order to avoid unnecessary repetition, authors are generally advised to present only "the bare facts" in the Clinical History section and then discuss the topics in detail in the Cultural Formulation.

The Cultural Formulation should compose the bulk of the submission. The main goal of every Formulation should be to enable the reader to locate

TABLE 8.1
Items to Be Included in *CMP* Clinical Cases

I. Clinical History
   1. Patient identification
   2. History of present illness
   3. Psychiatric history and previous treatment
   4. Social and developmental history
   5. Family history
   6. Course and outcome
   7. Diagnostic formulation (Axes I-V)

II. Cultural Formulation
   A. Cultural Identity
      1. Cultural reference group(s)
      2. Language
      3. Cultural factors in development
      4. Involvement with culture of origin
      5. Involvement with host cult
   B. Cultural Explanations of the Illness
      1. Predominant idioms of distress and local illness categories
      2. Meaning and severity of symptoms in relation to cultural norms
      3. Perceived causes and explanatory models
      4. Help-seeking experiences and plans
   C. Cultural Factors Related to Psychological Environment and Levels of Functioning
      1. Social stressors
      2. Social supports
      3. Levels of functioning and disability
   D. Cultural Elements of the Clinician-Patient Relationship
   E. Overall Cultural Assessment

the sufferer within his/her most relevant cultural context and to clarify the essential cultural determinants that shape the form of the clinical variables. To this end, succinct summaries of pertinent ethnic group history and of past research on the indigenous idioms of distress or the help-seeking options used by the patient may be useful at times, especially for purposes of comparison. Some Formulations will also require a subtle reflexive analysis of the author-patient interaction, including a discussion of cultural factors impacting the process of diagnostic assessment and ethnographic writing. Every submission should discuss all the elements in table 8.1, but the relative length and importance of each Formulation item will of course vary with the case. Some cases will present a diagnostic dilemma exclusively, or mostly an issue in health services utilization, and each Cultural Formulation should also emphasize the main aspect of the case. Readers should expect to find in the Formulation specific cultural commentaries on the key facts mentioned in the Clinical History. The DSM-IV outline and the two cases published below may serve as further guides for future submissions.

Finally, we are especially interested in cases that justify the need for improvements to the Cultural Formulation format itself. Perhaps the main benefit the section can produce is to develop an iterative process of revision around the Formulation proposal. Tentative areas for exploration may be: how can we make the Formulation more responsive to the particular exigencies of working with children? Do some sections, like the one on cultural identity, require a framework that distinguishes the information obtained from the child from the input received from additional sources, such as parents and teachers? Also, how can the Formulation move beyond the person in order to focus more directly on the social environment that structures differential exposures and responses to stress and trauma (Manson 1995)? Authors are encouraged to think critically about the Formulation as currently elaborated and to develop their ideas in the form of cases.

In sum, the Cultural Formulation presents an exciting challenge: will it provide the space for some of the "thick description" (Geertz 1973) that raises the real-world cultural complexity of clinical work? With more elaboration, the Formulation could grow into a comprehensive format that facilitates many of the goals of cultural psychiatry and psychology: expanding the established nosology used for diagnostics and epidemiology; providing clinicians with a concrete methodology for incorporating cultural analysis into evaluations and treatments; teaching psychiatric residents and other mental health trainees how to develop a contextualizing and processual understanding of their patients' suffering; and operationalizing the cultural assessment of clinical effectiveness required for valid outcome research. The *CMP* Clinical Cases Section invites you to participate in the evolution of this promising new framework for clinical cultural analysis.

References

Alarcón, Renato D. (1995). Culture and psychiatric diagnosis: Impact on DSM-IV and ICD-10. *The Psychiatric Clinics of North America* 18(3): 449–465.

American Psychiatric Association. (1994). *Diagnostic and statistical manual of mental disorders*, 4th Edition (DSM-IV). Washington, DC: American Psychiatric Press.

Canino, G. J., Lewis-Fernández, R., and Bravo, M. (1997). Methodological challenges in cross-cultural mental health research. *Transcultural Psychiatric Research Review* 34(2):163–184

Carstairs, G. M., and Kapur, R. L. (1976). *The great universe of Kota: Social change and mental disorder in an Indian village*. Berkeley: University of California Press.

Frances, A. J., Pincus, H. A., Widiger, T. A., et al. (1990). DSM-IV. Work in progress. *American Journal of Psychiatry* 147: 1439–1448.

Friedman, R. S., and Lister, P. (1987). The current status of psychodynamic formulation. *Psychiatry* 50(2):126–141.

Geertz, C. (1973). Thick description: Towards an interpretive theory of culture. In *The interpretation of culture*, pp. 3–30. New York: Basic Books.

Good, B. J. (1994). *Medicine, rationality, and experience: An anthropological perspective.* Cambridge: Cambridge University Press.

Good, B. J., Good, M-J. D. (1986). The cultural context of diagnosis and therapy: A view from medical anthropology. In M. R. Miranda and H. H. L. Kitano (Eds.), *Mental health research and practice in minority communities.* U.S. Department of Health and Human Services Publication No. (ADM) 86-1466. Washington, DC: U.S. Government Printing Office.

Guarnaccia, P. J. (1996). Comments on culture and multiaxial diagnosis. In J. E. Mezzich, A. Kleinman, H. Fábrega et al. (Eds.), *Culture and psychiatric diagnosis.* Washington, DC: American Psychiatric Press.

Guarnaccia, P. J., Canino, G. J., Rubio-Stipec, M., et al. (1993). The prevalence of *ataques de nervios* in the Puerto Rico disaster study: The role of culture in psychiatric epidemiology. *J Nerv and Ment Dis* 181: 159–167.

Guarnaccia, P. J., Good, B. J. and Kleinman, A. (1990). A critical review of epidemiological studies of Puerto Rican mental health. *Am J Psychiatry* 147: 1449–1456.

Herschbach, L. (1995). True clinical fictions: Medical and literary narratives from the Civil War hospital. *Culture, Medicine, and Psychiatry* 19(2):183–205.

Kleinman, A. (1986). *Social origins of distress and disease: Neurasthenia, depression, and pain in modern China.* New Haven, CT: Yale University Press

———. (1988). *The illness narratives: Suffering, healing, and the human condition.* New York: Basic Books.

Lewis-Fernández, R., and Kleinman, A. (1993). Culture, personality, and psychopathology. *J Abnormal Psychology* 103: 67–71.

———. 1995 Cultural psychiatry: Theoretical, clinical, and research issues. *The Psychiatric Clinics of North America* 18(3): 433–448.

Lin, K-M. (1995). Asian American perspectives on cultural formulation. Panel presentation, Symposium 60, DSM-IV Cultural Formulation and ethnic diversity. In *Syllabus and proceedings summary of the 148th annual meeting of the American Psychiatric Association*, p. 110. Washington, DC: American Psychiatric Press.

Manson, S. M. (1995). Personal communication. San Diego meeting of the Group on Culture and Diagnosis. February 18.

Manson S. M., Shore, J. H., and Bloom, J. D. (1985). The depressive experience in American Indian communities: A challenge for psychiatric theory and diagnosis. In A. Kleinman and B. J. Good (Eds.), *Culture and depression: Studies in the anthropology and cross-cultural psychiatry of affect and disorder*, pp. 331–368. Berkeley: University of California Press.

Mezzich, J. E. (1995a). Cultural formulation and comprehensive diagnosis: Clinical and research perspectives. *The Psychiatric Clinics of North America* 18(3): 649–657.

———. (1995b). Development of the DSM-IV Cultural Formulation. Panel presentation, Symposium 60, DSM-IV Cultural Formulation and ethnic diversity. In *Syl-*

labus and proceedings summary of the 148th annual meeting of the American Psychiatric Association, pp. 109–110. Washington, DC: American Psychiatric Press.

———. (1996). Culture and multiaxial diagnosis. In J. E. Mezzich, A. Kleinman, H. Fábrega, et al. (Eds.) *Culture and psychiatric diagnosis.* Washington, DC: American Psychiatric Press.

Mezzich, J. E., Good, B. J., Lewis-Fernández, R., et al. (1993). Cultural formulation guidelines. In J. E. Mezzich, A. Kleinman, H. Fábrega, et al., eds. *Revised cultural proposals for DSM-IV.* pp. 161–168. Technical Report, NIMH Group on Culture and Diagnosis, Pittsburgh. PA.

Mezzich, J. E., and Good, B. J. (1996). On culturally enhancing the DSM-IV multiaxial formulation. In T. A. Widiger, A. J. Frances, H. A. Pincus, R. Ross, M. B. First, and W. Wakefield Davis (Eds.), *DSM-IV sourcebook.* Vol. 2. Washington, DC: American Psychiatric Press.

Perry, J. C. (1989). Scientific progress in psychodynamic formulation. *Psychiatry* 52(3): 245–249.

Perry, S., Cooper, A. M., and Michels, R. (1987). The psychodynamic formulation: Its purpose, structure, and clinical application. *Am J Psychiatry* 144(5):543–550.

Rubel, A. J. (1964). The epidemiology of a folk illness: Susto in Hispanic America. *Ethnology* 3: 268–283.

Russell, J. G. (1989). Anxiety disorders in Japan: A review of the Japanese literature on shinkeishitsu and taijinkyofusho. *Culture, Medicine, and Psychiatry.* 13: 391–403.

Saris, A. J. (1995). Telling stories: Life histories, illness narratives, and institutional landscapes. *Culture, Medicine, and Psychiatry* 19(1):39 72.

9

Cultural Formulation and Comprehensive Diagnosis

Clinical and Research Perspectives

Juan E. Mezzich

THE PAST TWO DECADES have witnessed important gains in the systematization of psychiatric nosology and the explicitation of categoric definitions, both leading to the improvement of diagnostic reliability. The main emerging challenge is now to advance the validity or usefulness of psychiatric diagnosis. Two interrelated responses to this challenge are the proposal of a comprehensive diagnostic model and the development of a cultural formulation.

The comprehensive diagnostic model being explored by a workgroup of the World Psychiatric Association (13) enriches the standardized diagnostic statement with an idiographic or personalized complement. The Cultural Formulation Outline recently incorporated into DSM-IV (1) represents an idiographic statement intending to supplement standardized diagnostic ratings with a narrative description of the cultural framework of the patient's identity, illness, and social context and of the clinician-patient relationship. This cultural formulation first stimulated the development of a broader, standardized, *and* idiographic diagnostic formulation, and then became an example or facet of this broader model's idiographic component. These two contributions to the upgrading of diagnostic validity are discussed separately in the following two sections. Their presentation back to back intends to clar-

From *The Psychiatric Clinics of North America* 18, no. 3 (September 1995)

ify their interrelationships. Their joint implications are the subject of the final section of this article.

Comprehensive Diagnostic Model

The need for diagnostic formulations that would bring greater justice to the complexity of clinical conditions has been recognized for some time (e.g., Strauss [23]). More recently, a comprehensive diagnostic model that contextualizes the patient's illness and encompasses both standardized and personalized elements has emerged and is articulating the International Guidelines for Diagnostic Assessment under development by the World Psychiatric Association Section on Classification, Diagnostic Assessment and Nomenclature (13). The three components of this comprehensive diagnostic model are outlined in the following sections.

Nosologic Classification

This is the hierarchical ordering of illnesses that traditionally has constituted the core of standard classification systems such as the various versions of the World Health Organization's International Classification of Diseases, including its current tenth revision, ICD-10 (26). Nosologic classification is also the core of nationally produced instruments, such as the various editions of the American Psychiatric Association's *Diagnostic and Statistical Manual of Mental Disorders* as well as the first and second editions of the *Chinese Classification of Mental Disorders* (2). Although nosologic description has been formulated conventionally in typologic or categoric terms, attempts are being made to use dimensional scales for the description of certain areas of psychopathology, such as schizophrenic phenomenology and personality disorders (25). A sizable portion of clinical research in psychiatry is aimed at studying the phenomenology of mental disorders, their etiopathogenic factors, as well as their longitudinal unfolding. Findings from such research should promote the refinement of nosologic classification.

Standardized Multiaxial Formulation

This formulation generically represents an attempt to characterize the plurality of mental and physical disorders presented by many patients, contextualized in terms of the psychosocial environment in which the illnesses appear as well as of their effect on adaptive functioning. This contextualization is implemented through standardized instruments either of categoric or dimensional types. Multiaxial evaluations, along with syndromic description and operationalized diagnostic criteria, have been recognized in international surveys (12, 16) as the most important contemporary innovations in diagnostic methodology. Multiaxial schemas are, in fact, a regular feature of the new standard diagnostic systems, such as ICD-10 and DSM-IV.

Illustratively, the DSM-IV multiaxial assessment schema includes the following axes: I. Clinical Disorders, II. Personality Disorders and Mental Retardation, III. General Medical Conditions, IV. Psychosocial and Environmental Problems, and V. Global Assessment of Functioning. A Multiaxial Presentation of ICD-10 is being developed by the Mental Health Division of the World Health Organization, and contains the following axes: I. Clinical Diagnoses; II. Disablements (divided into four areas: personal care, occupational functioning, functioning with family/household, and broader social functioning); and III. Contextual Factors. Exemplifying a growing interest for the preparation of national adaptations of standard international classification instruments, and as part of the Third Cuban Glossary of Psychiatry, an adaptation of the ICD-10 multiaxial schema through complementary axes recently has been published (19).

Idiographic Formulation

This personalized and flexibly articulated component of a comprehensive diagnostic model has emerged as a complementing response to the limitations of the standardized components of the model. First are *content* limitations. There are a number of aspects relevant to understanding a case and conducting clinical care that are not part of a nosologic classification or a multiaxial formulation. For example, in a literature review of components of a flexible psychiatric formulation, Faulkner et al. (3a) identified the following elements as the most frequently considered: genetic factors, constitutional factors, psychological processes, ego functioning, and sociocultural factors. Important information in these areas is not standardizable, and this calls for a nonstandardized, flexibly organized, and narratively presented complement to standard diagnostic ratings.

A second major limitation of standardized nosologic classifications and multiaxial formulations is that they represent the clinician's perspectives or views. Increasingly recognized is the need to attend also to the *perspectives of the patient and the patient's family*. Kleinman (11) has demonstrated compellingly the importance of carefully examining the experience of the patient and his or her explanatory models and those of the pertinent reference group. Strauss (22) has proposed a focus on the person of the patient as key to understanding mental illness. Van Praag (24) has argued for a reconquest of the subjective as a way of fertilizing psychiatric diagnosis.

Cultural Formulation

The cultural formulation, particularly the proposal prepared for the DSM-IV, is discussed with regard to its conceptual background, key features of its development, and the actual outline published in DSM-IV.

Clinical Anthropologic Bases

General recommendations toward a cultural statement to upgrade or potentiate standard psychiatric diagnosis have been offered repeatedly over the past decade in the professional literature (3, 5, 8, 11, 14). Furthermore, concentration on the personal experience of the patient is becoming a focus of convergence between anthropologic considerations on the cultural matrix of psychopathology and a particular movement within clinical and social psychiatry. In effect, Strauss (22) has pointedly argued that psychiatrists, more than treating mental disorders, care for people who happen to experience such disorders. This coincides with the anthropologic emphasis made by Geertz (4) on the "native point of view."

A review of the recent literature on cultural formulation revealed that a focus on the *patient's personal perspective* is, in fact, recognized as fundamental (5, 7, 9, 10). In terms of themes or elements for a cultural formulation, four of the seven papers offering specific recommendations spoke of several facets of the *cultural identity of the individual*, that is, behavioral or ideologic ethnicity (10) and spiritual or religious involvement (6, 7, 21). Another major theme was *cultural factors pertinent to the patient's illness*, recommended by both Good and Good (5), in terms of idioms for experiencing and communicating illness, culture-specific illness categories, explanatory models, and predominant care-seeking patterns, and by Kleinman (10), who considered the cultural significance of symptoms, culturally salient illnesses, and explanatory models of illness. A third major theme corresponds to *cultural factors on social environment and functioning*, articulated by Good and Good (5) with regard to perceived level of disability, as well as by Ramírez (21) in terms of three elements in his Puerto Rican Octagonal Assessment Schema (i.e., perceived social stress, connectedness to sociocultural supports, and acquired maturity). A fourth theme involves *intercultural elements of the clinician-patient relationship*, represented by negotiation between patient/family and professionals and the consideration of the clinician's biases.

Constructing Cultural Formulation Guidelines

The opportunity for crystallizing specific guidelines for a cultural formulation appeared in 1991 within the framework of a project to develop proposals for enhancing the cultural validity and suitability of DSM-IV. A National Institute of Mental Health (NIMH) conference held in Pittsburgh in April 1991 for a meeting of minds between a group of cultural experts and representatives of the American Psychiatric Association's DSM-IV Task Force and Work Groups identified a number of structural elements in the new manual as foci for a cultural development program. These included the introduction to the manual, cultural considerations sections for the text of the various diagnostic categories, a glossary of culture-bound syndromes, and guidelines for a cultural formulation.

The idea for a cultural formulation appeared upon discussing the possibility of a "cultural axis." Diagnostic axes, as incorporated in official diagnostic systems such as ICD-10 and DSM-IV, are contextualizing schemas that involve domains assessed with standardized instruments (typologies or dimensional scales). Diagnostic axes, therefore, were not considered appropriate for articulating a cultural statement, which, given the complexity of the cultural matrix, requires organizational flexibility and the use of all the resources of natural language.

A Culture and Diagnosis Group established with the support of the NIMH Office for Special Populations undertook the preparation of the various cultural proposals for DSM-IV agreed to at the 1991 Pittsburgh conference, including a cultural formulation guideline. The process of conceptualizing a cultural formulation was informed by the literature review summarized in the preceding section. To the first four elements supported by the literature review (cultural identity of the patient, cultural factors in the patient's illness, cultural factors pertinent to social environment and functioning, and intercultural elements in the clinician-patient relationship) was added a summary: overall cultural statement for diagnosis and care.

A draft of the Cultural Formulation Guideline was presented in January 1992 to the DSM-IV Task Force, which received it warmly and recommended its experimental piloting. This pilot project, aimed at appraising the feasibility and suitability of the Guideline, was carried out by a subgroup of the NIMH Culture and Diagnosis Group. The project included the application of the draft of the Guideline to sets of cases from the four main ethnically identified minorities in the United States, that is, African Americans, American Indians, Asian Americans, and Latinos or Hispanic Americans. For each case, a succinct clinical history, a multiaxial diagnosis, and a cultural formulation were prepared. The results of the pilot project led to the revision of the Cultural Formulation proposal (17), which included three parts: an introduction, the key five elements of the formulation, and four illustrative cases. Finally published in DSM-IV (1) were the first two sections of the proposal. They were included without the illustrative cases in Appendix I of the DSM-IV, along with the Glossary of Culture Bound Syndromes (see chapter 7 for text of the Cultural Formulation Outline).

Impact on Clinical Care and Research

The possibilities offered by the Cultural Formulation (CF) to enhance patient care, professional training, and clinical and epidemiologic research, particularly from a comprehensive diagnosis model viewpoint, are outlined in the following sections.

Clinical Care and Training

Regarding patient care, the first potential impact of the CF is on greater understanding of the patient condition. In fact, the first three elements of the CF involve a sensitive and detailed exploration of the patient's identity, illness, and context. In this regard, the CF may constitute a "golden gate" to approach and better understand the patient's condition and experience. A second important implication of the CF for patient care refers to the enlarged data base it may yield for use in treatment planning, adding to what standardized multiaxial diagnostic ratings have been shown to offer (15). Relevant here is not only the potentially more accurate information that can be obtained through the CF on psychopathologic syndromes, the psychosocial environment in which they emerge, and their impact on the performance of crucial social roles, but also information on the meaning of these clinical problems and issues for the patient and family. This leads to the third potential benefit of the CF, namely the likelihood of a more enthusiastic engagement of the patient in the clinical care process. This greater engagement, crucial for treatment effectiveness, is predicated on the expectation that the patient assessed with the CF and a comprehensive diagnostic model may feel more fully understood and respected.

Culturally competent and sensitive professional training is being endorsed widely as highly desirable on the grounds that it leads to better treatment outcomes. More clarity is needed, however, on how to conceptualize and organize such professional training. The CF offers here a contribution by emphasizing the need to attend to the patient's perspectives and some of the key content areas on which proficiency is required.

Several educational projects are being planned by the NIMH Culture and Diagnosis Group to facilitate the full use of the CF in patient care and professional training. These include an *Introduction to the Cultural Formulation*, as a short booklet intended for wide and prompt circulation, and a *Cultural Casebook*, which will illustrate the competent use of the CF with a large variety of cases reflecting the cultural and social plurality of U.S. society.

Potentiating these efforts with the CF, plans are being considered for the NIMH Culture and Diagnosis Group to interact with pertinent national and international groups. These include the American Psychiatric Association Work Group on Psychiatric Evaluation Practice Guidelines and the World Psychiatric Association Work Group on International Guidelines for Diagnostic Assessment.

Clinical and Epidemiologic Research

One important research line would be to carry out further work on the CF itself. This should include refinement of the schema's content and organization as well as the preparation of additional, more specific assessment instructions. Also of interest would be to explore the standardization of selected components of the CF. Illustrative of pertinent possibilities are acculturation and biculturality scales (20) and the World Health Organization project on standardizing a subjective and multidimensional concept of quality of life (18).

Another promising research line would investigate the value of the CF to enhance treatment effectiveness and the prediction of illness course. These studies, particularly pertinent to naturalistic settings as opposed to laboratory circumstances, would be highly valuable for a contextualized understanding of psychopathology as well as for health services research. Also heuristically promising would be to use the CF for the development of contextualized epidemiologic methods. This might offer a second-generation development beyond the well-known contributions of syndromatic clinical nosology and explicit diagnostic definitions for the instrumentation of modern epidemiologic surveys (8a).

Summary

The Cultural Formulation constitutes a distillation of the new cross-cultural psychiatry, designed by the NIMH Culture and Diagnosis Group, and incorporated into DSM-IV as one of its significant innovations. The role of the Cultural Formulation in clinical care, training, and research can be better understood and its impact extended when considered within the framework of a comprehensive diagnostic model.

References

1. American Psychiatric Association. (1994). *Diagnostic and statistical manual of mental disorders.* 4th edition. Washington, DC: American Psychiatric Association.

2. Chinese Medical Association. (1989). *Chinese classification of mental disorders.* 2nd edition. Hunan: Hunan Medical University Press.

3. Fabrega, H. (1987). Psychiatric diagnosis: A cultural perspective. *J Nerv Ment Dis* 175:383–394.

3a.Faulkner, L. R., Kinzie, J. D., Angell, R., et al. (1985). A comprehensive psychiatric formulation model. *J Psychiatric Ed* 9:189–203.

4. Geertz, C. (1983). *Local knowledge.* New York: Basic Books.

5. Good, B. J., Good, M-J. D. (1986). The cultural context of diagnosis and therapy: A view from medical anthropology. In M. R. Miranda and H. H. L. Kitano (Eds.), *Mental health research and practice in minority communities,* pp. 165–198. U.S. Department of Health and Human Services Publication No. (ADM) 86–1466. Washington, DC: U.S. Government Printing Office.

6. Guarnaccia, P. J. (1996). Comments on culture and multiaxial diagnosis. In J. E. Mezzich, A. Kleinman, H. Fábrega et al. (Eds.), *Culture and psychiatric diagnosis.* Washington, DC: American Psychiatric Press.

7. Hughes, C. C. (1993). Culture in clinical psychiatry. In A. Gaw (Ed.), *Culture, ethnicity, and mental illness,* pp. 3–41. Washington, DC: American Psychiatric Press.

8. Hughes, C. C. (1985). Culture-bound or construct-bound? In R. C. Simons and C. C. Hughes (Eds.), *The Culture-bound syndromes,* pp. 3–24. Dordrecht, Netherlands: D Reidel.

8a.Jablensky, A. (1993). Impact of the new diagnostic systems on psychiatric epidemiology. In J. A. Costa e Silva and C. C. Nadelson (Eds.), *International review of psychiatry,* pp. 13–43. Washington, DC: American Psychiatric Press.

9. Jones, E. E., and Thorne, A. (1987). Rediscovery of the subject: Intercultural approaches to clinical assessment. *J Consult Clin Psychol* 55:488–495.

10. Kleinman, A. (1988). *The illness narratives: Suffering, healing, and the human condition.* New York: Basic Books.

11. Kleinman, A. (1988). *Rethinking psychiatry: From cultural category to personal experience.* New York: Free Press.

12. Maser, J. D., and Kaelber, C. (1991). International use and attitudes toward DSM-III and DSM-III-R: Growing consensus in psychiatric classification. Special issue: Diagnosis, dimensions, and DSM-IV: The science of classification. *J Abnorm Psychol* 100:271–279.

13. Mezzich, J. E. (1995). International perspectives on psychiatric diagnosis. In H. I. Kaplan and B. J. Sadock (Eds.), *Comprehensive textbook of psychiatry.* 6th edition, pp. 692–703. Baltimore: Williams and Wilkins.

14. Mezzich, J. E., and Berganza, C. E. (1984). Culture and psychopathology. New York: Columbia University Press.

15. Mezzich, J. E., and Schmolke, M. M. (1995). Multiaxial diagnosis and psychotherapy planning: On the relevance of ICD-10, DSM-IV and complementary schemas. *Psychother Psychosom* 63:71–80.

16. Mezzich, J. E., Fabrega, H., Mezzich, A. C. (1985). An international consultation on multiaxial diagnosis. In P. Pichot, P. Berner, R. Wolf, et al. (Eds.), *Psychiatry: The state of the art*, pp. 51–56. London: Plenum Press.

17. Mezzich, J. E., Good, B. J., Lewis-Fernández, R., et al. (1993). Cultural formulation guidelines. In J. E. Mezzich, A. Kleinman, H. Fabrega, et al. (Eds.), *Revised cultural proposals for DSM-IV*. Technical report, NIMH Group on Culture and Diagnosis, pp. 161–168. Pittsburgh, PA, September.

18. Orley, J., and Kuyken, W. (1994). *International quality of life assessment*. Heidelberg: Springer-Verlag.

19. Otero-Ojeda, A. A. (1994). *Adaptación cultural del esquema multiaxial de la CIE-10 a través de ejes complementarios*. La Habana: Editorial Científico-Técnica.

20. Padilla, A. M. (1994). Bicultural development: A theoretical and empirical examination. In R. G. Malgady and O. Rodriguez (Eds.), *Theoretical and conceptual issues in Hispanic mental health*. Malabar, FL: Krieger Publishing.

21. Ramírez, E. (1991) *Octagonal assessment schema*. San Juan: Technical Report, Department of Mental Health of Puerto Rico.

22. Strauss, J. S. (1992). The person—key to understanding mental illness: Towards a new dynamic psychiatry, III. *Br J Psychiatry* 161 (Suppl. 18): 19–26.

23. Strauss J. S. (1975). A comprehensive approach to psychiatric diagnosis. *Am J Psychiatry* 132:1193–1197.

24. Van Praag, H. M. (1992). Reconquest of the subjective: Against the waning of psychiatric diagnosing. *Br J Psychiatry* 160:266–271.

25. Widiger, T. A. (1991). Personality disorder dimensional models proposed for DSM-IV. *J Personality Dis* 5:386–398.

26. World Health Organization. (1992). *Tenth revision of the International Classification of Diseases and Related Health Problems* (ICD-10). Geneva: WHO.

10

Issues in the Assessment and Diagnosis of Culturally Diverse Individuals

Francis G. Lu, Russell F. Lim, and Juan E. Mezzich

A CONSIDERATION OF CULTURE is essential in the process of the interview, case formulation, diagnosis, and treatment of culturally diverse individuals. The evaluation of these individuals raises many issues that clinicians need to address to formulate an accurate diagnosis and treatment plan that will be acceptable to the patient. The assessment of minority patients has additional layers of complexity when compared with assessment of nonminority patients, especially when the patient has a different cultural or ethnic background from the clinician. Thus, clinicians need to develop culturally competent knowledge, attitudes, and skills. The clinician should have some knowledge of the patient's cultural identity, and the use of a cultural consultant may be appropriate to avoid biases and misdiagnosis (Budman et al. 1992), even if the clinician and patient are of the same culture and ethnicity (Comas Diaz and Jacobsen 1991; T. L. Cross et al. 1989; Pinderhughes 1989). Also, clinicians need to be aware of their own cultural identity and their attitudes and beliefs toward ethnic minorities, because these will affect their relationships with patients. Finally, clinicians need additional skills because traditional methods of interviewing the patient may not be effective and psychological tests may not be adequate or appropriate. Clinicians may need to use an interpreter (Westermeyer 1990) or may need to conduct family interviews, and psychological tests may need modification (Marsella 1989).

Many organizations have begun to address these issues in the assessment

From *The American Psychiatric Association Review of Psychiatry* 14 (1995)

and diagnosis of culturally diverse individuals. Both the American Psychological Association and the American Counseling Association have recognized the importance of considering the effect of culture on diagnosis and treatment. These organizations have published similar guidelines for clinical competence with culturally diverse individuals. The American Psychological Association (1993) guidelines acknowledge the necessity of assessing individuals in the context of their ethnicity and culture, respecting their indigenous beliefs and practices (including those involving religion and spirituality), assessing the patients' support system, evaluating the patients in their primary language, and taking a history that accounts for immigration and acculturation stresses. The American Counseling Association guidelines stress the awareness of both patient and clinician beliefs, the attainment of background knowledge about the patient (including his or her worldview), and the development of culturally competent skills (Sue et al. 1992). In addition, the ICD-10 (World Health Organization 1992) incorporated major methodological developments such as a phenomenological organization of nosology, use of more specific definitions for diagnostic categories, the employment of a multiaxial framework, and the development of an international psychiatric lexicon (containing a description of culture-bound syndromes) as well as an international casebook. Finally, the American Psychiatric Association acknowledged the impact of culture and ethnicity on diagnosis and treatment, as stated in the introduction to DSM-IV (American Psychiatric Association 1994a):

> Special efforts have been made in the preparation of DSM-IV to incorporate an awareness that the manual is used in culturally diverse populations in the United States and internationally. Clinicians are called on to evaluate individuals from numerous different ethnic groups and cultural backgrounds (including many who are recent immigrants). Diagnostic assessment can be especially challenging when a clinician from one ethnic or cultural group uses the DSM-IV Classification to evaluate an individual from a different ethnic or cultural group. A clinician who is unfamiliar with the nuances of an individual's cultural frame of reference may incorrectly judge as psychopathology those normal variations in behavior, belief, or experience that are particular to the individual's culture. (p. xxiv)

Whereas in DSM-III-R (American Psychiatric Association, 1987) the importance of culture was only briefly acknowledged, DSM-IV has an appendix that contains an outline for cultural formulation and a glossary of culture-bound syndromes. In addition, "specific culture features" are considered where appropriate in the actual diagnostic categories. In summary, the consideration of cultural factors in the assessment, diagnosis, and treatment of culturally diverse individuals has gained recognition in a variety of disciplines in the last decade.

In this chapter, we present a brief history of psychiatric case formulation; define culture, ethnicity, and race; and focus on an explication and elaboration of the DSM-IV outline for cultural formulation. Aspects of cultural formulation include assessing a patient's cultural identity and understanding how culture affects the explanation of the individual's illness, support system, and the clinician-patient relationship as well as understanding how culture affects the assessment and diagnosis of culturally diverse individuals.

Case Formulation: Background History

The formulation of cases has been essential to the assessment, diagnosis, and treatment of patients since Freud's time, and many models have been proposed to organize patient data and inform treatment. These models include the psychodynamic, the biological, the behavioral, and the biopsychosocial (Sperry et al., 1992). Earlier in this century, the psychodynamic model was the most prominent; it begins with the assumption that the patient's problems can be understood as a result of conflicts that result in anxiety (Perry et al., 1987). The biological model, which posits an organic basis for psychopathology, was more commonly associated with other medical specialties and has become more prominent since 1950 with the advent of psychotropic medications (Ayd and Blackwell, 1984), the discoveries of sensitive receptor assays resulting in more specific drugs (Snyder, 1985), and the development of improved structural and functional brain-imaging techniques (Andreason, 1989). The behavioral model operates on the premise that an individual's behavior is determined by learning patterns such as disordered thoughts from an event, which then result in behaviors that are self-reinforcing (Cohen and Farrell, 1988). The biopsychosocial model, which is based on systems theory, states that patients' biological state, psychological makeup, and environment all affect their illness presentation and treatment (Engel 1980).

We believe that focusing on the cultural formulation enhances the usefulness of the biopsychosocial model, especially for culturally diverse individuals. The cultural formulation highlights the effect of culture on the expression of symptoms, definition of illness, and treatment. In the past, many authors have discussed the importance of considering the effect of culture on diagnosis and treatment. Fabrega (1987) and Kleinman (1988) agreed that culture affects the clinician's impressions of normality and categories of illness. Rogler and Cortes (1993) stated that culture affects the patient's access to mental health care. Sue and Sue (1990) stated that the impetus for the increasing interest in cultural issues lies in the recognition that our society is becoming multiracial, multicultural, and multilingual, whereas the training of mental health professionals has not reflected this trend, preferring to remain monocultural.

Cultural Formulation

Hinton and Kleinman (1993) discussed a practical approach to making culturally appropriate formulations. The first step is to show empathy during the interview and then to elicit the patient's perspective on the illness. Next, the patient's experience can be assessed in the context of the patient's family, workplace, health care systems, and community. Finally, the patient's illness can be diagnosed both through DSM-IV categories and through the patient's cultural idioms of distress. Hinton and Kleinman's overall schema is similar to the one developed by the National Institute of Mental Health (NIMH) Culture and Diagnosis Group (Mezzich et al., 1993). (See chapter 7 for the text of the DSM-IV Cultural Formulation Outline.) Before reviewing each of the outline's topics, we need to define some key terms.

Definitions

Culture

As described by the NIMH Culture and Diagnosis Group (Mezzich et al., 1993) for incorporation into DSM-IV, culture and ethnicity are related concepts. According to that group:

> Culture refers to meanings, values, and behavioral norms that are learned and transmitted in the dominant society and within its social groups. Culture powerfully influences cognitions, feeling, and "self" concept, as well as the diagnostic process and treatment decisions. Ethnicity, a related concept, refers to social groupings which distinguish themselves from other groups based on ideas of shared descent and aspirations, as well as to behavioral norms and forms of personal identity associated with such groups. (p. 7)

Culture has many meanings and can be thought of as the beliefs, customs, technologic achievements, language, and history of a group of similar people (Johnson 1988). Alternatively, it can be thought of as the values, meaning, and behaviors that are transmitted by the dominant group. Its precise definition is poorly agreed on; Kroeber and Kluckhohn (1963) listed more than 150 definitions. Linton (1945) defined *culture* as being a shared, learned behavior transmitted from one generation to another, having both external and internal components. The external components include beliefs, laws, traditions, customs, morals, and habits; the internal components consist of norms, rules, standards, ideals, and values.

Cultures also differ in their conception of personal identity. In general, Eastern cultures favor a group identity, whereas Western cultures favor individual autonomy. Another significant difference is the concept of the body. Western societies tend to see the mind and body as separate, whereas Eastern societies tend to see the mind and body as a whole. Cultural expectations and norms determine if a constellation of symptoms is judged as pathological or not. Various disorders have differing prevalences in different ethnic groups, and each group has variations in the expression of the illness (Burnam et al., 1987; Canino et al., 1987; Karno et al., 1987). For example, many Australians, who typically value independence, may have a more difficult time with depression because it makes them more dependent on others, whereas many Japanese, who value community-based decisions, may have less difficulty with depression (Radford et al., 1991). Each culture has its own range of communication style (e.g., language, gestures, and rituals), eating behaviors, family roles (e.g., marital, gender, and leadership roles), beliefs and rituals (e.g., child rearing and sexual practices), and ways of regulating aggressive and sexual drives. In summary, culture can be understood as a complex construct of socially transmitted ideas, feelings, and attitudes that shape behavior, organize perceptions, and label experiences.

Ethnicity

Ethnicity refers to an individual's sense of belonging to a group of people sharing a common origin and history, along with similar cultural and social beliefs (Group for the Advancement of Psychiatry, 1987). It is thus closely linked to the individual's self-image. *Ethnicity* also refers to shared descent and aspirations, as well as behavioral norms and personal identity. Finally, *ethnicity* may imply national and geographical origin, as well as religious beliefs. Incorrect assumptions about ethnicity, based on language or appearance alone, can lead to misunderstanding and misdiagnosis of culturally diverse minority individuals (Del Castillo, 1970; Hughes, 1993).

Race

In contrast to ethnicity and culture, *race* is not mentioned in DSM-IV; it refers to the biologically determined similarities of a group, which affect the interactions with others when perceived differences lead to the use of value hierarchies embodied in bias or prejudice. According to Pinderhughes (1989), *race* has "a different level of cultural meaning than ethnicity" (p. 71). For example, a West Indian black is ethnically and culturally different from an African American, yet both may be treated with the same prejudiced attitudes by whites. Pinderhughes stated that race has social meaning, assigns status, limits opportunities, and influences interactions between patients and clinicians. For example, the psychological effect of a person's facial complexion can be traced to the racism that has as its roots the history of conflicts between certain social groups in the United States. Racial prejudices influence the expectations that people have of one another and can lead clinicians to stereotype individuals.

Cultural Identity

These are many components to a patient's cultural identity that go beyond the concepts of ethnicity and race, because a person may have several cultural reference groups. For example, two Hispanic persons may come from Mexico but may have different cultural identities depending on the socioeconomic status and geographical region from which they originated. Multiple factors affect an individual's cultural identity (table 10.1).

It is vital to know these multiple aspects about patients' cultural identity to avoid misconceptions based on ignorance or stereotypes related to ethnicity and race or any one aspect of cultural identity. Clinicians need to explore the patient's developmental history to understand what makes him or her either different from or similar to a person born and raised in the predominant host culture in the United States. These characteristics may include country of origin, family structure, customs, values, and beliefs, as well as attitudes about medicine and psychiatry. If patients are recent immigrants, clinicians need to explore the immigration experience, including any trauma, separation, losses, alienation, class displacements, or disappointments. If the patients are not recent immigrants but belong to later generations, focus can

TABLE 10.1
Aspects of Cultural Identity Development

Ethnicity	Gender
Race	Age
Country of origin	Sexual orientation
Language	Religious and spiritual beliefs
Acculturation	Socioeconomic class and education

be placed on the level of their acculturation, which refers to the degree to which they have adopted the beliefs, values, and practices of the host culture (Westermeyer, 1993).

Previous work on the concept of cultural identity includes the concept of worldview, whether Eurocentric or multicultural, which avoids the use of labels that can oversimplify and stereotype (Ivey et al., 1993). Patients' histories can be thought of in terms of their personal, family, and cultural histories. These histories are held by the patients as constructs, which can be detected by their use of key words or words that they use over and over as they interact with the clinician. Kelly (1955) stated that constructs are not the concrete reality, but the individual's personal explanation and meaning. Family constructs can be elicited with a genogram and a developmental history. Finally, cultural constructs can be assessed by asking about gender, religious, or ethnic and racial issues among other aspects (table 10.1).

Another method of conceptualizing cultural identity is through an interpersonal grid, which involves assessing the patient's worldview by using system variables. The clinician attempts to discuss particular topic areas—such as demographic (age, gender, and location), status (social, educational, and economic), and affiliations (ethnic, religious, and family)—and the behaviors, expectations, and values associated with these factors (Pedersen and Ivey, 1993). Thus, clinicians are better able to interpret and predict their patients' behaviors if they are aware of the differences between their own and their patients' explanations of behaviors. This model helps the clinician to understand that the same behavior can have different meanings to others and that behavior needs to be interpreted in the context of these topic areas.

Finally, another schema for understanding cultural identity is the multicultural cube, which adds the dimension of level of "cultural identity development" (Ivey et al., 1993, p. 100). Cultural identity development refers to how the culturally diverse individual sees himself or herself in respect to the host culture. The least developed level is acceptance or conformity, which describes a compliant position. Following that level is one of dissonance, where the individual is in conflict with his or her own cultural identity and that of society. The next level is resistance, in which the individual rejects all that is the host culture. Following that level is one of introspection, which implies that both cultures can coexist, but that the host culture is irrelevant. Finally, there is the level of integrative awareness, in which individuals can accept the best and worst aspects of both cultures (Atkinson et al. 1989). Similar well-researched schema of racial and ethnic identity development has focused on African Americans (Cross, 1991), African Americans and whites (Helms, 1990), Asian Americans (Sue and Sue, 1990), and Hispanics (Bernal and Knight, 1993).

Assessment of Ethnicity

The ethnicity of a patient can be assessed by taking a careful history of the patient's development and family. Clinicians can ask patients to describe their grandparents' and parents' country of origin, religion, primary language, traditional roles, and traditional skills. Patients should be asked about their socialization experiences (such as their proficiency with their culture's native language), their role in their family constellation, special rituals during certain ages (rites of passage), religious practices, holiday observances, or preparation of ethnic food that they have observed with their families. Finally, patients should be asked to what extent they are following the ceremonies, rituals, customs, and hobbies of their ancestors and the level of contact they have with their relatives or ethnic organizations.

Language

Language identifies and codifies an individual's experience, which is not readily translated from one language to another without distortion. Because culturally diverse patients sometimes speak more than one language, it is important to determine what language they consider their primary language. Usually this is the language first learned; however, it may not be the language of their ethnic culture, but of their host culture. It is the one in which they feel the most comfortable expressing themselves. If a secondary language is used, a more limited, and possibly inaccurate, history can result in misdiagnosis (Del Castillo, 1970; Marcos et al., 1973). Advanced forms of communication—such as humor; assertiveness; and the expression of displeasure, frustration, and love—are hampered by the patient's lack of fluency in the new language (Westermeyer 1989). In addition, communication includes nonverbal communication, such as distance between speakers, eye contact, physical touch, and local forms of gesticulation. Different ethnicities also communicate in different styles. For example, Sue and Sue (1990) stated that there are high-content groups, such as African Americans, Asians, Hispanics, and Native Americans, who use different nonverbal communication than other ethnicities, such as whites.

Migration History

For recently immigrated patients, an important part of their cultural identity relates to their migration history, which should be recorded in the psychosocial history section of the written evaluation. As described by Lee (1990) (table 10.2), the purpose of a migration history is to determine the patient's

TABLE 10.2
Migration History

Premigration history	Country of origin, family, education, socioeconomic status, community and family support, political issues, war, trauma.
Experience of migration	Migrant versus refugee: Why did they leave? Who was left behind? Who paid for their trip? Means of escape, trauma.
Degree of loss	Loss of family members, relatives, friends. Material losses: business, careers, properties. Loss of cultural milieu, community, religious, spiritual support.
Traumatic experience	Physical: Torture, rape, starvation, imprisonment. Psychological: Rage, depression, guilt, grief, post-traumatic stress disorder.
Work and financial history	Original line of work, current occupation, socioeconomic status.
Support systems	Community support, religion, family.
Medical history	Beliefs in herbal medicine, somatic complaints.
Family's concept of illness	What do family members think the problem is? Its cause? What do they do for help? What result is expected?
Level of acculturation	First or second generation.
Impact on development	Level of adjustment, assess developmental tasks.

Source: Adapted from Lee (1990).

background history and to measure their baseline functional level as well as the generational status of the patient. These are actually two parts to the migration history: the premigration history and the immigration history.

A premigration history includes country of origin, position in the family, education, employment status, level of support, political issues, experiences of war, and traumatic events. It may be helpful to know the recent history of the region, common religious beliefs, and from which social class the patient originated. The clinician's goal is to understand the patient's former baseline life experience in his or her native country prior to migration.

The immigration history includes the reasons for leaving, who was left behind, who paid for the trip, and hardships endured and trauma suffered, including experiences of torture, beatings, starvation, rape, and imprisonment in a refugee or detention camp. Patients can be described as "migrants" or "refugees"; migrants leave their county voluntarily and often easily, whereas refugees are either forced out or flee the country surreptitiously, encountering many traumas and losses. Clinicians need to explore the extent of loss and traumatic experiences. These can include the loss of family members, relatives, and friends; material losses of property, financial resources, businesses, and careers; and loss of their cultural milieu, community support, and religious and spiritual support.

Degree of Acculturation

Immigrants routinely experience some degree of culture shock, and clinicians can assess the patient's level of adjustment by inquiring about his or her competence in the English language and in negotiating the tasks of learning to live in this country. This can be seen in activities such as the successful attainment of housing, employment, and child care and a mastery of public transportation. Demographic information can help assess the rate of acculturation. Important variables include the number of years spent in the United States, the age at the time of immigration, exposure to Western culture in the country of origin, and contacts with native-born Americans. Younger immigrants acculturate more quickly and learn English faster than older immigrants. Standard parts of the psychosocial history should be utilized to assess the rate of acculturation; these include occupational and social histories. The occupational history should survey the difference between the patient's work status in the United States and in the patient's home country.

A patient with a history of downward mobility in his or her occupational status could develop lowered self-esteem and insecurity, which might precipitate a mental disorder. The social history can also help determine how much support the patient can rely on from family or an extended network, such as family organizations or churches. Living in an ethnic community can also buffer the acculturation process. The patient's proficiency in English and contact with others outside of the cultural enclave are useful measures of acculturation. Of note is that DSM-IV has a new category for "acculturation problem" in the section titled "Other Conditions That May Be a Focus of Clinical Attention," indicating that distressing acculturation experiences can occur without necessarily labeling them as symptoms of a mental disorder.

Another way of assessing the degree of acculturation of patients is by a framework that is numerative (i.e., first generation, second generation, third generation) or descriptive (i.e., traditional, transitional, bicultural, Americanized) (Lee, 1990). Traditional families are born and raised in their country of origin. In general, these immigrants speak only their native language, live in ethnic enclaves (like Chinatown or "Little Italy" in New York City), and could have a rural background. They tend to approach problems in a more concrete manner and are more likely to have adjustment disorders and major depression and to describe their problems in somatic terms. Transitional families have parents that speak very little English, whereas their children are better acculturated. They commonly have parent-child conflicts, role confusion, and marital difficulties. These families suffer from the erosion of the authority of the parents by their dependence on their children for linguistic and cultural translation. The most effective therapies for these patients are cognitive and behavioral. Bicultural families have parents who are professionals or business owners and are primarily English speaking. The parental authority is egalitarian as opposed to patriarchal. These families traditionally live in the suburbs. They are often more stable than the above two family structures. Finally, Americanized families are usually several generations removed from immigration. Often the original native culture is lost, because parents and children speak only English. Interethnic marriage is more common, and families are individualistic, competitive, and egalitarian. They are usually stable and present no significant differences from Westernized patients.

A final way of looking at acculturation was described by Padilla (1980), who suggested both that acculturation can be thought of in more than one dimension and that the clinician should assess separately degrees of identification with the host culture and with the original culture. In connection with this, bicultural individuals seem to have better social adjustment and performance than those who either identify only with the new culture and lose affiliation with their family origins or identify only with the original culture and seclude themselves into cultural ghettos.

Gender

Gender identity issues also interact synergistically with ethnic identity to shape one's cultural identity and have many implications for assessment and treatment. Notman et al. (1991) and Myers (1991) concisely reviewed the impact of both female and male gender identity or development across the life cycle. They pointed out the complex interaction of gender identity and age on one's cultural identity. Fullilove (1993) outlined how minority women's status affects health status, sexual practices, and treatment settings. Comas-Diaz and Greene (1994) stressed the heterogeneity among women of color by integrating culturally relevant and gender-sensitive issues into guidelines for clinical practice with African American, Latina/Hispanic, Asian American, American Indian, and West and East Indian women.

Age

Psychiatry has long acknowledged the impact of age on one's identity formation. As with gender, age interacts with the other aspects of cultural identity to influence development and psychiatric assessment and treatment. For example, Canino and Spurlock (1994) offered clinical guidelines for working with economically disadvantaged children and adolescents from culturally diverse backgrounds that recognize the significance of cultural variations in help-seeking behavior, discrimination, and socioeconomic pressures on children's adaptive responses and mental health. The American Psychiatric Association (1994b) Task Force on Ethnic Minority Elderly also presented specific outlines for clinical care of the elderly from the four major ethnic minority groups.

Sexual Orientation

Sexual orientation defines an essential aspect of one's cultural identity. Stein (1993) extensively reviewed the development and meaning of lesbian, gay, and bisexual identities. Furthermore, assessment and treatment implications are outlined for persons with these sexual orientation identities across ethnic, age, and class groups to acknowledge the synergistic impact of these aspects of cultural identity. This work is greatly expanded on by Cabaj and Stein (1996).

Religion and Spirituality

Diverse cultures possess diverse religious and spiritual beliefs that are an important aspect of cultural identity and that affect health (Numbers and Amundsen, 1986; Sullivan, 1989) and mental health. Fitchett (1993) reviewed twenty-eight methods of spiritual assessment in pastoral care, some of which can be applied to both hospital and outpatient contexts. Most significantly, for religious and spiritual identity development, is the work of Fowler (1981) on the stages of faith.

Cultural Explanations for Illnesses

From a clinical point of view, understanding the patient's view of his or her illness helps determine our assessment and our treatment plan. Different cultures express their symptoms differently (Kleinman, 1988), and concepts of illness also vary with culture. For example, for the Chinese in Hong Kong, Cheung (1987) found that patients had three explanatory models for mental disorders. They could explain their illness as based on psychological, somatic, or mixed factors. Their explanation of the illness influenced how they went about getting help. The patients who had purely psychological explanations were the least likely to seek help. Because of this, Cheung recommended that clinicians specifically inquire about psychological symptoms, because these patients were not likely to volunteer them.

Idioms of Distress

Idioms of distress were defined by Nichter (1981) as the ways in which individuals "express, experience, and cope with feelings of distress" (p. 399). These are further described as "culturally constituted in the sense that they initiate particular types of interaction and are associated with culturally pervasive values, norms, generative themes, and health concerns" (p. 379).

In the DSM-IV appendix on culture-bound syndromes, there is a glossary listing "some of the best-studied culture-bound syndromes and idioms of distress that may be encountered in clinical practice in North America" (pp. 844–845). An example listed is *ataque de nervios*, a syndrome of uncontrollable shouting, crying, trembling, and aggression typically triggered by a stressful event involving family and followed by amnesia. Also included is *nervios*, a state of vulnerability to stress, marked by headaches, irritability, stomach problems, inability to concentrate, and dizziness. These two idioms are typically seen in Latino patients. Another example is *zar*, a syndrome of being possessed by spirits, evidenced by shouting, singing, crying, and a withdrawal from daily tasks.

A final example of a common idiom of distress is somatization, which can be seen in Hispanics, Asians, and people from Islamic cultures, among others, who can present with somatic complaints. In these cultures, most difficulties are conceptualized as somatic, and mental difficulties are either not conceptualized or are stigmatizing and therefore not even talked about (Angel and Guarnaccia, 1989; Blue and Gonzalez, 1992). It is important to remember that idioms of distress are not limited to one ethnic group, but can be seen in many ethnic groups. Finally, any of the idioms of distress can be pathological, depending on the level of disability. Without a knowledge of idioms (e.g., *ataque de nervios*), clinicians could make an erroneous diagnosis of panic disorder or somatization disorder (Guarnaccia et al., 1990).

Norms

Clinicians need to realize that cultural norms will influence how particular behaviors are judged. What may be abnormal and psychopathological in

Western culture may be considered normal and culturally acceptable in a non-Western society, and vice versa. Egland et al. (1983) studied bipolar illness in the Amish people, a culture that is known for its restraint in the expression of emotions. The Amish definitions of *grandiose* described behavior within the host culture's norms of behavior, such as driving a car or planning a vacation during the "wrong season," yet exceeded their norms sufficiently to meet criteria for bipolar disorder, because they were Amish. Individuals from diverse cultures present difficulties in diagnosis and treatment because the norms and expectations that are used to evaluate them may be different for different cultures.

Idioms of distress or culture-bound syndromes in other cultures may be considered outside the boundaries of expected illness behavior of the predominant culture. It is imperative that clinicians judge possible symptoms and syndromes of psychopathology against a knowledge of the cultural norms of the patient's cultural identity. If one is not aware of one's lack of understanding, errors can be made either by overpathologizing what is considered normal in that culture or by ascribing to cultural normality what is actually considered psychopathological in that culture.

Newhill (1990) described a series of guidelines for interpretation of "psychotic" symptoms for clinicians in culturally diverse individuals. First, the clinician should determine if there is any factual basis for ideas of persecution. Next, the clinician must determine if the patient's behavior is present in other members of their community, and if the behavior is explicable in terms of past experiences or as a belief of the patient's community. The clinician should consider the possibility that the patient's description is a figure of speech. Often, the presentation is one between an explainable model and psychosis. A cultural consultant may be needed to help with this process of understanding (Budman et al., 1992).

Culture-Bound Syndromes

Culture-bound syndromes represent conditions that tend to emerge or adopt a distinct presentation in specific cultures. They often incorporate local symptom constellations. They are important to identify, because the patient's definition of the illness has an impact on the effectiveness of the treatment, which must optimally operate within the patient's belief system. DSM-IV defines culture-bound syndromes as "recurrent, locality-specific patterns of aberrant behavior and troubling experience that may or may not be linked to a particular DSM-IV diagnostic category" (p. 844). An example of a culture-bound syndrome is *taijin kyofusho*, a Japanese syndrome that refers to an individual's intense fear that his or her body or its functions are offensive to other people. Of note is that this syndrome is listed as a diagnosis in the Japanese clinical modification of ICD-10. Neurasthenia or *shenjing shuairuo*, another culture-bound syndrome, is characterized by mental and physical exhaustion and may fit DSM-IV criteria for mood or anxiety disorder, as well as neurasthenia in ICD-10. Culture-bound syndromes are discussed further by Hughes (1993) and Wintrob (1996).

Explanatory Models

According to Helman (1990), explanatory models are how a patient explains his or her illness. It consists of the patient's notions of the illness's etiology, timing, mode of onset, pathophysiology, natural history, severity, and appropriate treatments, and it is specific to a single episode of the illness. Clinicians can elicit the patient's explanatory model by asking what the patient thinks has happened, why, and why now. Next, the clinician asks what will happen if nothing is done, and what effect it will have on others. Finally, the patient is asked what should be done about it. An example of an explanatory model that some Westernized patients are comfortable with may be the psychodynamic, whereas some traditional Native Americans may be more comfortable with an explanation from their witch doctor that they have "broken a taboo" of their family. In addition, they may also believe that they can hear the voice of a dead person calling to them as the spirit travels to the afterworld. If a clinician was unaware of this belief, the patient could be diagnosed as psychotic. In summary, to avoid such misconceptions, clinicians should ask patients what they believe is causing their illness, why it is a problem now, what will happen if they get no treatment, and what type of treatment they desire (Kleinman 1988).

Help-Seeking Behavior

Culture also affects help-seeking behavior; the definition of the patient's problem, how it will be expressed (somatically, behaviorally, or affectively), who should be consulted, and the preferred treatment strategies depend on the patient's explanatory model of illness (Kleinman, 1988; McGoldrick et al., 1982; Rogler and Cortes, 1993). For example, because some patients tend to act healthier than they appear to avoid the stigma of illness, a collateral history is sometimes necessary to obtain an accurate history. However, families and other informants also may minimize symptoms because there may be a stigma involved in even seeking assistance with mental disorders. Finally, culture affects patients' expectations of treatment. Many first-generation ethnic minority patients, such as recently immigrated Asians, expect their clinicians to be authoritarian, not egalitarian, and are confused by a nondirective stance (Schlesinger, 1981).

Indigenous healing practices may be utilized; examples include curanderos, shamans, medicine men, and fortune tellers (Gaines, 1991). A typical sequence of coping and help-seeking in a traditional Chinese family might include intrafamilial coping, followed by consultation with trusted elders and friends. The family would then seek outside help, going to herbalists and acupuncturists. They might then consult a religious person, or a physician, but would present with somatic complaints. Finally, as the patient deteriorates, the family reaches its limit and can no longer maintain the patient at home. There often is a rejection and scapegoating of the patient to decrease the shame and humiliation to the patient's family. The last resort is often hospitalization in a Western hospital (Lin and Lin, 1981).

Cultural Factors Related to the Psychosocial Environment

Thus far we have discussed the patients' cultural identity and their corresponding models of illness. The clinician's understanding of these areas will guide them to explore patients' particular stresses and coping mechanisms, including their support systems. The next section will discuss each of these topics in turn.

Stressors

In addition to the premigration and migration stressors, recent immigrants face a specific set of postmigration stressors. The immigrant must confront the need to learn the host language and customs and to negotiate the tasks of procuring housing, transportation, employment, and child care. In addition, the new migrant must cope with losses, the sequelae of traumatic experiences, and experiences with racism, sometimes without the benefit of their familiar support systems. For some ethnic groups, asking for help is an admission that one has failed, and developing a psychiatric illness would be an additional stigma. Asian ethnic groups face an additional stressor in that any failure of an individual in the family reflects on the reputation of the entire family, causing a "losing of face" leading to shame and embarrassment. Children of immigrants may face other stressors such as role confusion.

Specific problems are associated with specific ethnic groups. For example, Hispanics encounter particular difficulties with some stressors. Cullen and Travin (1990) discussed the resistances that would inhibit Spanish-speaking sex offenders from participating in group therapy. First, they found that patients expressed themselves better in Spanish than in English, thus not being understood is a stressor. Next, their expected sex role was in conflict with their crime. For men, they were expected to be independent, strong, and aggressive and to identify with virility. To be homosexual or a child molester is a display of "lack of shame," and an open discussion of sexuality would show a lack of respect to the therapist, adding to the patient's shame. Finally, Hispanics derive their self-worth from how successfully they can accomplish their cultural role obligations, such as providing for the security and well-being of their family, and not their social status. Thus, for multiple reasons, a Hispanic convicted of a sex offense would be reluctant to participate in therapy because of his or her cultural beliefs.

Developmental, Family, and Psychosocial History

An understanding of family dynamics and cultural values is crucial in assessing the patient's psychosocial environment. McGoldrick et al. (1982) described an approach to the assessment of the family, concentrating on the culture's definition of family and changes in the life cycle of the family. To prevent stereotyping, generalizations about traditional ethnic groups must be used only as a backdrop to the assessment of a particular family.

A culturally diverse individual's expectations of their life course is affected by their stage of development and age at immigration. Expectations of the achievement of milestones and definitions of family roles change when people migrate to different cultures. Assessing the expectations for the patient's stage of development in the family life cycle is important because this is often disrupted by migration or influenced by experiences with racism. For example, children who ordinarily would be expected to have few responsibilities often suffer from role reversal when they are pressed into service as linguistic and cultural translators for their parents. Further, poverty related to race and social status will limit their opportunities and expectations. For example, in a major textbook on the psychosocial development of minority group children, Powell (1983) observed that African-American children are affected by racist beliefs that they are substandard human beings. Hispanic children are often subjected to differing sets of expectations from their parents and their white teachers. Native American children are often separated from their families, going against their custom of making the child the center of tribal life. Adolescents who migrate have difficulties because of multiple transitions. Young adults in the stage of identity formation can be cut off from their heritage and feel alienated. New families could lose their support networks.

Elderly persons feel the losses of migration more keenly because they leave behind more memories and connections than the younger immigrants. They often migrate at a later stage of life, making them less able to acculturate, and they have a higher risk of culture shock (Sakauye, 1992). They are more likely to develop culture-bound syndromes and create difficulties in diagnosis because they typically speak only their native language. Ethnic minority elderly persons may feel displaced in Western societies in which elderly persons may be abandoned or placed in nursing homes.

Some specific issues with other ethnic minority elderly groups include (1) the overdiagnosis of schizophrenia and dementia in African Americans; (2) the undertreatment of Asian elderly due to poor education, superstition, and their fear of Western medications; (3) the underutilization of services by Hispanic elderly, secondary to their concerns about social stigma; and (4) the tendency of Native American elderly to rely on traditional healers, whose beliefs are poorly understood by Western clinicians (American Psychiatric Association, 1994b).

Lee (1990) described other problems in the family associated with immigration. These include changes in family dynamics, sometimes seen in the developmental crises of relocated children. Thus, an analysis of the family structure is an important part of the assessment. The clinician should know which family member has the most power and makes most of the major decisions. Changes in the balance of power in the family often caused by immigration can make children more powerful by virtue of speaking the language of the new culture. This potential role reversal caused by differing English-language ability between generations creates difficulties between parents and children and can lead to a split in loyalties. Some fathers may not be able to work, and their wives may have to go to work. The father may have to share his role with his children and his wife, and he may experience shame. Other types of family problems include intergenerational conflicts, pivoting on age, education, and language. Conflicts may also develop with in-laws, marital partners, siblings, or a hostile-dependent relationship with a sponsor.

The family's concept of illness is also important in treatment. Clinicians need to understand the family's explanatory models and treatment expectations. A thorough medical history may help the clinicians to understand if their patients consider herbal medicine useful, or if they tend to express their distress in somatic symptoms.

Religion and Spirituality

Religion and spirituality have tended to be either ignored or pathologized by mental health practitioners. Reviews by Lukoff et al. (1992a, 1992b, 1993), Matthews et al. (1993), and Larson (1993) underscored the complex interaction religious and spiritual beliefs can have on an individual's mental health status, assessment, and treatment. These interactions point to often positive correlations with mental health status; the importance of a wide differential diagnosis during assessment, including the new DSM-IV "non-illness" category of religious or spiritual problem; and the importance of the acknowledgment of and working with these beliefs as possible supports for the person rather than just manifestations of psychopathology. Browning et al. (1990) presented information on the historical interactions between psychiatry and the Protestant, Jewish, and Roman Catholic religious perspectives. Religious institutions can provide support for culturally diverse individuals. For example, Griffith and Young (1988) described the therapeutic aspects of Christian religious ritual in African Americans. In addition, the interaction between religion and family can provide a source of support or stress that must be assessed, utilized, and addressed (Burton, 1992).

Impact of Culture on the Clinician-Patient Relationship

Influence of Clinician and Patient Ethnicity and Cultural Identity

Race, ethnicity, and culture also affect the clinician-patient relationship, which, in turn, affects diagnosis and treatment (Rogler, 1993). Both to avoid biases based on stereotypes of ethnicity or any one aspect of cultural identity and to understand how it impacts their interactions with patients, clinicians need to understand and appreciate their own multiple aspects of cultural identity development, and then that of their patients. They also need to be aware of their attitudes toward their patient's particular ethnicity to assist in engaging and understanding the patient (Spiegel, 1976). Hughes (1993) described methods for clinicians to attain self-knowledge; he suggested that clinicians first examine their assumptions about their patients based on their first impressions during the interview and then critically analyze those signs (appearance, mannerisms, or behavior) that they are using to define "pathology." By looking for stereotypes that may be influencing their judgment and behavior toward patients, clinicians have an opportunity to confront their own biases and prejudices.

Pinderhughes (1989) advised clinicians who work with ethnic minorities to form experiential groups in which clinicians can freely discuss their own feelings, perceptions, and experiences of race, ethnicity, and power. She stated that clinicians can explore their own ethnic background by considering its historical influence on their attitudes, feelings, and behaviors. This personal exploration is maximized in groups, where individuals can confront the meaning and values of their ethnicity, along with their feelings about "difference," experiences of racism, and feelings of powerlessness. Discussion questions that may be asked in these groups can be found in table 10.3.

Unacknowledged differences between aspects of the cultural identities of patient and clinician can result in assessment and treatment that is not optimally respectful of the patient and can be inadvertently biased or prejudiced. For example, the American Psychiatric Association's (1993) position statement on bias-related incidents noted that "bias-related incidents, arising from racism, from sexism, from intolerance based on religion, ethnicity, and national/tribal origin, and anti-gay and antilesbian prejudice, are widespread in society and continue to be a source of social disruption, individual suffering, and trauma" (p. 686). Mental health clinicians need to guard against letting such possible biases affect their work. In fact, the American Psychiatric Association (1990) issued "guidelines regarding possible conflict between psychiatrists' religious commitments and psychiatric practice." They stated that "psychiatrists should maintain respect for their patient's beliefs" (p. 542) and "should not impose their own religious, antireligious, or ideologic systems of belief on their patients" (p. 542).

Pedersen and Ivey (1993) suggested examining the assumptions inherent in the clinician about other cultures and challenging them. In addition, the way that the patient sees the clinician will affect the alliance, through the information shared or not shared, both by client and clinician (McDonald-Scott et al., 1992). Finally, it is important for clinicians to realize that cultural

TABLE 10.3
Discussion Group Questions for Cultural Identity Awareness Exercise

1. What is your ethnic background? What has it meant to belong to your ethnic group? How has it felt to belong to your ethnic group? What do you like about your ethnic identity? What do you dislike?
2. Where did you grow up, and what other ethnic groups resided there?
3. What are the values of your ethnic group?
4. How did your family see itself, as similar to or different from other ethnic groups?
5. What was your first experience with feeling different?
6. What are your earliest images of race or color? What information were you given about how to deal with racial issues?
7. What are your feelings about being white or a person of color? To whites: How do you think people of color feel about their color identity? To people of color: How do you think that whites feel about their color identity?
8. Discuss your experiences as a person having or lacking power in relation to the following: ethnic identity, racial identity, within the family, class identity, sexual identity, professional identity.

Source: E. Pinderhughes, *Understanding Race, Ethnicity, and Power: Efficacy in Clinical Practice* (New York: Free Press, 1989). Reprinted with permission of the publisher.

norms will influence how particular behaviors are judged according to consensual standards.

Transference and Countertransference

Comas-Diaz and Jacobsen (1991) explored how cultural, racial, and ethnic factors can arouse ethnocultural transference and countertransference when the clinician and the patient are of different ethnicities (interethnic) and when they share a common ethnicity (intraethnic) (table 10.4). An example of interethnic transference can be seen in a Native American's distrust of an authority figure from the dominant culture. Other examples include the patient being overly compliant and friendly in an attempt to negate a perceived power differential or denial when patients may naively think that racial or cultural differences have no effect in therapy.

TABLE 10.4
Ethnocultural Transference and Countertransference

- Interethnic transference
  - Overcompliance and friendliness
  - Denial of ethnicity and culture
  - Mistrust, suspicion, and hostility
  - Ambivalence
- Intraethnic transference
  - Omniscient-omnipotent therapist
  - The traitor
  - The autoracist
  - Ambivalence
- Interethnic countertransference
  - Denial of ethnocultural differences
  - Clinical anthropologist syndrome
  - Guilt
  - Pity
  - Aggression
  - Ambivalence
- Intraethnic countertransference
  - Overidentification
  - Us and them
  - Distancing
  - Cultural myopia
  - Overidentification
  - Anger
  - Survivor guilt
  - Hope and despair

Source: Adapted from Comas-Diaz and Jacobsen (1991).

Ethnocultural countertransference can also be seen. An example of interethnic countertransference is the cultural anthropologist syndrome, where the therapist may react to cultural differences by becoming an amateur anthropologist on an intrusive fact-finding mission, quite distinct from the relevant clinical concerns. Clinicians may have experienced trauma at the hands of a person from the same race as their patient and may displace their feelings about the incident to the patient and behave either aggressively or defensively. The therapist may not ask some questions due to feelings of guilt or pity caused by overidentifying with the patient. Finally, the clinician may deny the importance of ethnic and cultural differences as they impact on the therapy.

Even sharing the same ethnicity with a patient may be problematic and bring up intraethnic transference and countertransference issues. An example of intraethnic transference, as cited by Comas-Diaz and Jacobsen (1991), may be seen in some Irish Americans, who may believe that Irish clinicians are less competent than other professionals and would think less of a clinician of their same ethnicity. On the other hand, a patient of the same ethnicity as the therapist may see the therapist as a kind of hero or heroine and expect to be rescued by the therapist. The patient may be critical of the therapist as a "sellout" to their ethnicity and not deserving of trust. Examples of intraethnic countertransference include a clinician's idealization of his or her own ethnicity's strengths and projection of these onto the patients, which could set them both up for disappointments. Collusion or misinterpretations may occur because of an assumption of sameness. That sameness may be too threatening, and the therapist may react with defensive distancing. The therapist may react to demands made by the patient with anger because it reminds them of issues in their own lives. Finally, therapists from a disadvantaged background may feel guilty about having left others of the same ethnicity behind when they became professionals (Comas-Diaz and Jacobsen 1991).

Clinical Methods

A variety of methods are available to the clinician that can be used to establish rapport during the interview. Westermeyer (1989) discussed the usefulness of demonstration of interest, facilitating the patient's story, clarifying the patient's explanatory models, and ensuring that the interviewer's questions are understood by the patient by having the patient restate the question. Clinicians can create rapport by assessing the symptoms that the patient is most comfortable expressing. These are usually the somatic symptoms; treating these with respect and appropriate concern often facilitates rapport with the patient. Patients presenting with somatic complaints should be evaluated as if they were presenting for medical evaluation, with an exploration of precipitants and ameliorating and aggravating factors. Next, the clinician should carefully review the patient's complaints (review of symptoms), looking for the somatic symptoms of depression and anxiety (e.g., sleep or appetite disturbances, weight change, decrease in energy level, tachycardia, shortness of breath, and tremors). Once the patient is engaged, other more sensitive topics can be broached, such as the psychological symptoms of irritability, fears, thoughts of a gloomy future, crying spells, and nightmares, and then personal or family problems. These psychological symptoms need to be assessed directly and include problems with concentration and memory, feelings of mistrust, hallucinations, intrusive thoughts, and suicidal or homicidal ideas (Cheung, 1987). When dealing with traditional Asian clients, a quiet respectful demeanor is helpful, along with an acceptance of traditional healers (Meyers, 1992).

Mental Status Examination and Psychological Assessment

The cognitive and descriptive aspects of the mental status examination have been developed in Western European, British, and American settings. Although it is an effective way of organizing clinical observations, the standard mental status measures must be elicited, described, and integrated in ways sensitive to the patient's cultural identity. Patient responses are affected by the patient's culture of origin, educational level, and level of acculturation, among other factors. For example, the measure of orientation, commonly checked by asking patients the date, is affected by the use of differing calendars by various cultures and the degree of attention or inattention to time per se. Seasons vary around the world, depending on latitude, and some cultures do not use clocks (Westermeyer, 1993). For some illiterate societies, a birth date is irrelevant information. The interpretation of tests of abstraction, such as proverb interpretation, are difficult to use because the meaning and wording of proverbs vary widely between different societies and language groups. Calculation ability among illiterate cultures is often limited to arithmetic with single digits. Also, the general usefulness of fund-of-information and geography questions can vary widely due to differences in educational backgrounds, even within the same cultural or ethnic group. It is often an incorrect assumption that all persons know much geography (Escobar et al., 1986). The naming of objects is affected by the patient's familiarity with the items chosen. Finally, short-term memory tests will be adversely affected if clinicians use unfamiliar items; thus it should be tested using familiar items. Similarly, three-step commands should be simple (Hughes, 1993). Escobar et al. (1986) concluded that the Mini-Mental State Exam (MMSE) was influenced by age, ethnicity, educational level, and the language of the interview and recommended that it should be revised to remove social, educational, and cultural artifacts if it is to be used in a Hispanic population.

Marsella (1989) observed that many of the tests and self-assessment questionnaires used in research have been developed on Western subjects and are not appropriate for use among ethnic minority patients because they lack equivalence. Merely translating the items was insufficient and resulted in linguistic "in-equivalence," as meanings and connotations changed and idioms of expression differed between languages. Rating scales of symptoms can be utilized if translated, "back-translated" (verification of adequacy of translation by translating a statement from language A to language B and then, independently, from language B to language A), and validated (Marin and Marin, 1991). Examples include the Hopkins Symptom Checklist 25, translated into Vietnamese, Laotian, and Cambodian (Mollica et al., 1987), and the Harvard Trauma Questionnaire, translated into the same three languages (Mollica et al., 1992). Finally, translated tests are often not standardized for the testing group and must be properly normed on a representative patient group. Other sources of error included poor or inaccurate assumptions and translation, biased analysis, and inappropriate instruments (Rogler, 1989). Mere translation of existing rating scales must be viewed with caution unless these concerns are addressed.

Translation versus Interpretation

Some culturally diverse individuals speak a language that is different from the clinician's primary language; thus, interpretation is needed, which is distinguished from translation in that it attempts to convey meanings that would be missed in translation, such as the connotation of particular words or the meaning of cultural idiomatic expressions. For example, when a patient is interviewed, the patient's intended message to the clinician could be lost if there is no direct translation in English. Likewise, if there are no equivalents for the clinician's question in the patient's language, the question may be answered in a misleading way. Terms for emotion may vary between cultures in radical ways. Some cultures do not have direct expressions for concepts such as "depression," "elation," and "love." If possible, the interview should be conducted in the language with which the patient is the most comfortable, because symptoms will be expressed more completely in the language in which the patient is most familiar. Likewise, if clinicians are not fluent in the patient's primary language, they will miss nuances that an interpreter might be able to explain, such as idiomatic expressions. The clinician's choice of the language for the interview can be unclear; some patients may speak more than one language. Often, the language chosen turns out to be a language common to both clinician and patient. Optimally, the patient's primary language should be utilized, however, because feelings can be left out because they are more difficult to express in a second language (Westermeyer, 1989).

An optimal interpreter is trained in the basic aspects of psychiatric assessment and care. Interpreters facilitate translated communication because they are familiar with the purpose and objectives of an interview, such as the determination of symptoms and diagnoses, and have techniques of eliciting pertinent clinical information. In general, family members should not be used as interpreters unless absolutely necessary because they commonly may not translate everything that the patient says because of concerns of family privacy and shame or family dynamics (Westermeyer, 1990).

Westermeyer (1990) described the relationships among the interpreter, patient, and clinician as points in a triangle. The clinician should face and speak directly to the patient; while the interpreter is speaking, the clinician can observe the patient's nonverbal communication. Other practical points for the interview include technique and content issues. One should allow adequate time, almost double of what would ordinarily be needed without an interpreter (Westmeyer, 1989). Lee (1987) also referred to the triangular relationship of patient, interpreter, and provider as the "therapeutic triad"; communication can be channeled in six directions, from provider to interpreter, from provider to the patient, or from interpreter to patient, and vice versa. It is important for the clinician to speak slowly and clearly, to avoid jargon and idioms, and to stick to one topic at a time. Providers can assist interpreters by having a preinterview meeting in which the objectives of the interview, topics to be covered, how much time is available, and so on are discussed. Before the interview, it is important to clarify the type of interpretation desired, be it word for word, summary, or a cultural explanation, when the meaning of a patient's answer may be related to the patient's cultural identity. During the interview, clinicians must pay attention to the nonverbal communication between the provider and the patient, because this is the only form of direct communication that they have. These include nodding, smiling, eye contact, personal space, and foot tapping. Caution must be used in interpreting observations about nonverbal indicators because they can be confusing (Westermeyer, 1989). It may be helpful to reserve interpretation until a better sense of their meaning can be obtained, perhaps with the help of a cultural consultant (Budman et al., 1992). Finally, a postinterview meeting can be helpful to clarify information and to share and discuss clinical impressions.

Cultural Consultants

To facilitate an accurate cultural formulation for patients whose cultural norms, idioms of distress, explanatory models, and family dynamics are unfamiliar to the clinician, the use of a cultural consultant may be most helpful. Certainly, if clinicians find that their assessment and treatment are not effective, having the services of a cultural consultant would be imperative. Such consultants would ideally be familiar with both the patient's cultural norms and basic psychiatric assessment skills. They are distinguished from an interpreter, as they are familiar with systems issues, and can often serve as a liaison between the staff and the patient. Budman et al. (1992) described the use of a clinical consultant in a case of an Arab adolescent who was hospitalized and was not improving. The consultant was able to provide insight into the patient's cultural values. For example, the adolescent was seen as overly dependent on his mother. In addition, he had symptoms of inappropriate responses to questions, excessive sensitivity to rejection, and social isolation. The consultant provided information that typical Arab families are enmeshed and that the patient's somatic symptoms were also a typical Arab method of expressing distress. Because the consultant was fluent in the patient's language and familiar with both Western and Arab paradigms of illness, the consultant was able to act as a liaison between the staff and the patient's family. With the aid of the consultant, the treatment team formulated an accurate diagnosis and devised an appropriate treatment plan.

Cultural Assessment: Culture and Its Effect on Diagnosis and Care

Cultural Competence

Another way clinicians can assess their ability to work with culturally diverse individuals it to assess their own "cultural competence." Cultural competence is a set of culturally congruent beliefs, attitudes, and policies that make cross-cultural work possible (Cross et al., 1989). Cultural competence exists as points along a continuum, ranging from cultural destructiveness, cultural incapacity, cultural blindness, and precompetence, to cultural competence, and finally, cultural proficiency. Although originally written to describe systems of mental health care for children, this scale can be applied generically both to systems of care for adults and to individual clinicians. Furthermore, individual clinicians need to be aware of the system in which they operate because this will affect their ability to work with culturally diverse patients.

The worst end of the continuum, cultural destructiveness, is exemplified by institutionalized or personal racism, where access to resources is denied on the basis of race and other aspects of cultural identity. The next stage is cultural incapacity, which can present itself in any helping relationship when an authority figure (teacher, counselor, or supervisor) has biased and lowered expectations of minority clients. The following stage is cultural blindness, which manifests itself in the "melting pot" attitude that "all people are the same" and that culture makes no difference in either their patient's or clinician's lives or experience. In this instance, ethnic clients are judged by the majority standards of performance and blamed if they are unable to accomplish the goals of the majority culture. The stage following cultural blindness is precompetence, where an agency realizes its weaknesses in serving minority groups and attempts to improve some aspect of its service. Cultural competence, however, is marked by the genuine and informed acceptance and respect of cultural differences. To achieve this, clinicians should have done a self-analysis of their cultural identity and biases, should become aware of the dynamics of difference inherent in working with minority patients, and must seek additional knowledge and resources to work with patients. The final stage of cultural proficiency is used to describe agencies and individuals who are adding to the knowledge base of culturally competent practice through research and other activities.

Values that are essential for cultural competence include mutual respect and the belief that cultural issues are important, that social systems are fundamental and valuable in treatment, that the family is an integral part of the patient and varies according to culture, that diversity is valuable, and that self-knowledge is necessary to deal with ethnic minority patients (Cross et al., 1989).

In conclusion, the openness of the clinician's attitude is critical in avoiding biases in assessment and treatment. Clinicians must be willing to suspend judgment; accept new lifestyles; and approach ethnic minority patients with flexibility, warmth, understanding, and empathy (Cross et al., 1989).

Culture's Effect on Diagnosis

A Western clinician using DSM-IV may naively assume that all individuals are equal; however, most clinicians believe that a relativist position is more appropriate (Hinton and Kleinman, 1993). In fact, DSM-IV includes a section on specific culture features in the narrative description of diagnostic categories where appropriate. Because the nature of diagnosis is to distinguish abnormal from normal, clinicians need to consider cultural norms of behavior. Clinicians need to gather information, put the data in a historical perspective to help determine the stressors, and then make an assessment of the patient's strengths and resources; all of these are affected by culture. Most culturally competent clinicians are familiar with the principle of cultural relativism, which holds that the language and customs of a people have to be examined in the context of that particular culture and judged primarily in terms of their utility to that culture (Johnson, 1988). If principles of cultural relativism are not used, then the clinicians may fall prone to the "category fallacy," which refers to using a classification scheme developed for one culture and applying it inappropriately to another where there is no relevance and no equivalent meaning (Kleinman, 1988). For example, using the Diagnostic Interview Schedule in other cultures might lead to an erroneous diagnosis of psychopathology of otherwise normal behavior (Guarnaccia et al., 1990).

Conduct, adjustment, anxiety, somatoform, dissociative, personality, and dysthymic disorders can show great variation across cultures (Kleinman, 1988). On the other hand, certain schizophrenic and manic-depressive conditions show less variation across cultures, as do organic, metabolic, and substance-abuse disorders (Johnson, 1988). Further, clinicians need to be aware of differences in the prevalence of mental illness among various ethnic groups to make an accurate diagnosis based on the percentages of patients having a diagnosis (Burnam et al., 1987; Canino et al., 1987; Karno et al., 1987). For example, African Americans are more likely to have phobic disorder. However, epidemiological data must be interpreted carefully; although some studies have found a higher prevalence of schizophrenia in African Americans, once corrected for cultural differences, the prevalence appears to be the same as for the general population (Escobar, 1993).

Kleinman (1988) took an anthropological view to diagnosis of psychiatric illness across cultures. He described it as understanding the interface between personal experience and the person's social world, which is mediated by the patient's language, symbols, and values. DSM-IV is a system that is embedded in a social structure, in which a Western clinician is culturally congruent and competent both through professional training and personal socialization. He suggested that the DSM approach excludes certain diagnoses that are common in other cultures but not in the Western world. An example of a case formulation using both Eastern and Western guidelines may be useful to illustrate the differences (adapted from Kleinman, 1988).

> Mrs. A., a twenty-eight-year-old Chinese woman experiencing significant social stressors, presented to a local clinic complaining of feelings of guilt, suicidal ideation, insomnia, anorexia, anergia, anhedonia, as well as chronic headaches, dizziness, tiredness, easy fatigue, weakness, and tinnitus. She would qualify for a diagnosis of major depression by DSM-IV criteria. However, by ICD-10 criteria, she could be given a diagnosis of neurasthenia, with secondary depression, consistent with the Eastern view that much of the feelings experienced by indi-

viduals can be explained by somatic causes. They would explain her basic problem as a "lack of energy" in the central nervous system, where a Western evaluator might emphasize the presence of unusual stress or conflicts. Hence, Mrs. A. has one illness, but two diseases if one uses both systems of classification.

Mrs. A.'s illness is expressed through her culturally determined idioms and social relationships. Thus, she will tell her physician of her physical complaints and leave out the emotional distress. Further, Mrs. A. knows about the syndrome of neurasthenia and will describe her symptoms in a cluster to her physician to match that syndrome, providing some certainty and order for her.

Practically, clinicians can make culturally appropriate diagnoses if they can obtain some basic information such as the patient's expectations regarding different healing systems (folk healers), their models of illness and causality, and their cultural standards of normality and abnormality. An individual's cultural identity influences his or her particular pattern of disease expression, the manner in which the illness is experienced, as well as the type of help he or she will seek. It is important to be able to determine how much of the patient's presentation is due to acculturation issues and how much is due to a cultural explanation like *ataque de nervios.*

The NIMH Culture and Diagnosis Group (Mezzich et al., 1993) developed an outline for preparing a cultural formulation to be used with a multiaxial diagnostic system, which was incorporated into DSM-IV. Factors affecting Axis I and Axis II have already been discussed, in terms of consideration of norms and explanatory models. Pertinent to Axis III is the relationship between disease and culture, touching on illness distribution and course. Next, culture's impact on Axis IV was discussed on the influence of the family and the support system they afford. Finally, for Axis V, social and cultural expectations influence the patient's pattern of functioning, as well as the process of appraising functioning. Further information on the background of these contributions is available elsewhere (Mezzich et al., 1996).

In summary, culture influences self-monitoring and the initial experience of distress and dysfunction, idioms of expression, the individual's model of illness and healing, and the presentations of psychiatric disorders.

Conclusion

The assessment and treatment of culturally diverse individuals is facilitated by an appreciation of their cultural identity (including their immigration history), explanatory models for their illness and symptom expression, and their support system. The clinician must understand the impact of culture on the clinician-patient relationship and how it affects diagnosis and treatment. It is important to understand the culture of origin and how this culture differs from Western culture. We can then better appreciate how the process of acculturation creates conflicts. Clinicians can then use their knowledge of the patient's culture to direct and augment therapeutic efforts.

In this chapter, we have explored some of the factors that make up a cultural formulation; it constitutes an appreciation of the cultural identities of both the clinician and the patient. It also addresses the impact of culture on the therapeutic alliance, as well as the diagnosis and treatment of psychiatric disorders. It is hoped that in accordance with the guidelines in this chapter, clinicians can more appropriately diagnose culturally diverse individuals by using interpreters, family members, cultural consultants, and culturally appropriate psychological tests and can also design culturally informed treatment plans involving psychopharmacology, psychotherapy, and sociotherapy.

References

American Psychiatric Association. (1987). *Diagnostic and statistical manual of mental disorders*, 3rd Edition, Revised. Washington, DC: American Psychiatric Association.

American Psychiatric Association. (1990). Guidelines regarding possible conflict between psychiatrists' religious commitments and psychiatric practice. *Am J Psychiatry* 147:542.

American Psychiatric Association. (1993). Position statement on bias-related incidents. *Am J Psychiatry* 150:686.

American Psychiatric Association. (1994a). *Diagnostic and statistical manual of mental disorders*, 4th Edition. Washington, DC: American Psychiatric Association.

American Psychiatric Association. (1994b). *Ethnic minority elderly*. Washington, DC: American Psychiatric Press.

American Psychological Association. (1993). Guidelines for providers of psychological service to ethnic, linguistic, and culturally diverse populations. *Am Psychol* 48:45–48.

Andreason, N. A. (Ed.). (1989). *Brain imaging: Applications in psychiatry*. Washington, DC: American Psychiatric Press.

Angel, R. and Guarnaccia, P. J. (1989). Mind, body, and culture: Somatization among Hispanics. *Soc Sci Med* 28:1229–1238.

Atkinson, D. R., Morten, G., and Sue, D. W. (1989). *Counseling American minorities: A cross-cultural perspective*, 3rd Edition. Dubuque. IA: William C Brown.

Ayd, F., and Blackwell, B. (1984). *Discoveries in biological psychiatry*. Baltimore: Waverly Press.

Bernal, M. E., and Knight, G. P. (Eds.). (1993). *Ethnic identity*. Albany: State University of New York Press.

Blue, H. C., and Gonzalez, C. A. (1992). The meaning of ethnocultural difference: Its impact on and use in the psychotherapeutic process. *New Dir Ment Health Serv* 55:73–84.

Browning, D. S., Jobe, T., and Evison, I. S. (Eds.). (1990). *Religious and ethical factors in psychiatric practice.* Chicago: Nelson-Hall.

Budman, C. L., Lipson, J. G., and Meleis, A. I. (1992). The cultural consultant in mental health care: The case of an Arab adolescent. *Am J Orthopsychiatry* 62:359–370.

Burnam, M. A., Hough, R. L., Escobar, J. I., et al. (1987). Six-month prevalence of specific psychiatric disorders among Mexican American and Non-Hispanic Whites in Los Angeles. *Arch Gen Psychiatry* 44:687–694.

Burton, L. A. (Ed.). (1992). *Religion and the family.* New York: Haworth.

Cabaj, R. P., and Stein, T. S. (Eds.). (1996). *Textbook of homosexuality and mental health.* Washington, DC: American Psychiatric Press.

Canino, G. J., Bird, H. R., Shrout, P. E., et al. (1987). The prevalence of specific psychiatric disorders in Puerto Rico. *Arch Gen Psychiatry* 44:727–735.

Canino, I., and Spurlock, J. (Eds.). (1994). *Culturally diverse children and adolescents.* New York: Guildford.

Cheung, F. M. (1987). Conceptualization of psychiatric illness, and help-seeking behavior among Chinese. *Cult Med Psychiatry* 11:97–106.

Cohen, F., and Farrell, D. (1988). Models of the mind. In H. Goldman (Ed.), *Review of psychiatry,* 2nd Edition, pp. 20–33. Norwalk, CT: Appleton & Lange.

Comas-Diaz, L., and Greene, B. (Eds.). (1994). Women of color. New York: Guilford.

Comas-Diaz, L., and Jacobsen, F. M. (1991). Ethnocultural transference and countertransference in the therapeutic dyad. *Am J Orthopsychiatry* 61:392–402.

Cross, T. L., Bazron, B. J., Dennis, K. W., et al. (1989). *Towards a culturally competent system of care.* Washington, DC: CASSP Technical Assistance Center.

Cross, W. (1991). *Shades of black.* Philadelphia, PA: Temple University Press.

Cullen, K. and Travin, S. (1990). Assessment and treatment of Spanish-speaking sex offenders: Special considerations. *Psychiatr Q* 61:223–235.

Del Castillo, J. C. (1970). The influence of language upon symptomatology in foreign-born patients. *Am J Psychiatry* 127:242–244.

Egland, J. A., Hostetter, A. M., and Eschleman, S. K. (1983). Amish study, III: The impact of cultural factors of diagnosis of bipolar illness. *Am J Psychiatry* 140:67–71.

Engel, G. L. (1980). The clinical application of the biopsychosocial model. *Am J Psychiatry* 137:535–544.

Escobar, J. I. (1993). Psychiatric epidemiology. in A. C. Gaw (Ed.), *Culture, ethnicity, and mental illness,* pp. 43–73. Washington, DC: American Psychiatric Press.

Escobar, J. I., Burnam, A., Karno, M., et al. (1986). Use of the Mini-Mental State Examination (MMSE) in a community population of mixed ethnicity. *J Nerv Ment Dis* 174:607–614.

Fabrega, H. (1987). Psychiatric diagnosis: A cultural perspective. *J Nerv Ment Dis* 175:383–394.

Fitchett, G. (1993). *Spiritual assessment in pastoral care: A guide to selected resources.* Decatur, GA: Journal of Pastoral Care Publications.

Fowler, J. (1981). *Stages of faith.* New York: Harper & Row.

Fullilove M. (1993). Minority women: Ecological setting and intercultural dialogue.

In D. Stewart and N. Stotland (Eds.), *Psychological aspects of women's health care*, pp. 519–539. Washington, DC, American Psychiatric Press.

Gaines, A. (1991). *Ethnopsychiatry*. Honolulu: University of Hawaii Press.

Griffith, E., and Young, J. (1988). A cross-cultural introduction to the therapeutic aspect of Christian religious ritual. In L. Comas-Diaz and E. Griffith (Eds.) *Clinical guidelines in cross-cultural mental health*, pp. 69–89. New York: Wiley.

Group for the Advancement of Psychiatry. (1987). *Us and them: The psychology of ethnonationalism*. New York: Brunner/Mazel.

Guarnaccia, P., Good, B., and Kleinman, A. (1990). A critical review of epidemiological studies of Puerto Rican mental health. *Am J Psychiatry* 147:1449–1456.

Helman, C. G. (1990). *Culture, health, and illness*, 2nd Edition. Oxford, England: Butterworth-Heinman Limited.

Helms, J. (Ed.). (1990). *Black and white racial identity*. New York: Greenwood.

Hinton, I., and Kleinman, A. (1993). Cultural issues and international psychiatric diagnosis. In J. Costa de Silva and C. Nadelson (Eds.), *International review of psychiatry*, pp. 111–129. Washington, DC: American Psychiatric Press.

Hughes, C. C. (1993). Culture in clinical psychiatry. In A. C. Gaw (Ed.) *Culture, ethnicity, and mental illness*, pp. 3–41. Washington, DC: American Psychiatric Press.

Ivey, A. E., Ivey, M. B., and Simek-Morgan, L. (1993). *Counseling and psychotherapy: A multicultural perspective*, 3rd Edition. Needham Heights, MA: Allyn & Bacon.

Johnson, F. A. (1988). Contributions of anthropology to psychiatry. In H. Goldman (Ed.), *Review of psychiatry*, 2nd Edition, pp. 167–181. Norwalk, CT: Appleton & Lange.

Karno, M. Hough, R. L., Burnam, A., et al. (1987). Lifetime prevalence of specific psychiatric disorders among Mexican Americans and Non-Hispanic Whites in Los Angeles. *Arch Gen Psychiatry* 44:695–701.

Kelly, G. (1955). *The psychology of personal constructs*, Vols. 1 and 2. New York: W. W. Norton.

Kleinman, A. (1988). *Rethinking psychiatry*. New York: Free Press.

Kroeber, A. L., and Kluckhohn, C. (1963). *Culture: A critical review of concepts and definitions*. New York: Vintage Books.

Larson, D. (1993). *The faith factor, vol. 2: An annotated bibliography of systematic reviews and clinical research on spiritual subjects*. Rockville, MD: National Institute for Healthcare Research.

Lee, E. (1987). Working with interpreters: the therapeutic triad (executive producer E. Lee). San Francisco, CA: Calman Video Productions.

Lee, E. (1990). Assessment and treatment of Chinese-American immigrant families. In G. W. Saba, B. M. Karrer, and K. V. Hardy (Eds.), *Minorities and family therapy*, pp. 99–122. New York: Haworth.

Lin, T. Y., and Lin, M. C. (1981). Love, denial, and rejection: Responses of Chinese families to mental illness. In A. Kleinman and T. Y. Lin (Eds.), *Normal and abnormal behavior in Chinese culture*, pp. 387–401. Dordrecht, Netherlands: Reidel, 1981.

Linton, R. (1945). *The cultural background of personality*. New York: Appleton-Century-Crofts.

Lukoff, D., Lu, F., and Turner, R. (1992a). Toward a more culturally sensitive DSM-IV: Psychoreligious and psychosocial problems. *J Nerv Ment Dis* 180:673–682.

Lukoff, D., Turner, R., and Lu, F. (1992b). Transpersonal psychology research review: Psychoreligious dimensions of healing. *Journal of Transpersonal Psychology* 24:41–60.

Lukoff, D., Turner, R., and Lu, F. (1993). Transpersonal psychology research review: Psychospiritual dimensions of healing. *Journal of Transpersonal Psychology* 25:11–28.

Marcos, I. R., Urcuyo, L., Kesselman, M., et al. (1973). The language barrier in evaluating Spanish-American patients. *Arch Gen Psychiatry* 29:655–659.

Marin, G., and Marin, B. (1991). *Research with Hispanic populations.* Newbury Park, CA: Sage.

Marsella, A. J Ethnocultural issues in the assessment of psychopathology. In S. Wetler (Ed.), *Measuring mental illness: Psychometric assessment for clinicians*, pp. 231–256. Washington, DC: American Psychiatric Press.

Matthews, D., Larson, D., and Barry, C. (1993). *The faith factor: An annotated bibliography of systematic reviews and clinical research on spiritual subjects.* Rockville, MD: National Institute for Healthcare Research.

McDonald-Scott, P., Machizawa, S., and Satoh, H. (1992). Diagnostic disclosure: A tale in two cultures. *Psychol Med* 22:147–157.

McGoldrick, M., Pearce, I. K., and Giordano, J. (Eds.). (1982). *Ethnicity and family therapy.* New York: Guilford.

Meyers, C. (1992). Hmong children and their families: Consideration of cultural influences in assessment. *Am J Occup Ther* 46:737–744.

Mezzich, J. E., Kleinman, A., Fabrega, J., et al. (Eds.). (1993). *Revised cultural proposals for DSM-IV.* Technical report, NIMH Culture and Diagnosis Group. Pittsburgh, PA, September.

Mezzich, J. E., Kleinman, A., Fabrega, H., et al. (1996). *Culture and psychiatric diagnosis.* Washington, DC: American Psychiatric Press.

Mollica, R. G., Wyshak, G., De Marneffe, D., et al. (1987). Indochinese versions of Hopkins Symptom Checklist-25: Screening instrument for psychiatric care of refugees. *Am J Psychiatry* 144:497–500.

Mollica, R. G., Caspi-Yavin, Y., Bollini, P., et al. (1992). The Harvard trauma questionnaire: Validating a cross-cultural instrument for measuring torture, trauma, and post-traumatic stress disorder in Indochinese refugees. *J Nerv Ment Dis* 180:111–116.

Myers M. (1991). Men's unique developmental issues across the life cycle. In A. Tasman and S. M. Goldfinger (Eds.), *American Psychiatric Press review of psychiatry*, Vol. 10, pp. 578–593. Washington, DC: American Psychiatric Press.

Newhill, C. E. (1990). The role of culture in the development of paranoid symptomatology. *Am J Orthopsychiatry* 60:176–185.

Nichter, M. (1981). Idioms of distress: Alternatives in the expression of psychosocial distress: A case study from South India. *Cult Med Psychiatry* 5:379–408.

Notman, M., Klein, R., Jordan, J., et al. (1991). Women's unique developmental issues across the life cycle. In A. Tasman and S. M. Goldfinger (Eds.), American Psychiatric Press review of psychiatry, Vol. 10, pp. 556–577. Washington, DC: American Psychiatric Press.

Numbers, R. L., Amundsen, D. W. (Eds.). (1986). *Caring and curing: Health and medicine in the Western religious traditions.* New York: Macmillan.

Padilla, A. M. (Ed.). (1980). *Acculturation, theory, models, and some new findings.* Boulder, CO: Westview Press for the American Association for the Advancement of Science.

Pedersen, P., and Ivey, A. (1993). *Culture-centered counseling and interviewing skills.* Westport, CT: Praeger.

Perry, S., Cooper, A. M., and Michels, R. (1987). The psychodynamic formulation: Its purpose, structure, and clinical application. *Am J Psychiatry* 5:543–550.

Pinderhughes, E. (1989). *Understanding race, ethnicity, and power.* New York: Free Press.

Powell, G. J. (Ed.). (1983). *The psychosocial development of minority group children.* New York: Brunner/Mazel.

Radford, M. H. B., Nakane, Y., Ohta, Y., et al. (1991). Decision making in clinically depressed patients: A transcultural social psychological study. *J Nerv Ment Dis* 179:711–719.

Rogler, L. H. (1989). The meaning of culturally sensitive research in mental health. *Am J Psychiatry* 146:296–303.

Rogler, L. H. (1993). Culturally sensitizing psychiatric diagnosis: A framework for research. *J Nerv Ment Dis* 181:401–408.

Rogler, L. H., and Cortes, D. E. (1993). Help-seeking pathways: A unifying concept in mental health care. *Am J Psychiatry* 150:554–561.

Sakauye, K. (1992). The elderly Asian patient. *J Geriatr Psychiatry* 25:85–104.

Schlesinger, R. (1981). Cross-cultural psychiatry. *J Psychosoc Nurs Ment Health Serv* 19:9:26–29.

Snyder, S. H. (1985). Drug and endocrine receptors in the brain. *Science* 224:22–28.

Sperry, L., Gudeman, J. E., Blackwell, B., et al. (1992). *Psychiatric case formulation.* Washington, DC: American Psychiatric Press.

Spiegel, J. P. (1976). Cultural aspects of transference and countertransference, revisited. *J Am Acad Psychoanal* 4:447–467.

Stein, T. S. (Ed.). (1993). Changing perspectives on homosexuality. In J. M. Oldham, M. B. Riba, and A. Tasman (Eds.), *American Psychiatric Press review of psychiatry,* Vol. 12, pp. 3–129. Washington, DC: American Psychiatric Press.

Sue, D., and Sue, D. (1990). *Counseling the culturally different,* 2nd Edition. New York: Wiley.

Sue, D., Arredondo, P., and McDavis, R. J. (1992). Multi-cultural counseling competencies and standards. *Journal of Counseling and Development* 70:447–486.

Sullivan, L. (Ed.). (1989). *Healing and restoring.* New York: Macmillan.

Westermeyer, J. J. (1989). *Psychiatric care of migrants.* Washington, DC: American Psychiatric Press.

Westermeyer, J. J. (1990). Working with an interpreter. *J Nerv Ment Dis* 178:745–749.

Westermeyer, J. J. (1993). Cross-cultural psychiatric assessment. In A. C. Gaw (Ed.), *Culture, ethnicity, and mental illness,* pp. 125–144. Washington, DC: American Psychiatric Press.

Wintrob, R. M. (1996). Cultural comments on culture-bound syndromes. In J. E. Mezzich, A. Kleinman, H. Fabrega, and D. L. Parron (Eds.), *Culture and psychiatric diagnosis,* pp. 313–319. Washington, DC, American Psychiatric Press.

World Health Organization. (1992). The ICD-10 Classification of Mental and Behavioural Disorders. Geneva, Switzerland: World Health Organization.

Part III

Reflections and Prospects on the Cultural Formulation

SINCE THE INTRODUCTION of the DSM-IV Cultural Formulation, a number of authors have offered suggestions on the use and further refinement of this clinical and research tool. The following articles were selected for their analyses of the implications of the Cultural Formulation and related contributions and indications for future developments.

Rogler's (1996) paper on framing research on culture in psychiatric diagnosis proposes three levels progressively considering cultural influences in the diagnostic process: symptom assessment, configuring of symptoms into disorders, and the diagnostic situation. As for the first level, he demonstrates the cultural relativity of symptoms, whereby both their expression and their interpretation (by the patient and the clinician) are culturally mediated. The second level takes into consideration the configuration of symptoms into disorders that may be specific to a culture, as in the case of culture-bound syndromes, or value-bound and variable among different cultures, as in the case of anorexia nervosa. The third level, the diagnostic situation, examines cultural factors impacting on the clinician-patient interaction. The author offers useful suggestions for moving forward programmatically research on culture and diagnosis.

The Mezzich, Kirmayer, Kleinman, Fabrega, et al. (1999) paper on the place of culture in DSM-IV reviews the forces and the process that led to the incorporation of some cultural proposals in DSM-IV. The authors discuss how contextual factors interface with biological conceptualizations in recent diagnostic systems. It is clear however, that in spite of the progress made, much remains to be done in this area. Additionally, the authors cite the need to place more emphasis on the influence of class status, intracultural heterogeneity, and gender issues in mental health. Moreover, they recommend empirical research to evaluate the impact of the Cultural Formulation on the quality of diagnosis and care.

Caracci's (2000) paper finds an affinity between cultural and dynamic formulations and delineates the usefulness of the former to teach the latter. To this purpose a real case vignette drawn from a teaching course illustrates for each of the Cultural Formulation domains how information obtained to formulate the case culturally can help arrive at a deeper understanding of the case's dynamics. This article emphasizes the Cultural Formulation versatility and usefulness for psychotherapy beyond its application as a complement to standard multiaxial diagnosis.

11

Framing Research on Culture in Psychiatric Diagnosis

The Case of the DSM-IV

Lloyd H. Rogler

FOR OUR PURPOSES, Tylor's (1958, p. 1) classic definition of culture proposed in 1871 still suffices: "that complex whole which includes knowledge, belief, art . . . and any other capabilities and habits acquired by man as a member of society." Recent anthropological formulations of the concept, which are reflected in the cultural insertions in DSM-IV, orient the concept toward "local worlds of everyday experience" (Mezzich et al., 1994, p. 15). The formulations are consistent with Tylor's socially acquired "capabilities and habits," and are useful to cultural examinations of psychiatric diagnosis, such as those attempted here, because they attend to the proximal meanings, values, and norms enmeshing persons in "everyday experience."

A brief word about the context of this effort. Some years ago, I examined the meaning of culturally sensitive research in mental health (Rogler, 1989) and concluded that such research requires the continuing and finely calibrated interweaving of cultural components and cultural awareness throughout all phases of the research process. Subsequently, in anticipation of the publication of the DSM-IV, I focused this conclusion on psychiatric diagnosis and undertook the development of the framework presented here (Rogler, 1993) by examining research relevant to the evaluation of mental health. This article takes the next step by applying the framework to the cultural inser-

From *Psychiatry* 59 (May 1996)

tions in the DSM-IV. Here, the question is: Can the culturally oriented diagnostic issues appearing in the DSM-IV, which derive from a history of rich but dispersed studies in cross-cultural psychiatry and social psychiatry, be organized more or less systematically? Although at first sight the idea of cultural research on psychiatric diagnosis may appear so nebulous as to be daunting, I believe the framework being developed and the inclusion of some of my previously published analyses of research (Rogler, 1993) provide an affirmative answer.

Cultural Insertions in the DSM-IV

The DSM-IV (1994) treats cultural differences between the diagnostician and the client as "especially challenging" (p. xxiv). The basis for the challenge is presented throughout the text in discussions of cultural variations in the symptomatologies of familiar disorders and the diagnostic implications of such variations. For example, with respect to Axis I clinical disorders, such as schizophrenia and other psychotic disorders, the reader is advised about cultural variations in emotional expression, eye contact, and body language; and of tendencies to overdiagnose schizophrenia among some ethnic groups at the expense of underdiagnosing bipolar disorder (p. 281). Also, major depression may be experienced in some cultures in largely somatic terms, rather than with sadness or guilt (p. 324).

Axis II personality disorders receive similar cultural attention. For example, the behavior pertinent to paranoid personality disorder is to be considered contextually: minority group members, immigrants, and refugees often are guarded and defensive because of an unfamiliar or hostile social environment (p. 636). Religious beliefs and rituals—such as voodoo and shamanism, mind reading, the speaking of strange tongues—may erroneously appear to the uninformed outsider to be schizotypal (p. 643). Subsequently, the manual alerts the reader to the fact that the cultural variability of norms structuring interpersonal comportment, personal appearance, and emotional expressions could lead to an incorrect attribution of histrionic personality disorder (p. 656).

However, with the exception of a phrase calling attention to immigrants' "difficulty with acculturation" (p. 29) in the Axis IV outline of problems related to social environment, the manual's general statement on multiaxial assessment does not explicitly mention the concept of culture. The experts contributing to the DSM-IV recommended cultural annotations for the multiaxial assessments (Mezzich et al., 1994). Substantial bodies of cultural research are pertinent not only to the first two axes of clinical and personality disorders, which we address here, but also to the remaining three axes—general medical conditions, psychosocial and environmental problems, and global assessments of functioning. In the DSM-IV, these concerns are relegated to a brief supplement to the multiaxial statement in a cultural formulation outline of ways to evaluate and report the impact of cultural context on the client, which is followed by a glossary of culture-bound syndromes (pp. 843–849). These illustrations show how the DSM-IV attempts to meet the challenge of cultural sensitivity at home and abroad.

Framing Research

The framework proposed here is a hierarchy of three levels structuring the diagnostic process. From the bottom to the top, the levels are progressively more inclusive of cultural influences affecting the process: (1) the assessment of clinically relevant symptoms, (2) the configuration of such symptoms into disorders, and (3) the diagnostic situation composed of social interactions between clinician and client.

Symptom Assessment

The DSM-IV recognizes diagnostic errors stemming from the unqualified attribution of psychiatric significance to psychological experiences assumed to be symptomatic (p. xxiv): the voices of recently deceased relatives heard by some Native American groups (Kleinman and Good, 1985), or the religiously induced visual hallucinations of spiritualist mediums (Rogler and Hollingshead, 1985), or even culturally diffuse tendencies toward spiritualistic interpretations not rooted in organized religious ideologies (Guarnaccia et al., 1992).

Trances and fits of involuntary possession also have been documented cross culturally (Gonzalez et al., 1994). According to the DSM-IV, such behaviors "should not be considered inherently pathological" in the absence of knowledge about their distressful consequences and indigenous cultural definitions (p. 477). Nor should a symptom be routinely dismissed "merely because it is viewed as the 'norm' for a culture" (p. 324). Implicitly or explicitly, culture's relevance enters into such decisions because it is seen to mediate in a variety of ways the expression of symptoms.

A symptom treated in one culture as singular may well represent a plurality of symptoms in another culture. Thus, an anthropological study of depression among the Hopi Indians (Manson et al., 1985) discovered during pretesting that the concepts of guilt, shame, and sinfulness, treated as synonyms in the Diagnostic Interview Schedule (Robins et al., 1981), had to be kept separate. The pretesting adaptations required that the symptom items be made congruous with the respondents' culturally structured phenomenological experiences.

The adaptations based upon the Hopi's self-reports of guilt, shame, and sinfulness are instances of a much broader issue pertaining to the cultural significance and interpretation of subjective information. The issue was confronted directly in a large-scale epidemiological study of health status in a culturally pluralistic sample (Angel and Gronfein, 1988). The study sought to explain subjective self-reports of health and found that although actual physical health was correlated to the self-reports, it was far from being a sufficient explanation: using a succession of mathematical models, it concluded that "it is always necessary to begin with the assumption that a significant difference in culture or in social status affect [sic] subjective information and to proceed as if this were the case. Only empirical analyses can disprove the assumption" (p. 472).

The assumption is relevant to the DSM-IV's reliance on self-reports of subjective symptoms. Sometimes this reliance is acknowledged explicitly (pp. 349, 327, 332). But even when not acknowledged, the reliance is evident in the very nature of the symptoms: in mood disorders, the feelings of being sad or empty or worthless, the recurrent thoughts of death, and the suicidal ideation; in schizophrenia and the other psychotic disorders, the hallucinatory and delusional experiences; in personality disorders, the perceptions of hidden meanings, suspiciousness, bizarre thoughts, and fantasies.

Wilson's (1993) thoughtful historical analysis of the transformations resulting from DSM-III helps to clarify the role of subjective symptoms in diagnosis. The transformations succeeded in "narrowing of the psychiatric gaze in contemporary psychiatry" away from the concept of depth of mind and away from the concept of the unconscious, and toward "the methodology of explicit diagnostic criteria" (p. 408). The narrowing attempted, among other things, to rid the taxonomy of unverified assumptions about etiologies previously incorporated into definitions of disorders. But from my viewpoint, it did not expurgate from the language of Axes I and II the disorders' diagnostic reliance on the subjectivisms of mental phenomena. How these phenomena are constituted subjectively or mentally structured forms part of the hypothesis that culture mediates symptoms.

In whatever way symptoms are constituted, the proclivity to express them can be culturally influenced. Thus, the disproportionately high levels of epidemiologically assessed symptomatic distress among Puerto Ricans in comparison to other cultural groups (Dohrenwend, 1966; Haberman, 1976) could well be due to culturally shaped revelatory patterns of more readily admitting to such symptoms. When symptoms are culturally perceived as not strongly undesirable, they are more saliently divulged to the interviewer; the respondent then is classified, erroneously, as more ill. The point being emphasized is that culture, through its normative definitions of what is desirable or undesirable, performs a mediating function in the proclivity to express distress.

Culture's mediating function is evident, too, in the patterning of overt symptomatic behavior. A study of the Old Order Amish (Egeland et al., 1983) is illustrative. Seeking to operationalize the criterion of "excessive involvement in activities" (which formed part of the mania/hypomania concept in Spitzer et al.'s (1977) Research Diagnostic Criteria), the study had to rely on the behaviors the Amish themselves perceived as conspicuously excessive: dressing up in worldly clothes, treating the livestock too roughly, using the public telephone too often, or violating the norms of agrarian frugality by planning a vacation during the wrong season of the year.

The structuring and regulatory function of cultural norms, releasing or constraining expressions of distress, operate through the medium of significant others in the respondents' primary groups (Mechanic, 1968; Rogler and Cortes, 1993). Significant others' evaluations of distress shape the respondents' pathways to mental health care. For example, Chinese clients experience protracted delays in seeking professional help because of the stigma mental disorders impose upon the family (Lin et al., 1982); some Hispanic groups underutilize professional mental health care because their problems are contained within indigenous institutions (Rogler and Cortes, 1993). Epidemiological assessments of the clinical severity of symptoms to determine whether they are candidates for a psychiatric disorder sometimes are based upon whether or not help has been sought (Robins et al., 1981). Help seeking varies among cultural groups (Rogler and Cortes, 1993). Assessments of the severity of symptoms, consequently, are affected by culture.

In sum, the symptom variability recognized by the DSM-IV derives from culture's mediation in the subjective structuring of symptoms, the proclivity to express such symptoms, the patterning of overt symptomatic behaviors indicative of disorder, and, in epidemiological assessments, in treating help seeking as evidence of clinical severity. The basic point was stated succinctly by the experts contributing to DSM-IV: "What the patient reports is itself an interpretation of suffering based upon his or her own cultural categories, words, images and feelings for expressing (and thereby constituting) symptoms. The psychiatrist's view is, then, an interpretation, with its own cultural categories, of that interpretation" (Mezzich et al., 1994, p. 19).

Configuring Symptoms into Disorders

Culture-bound syndromes, the most conspicuous instances of culture's role in configuring symptoms, are defined by the DSM-IV as "recurrent, locality-specific patterns of aberrant behavior and troubling experience that may or may not be linked to a particular DSM-IV diagnostic category" (p. 844). Its glossary of the syndromes (pp. 844–849), based upon the observations of cultural experts (Hughes et al., 1992), includes the Indonesian *amok*, the Malaysian *koro* and *latah*, the West African and Haitian *boufee delirante*, and the Hispanic *ataque de nervios* and *susto*. They are presented not as alien exotic disorders but as part of the cultural landscape, including modern industrial societies.

Anorexia nervosa is not listed in the DSM-IV glossary of culture-bound syndromes, but references are made to its being conceptualized as a culture-bound syndrome in the cross-cultural literature. It appears in the DSM-IV text under "Eating Disorders" (pp. 539–545), along with what could be seen as the first premise of a culturally based epidemiological theory of the illness: noting the apparent increasing incidence of anorexia nervosa and its higher prevalence among women, the DSM-IV points to a cultural value: "being considered attractive is linked to being thin" (p. 542). Another premise could be added: as this cultural value diffuses into industrializing countries, and becomes integrated into the body-conscious commercialized interest reflected in the modern mass media, it provides the core for the configuring of psychotic and somatic symptoms built around beauty as body thinness. Thus, anorexia nervosa could well have been classified as a culture-bound syndrome.

However, in a significant departure from customary biomedical interpretations, the DSM-IV does not define each culture-based syndrome as an instance of a traditional disorder (p. 844). Interpretations of such syndromes usually derive from the "pathogenic/pathoplastic" model of looking upon biology as providing the structure of the disorder and upon social and cultural factors as shaping the content of the disorder. This model, according to Kleinman (1988), tacitly "has become close to a professional orthodoxy" (p. 24). It has promoted an almost routinelike reductionistic formulation of culture-bound syndromes. The assumption is that once culture is "stripped" away from a syndrome, a traditional disorder is at the source: *amok* is seen as a brief reactive psychosis; *susto* as a depressive disorder. The previously quoted DSM-IV definition of culture-based syndromes indicates, however, that the definitional "linkage" between a syndrome and a particular diagnostic category "may or may not" be appropriate. Some syndromes may retain an integrity not reducible to a traditional disorder. This integrity itself invites hypotheses such as: persons occupying the same set of statuses in the social structure—middle-class adolescent females who are acquiring modern concepts of beauty—share similar cultural experiences, including the values imparted by the mass media; the similarity of status-derived cultural experiences is conducive to similarities in symptom expression and in symptom configuration.

Precedents for the measurement of culture-based syndromes and for testing their relationship to the more traditional disorders are now being established. An epidemiological study in Puerto Rico is relevant because it focused upon *ataques de nervios* (Guarnaccia, 1992). The sudden seizures in this syndrome "include uncontrollable shouting, attacks of crying, trembling, heat in the chest rising into the head, and verbal and physical aggression" (DSM-IV, p. 845). The study found that persons identified as being at risk for *ataques* were significantly more likely to experience eight psychiatric disorders assessed by the Diagnostic Interview Schedule (DIS) (Robins et al., 1981), in particular, depressive episode, dysthymia, agoraphobia, and phobic disorder. Moreover, consistent with the previous hypothesis that persons occupying the same set of social structural statuses share symptomatologies mediated by common cultural experiences, the persons at risk for *ataque de nervios* were as follows: female, over forty-five years of age, less than a high school education, formerly married, and outside the laboring force or unemployed. Thus, this culture-bound syndrome is comorbid with other disorders and centers disproportionately on one of the most marginated segments of the Puerto Rican population.

The increasing cultural pluralism of American society, which is nurtured by immigration, means that culture-bound syndromes should be included in epidemiological studies assessing the comorbidity of mental disorders. Immigrants bringing their own culture bring, too, their traditional culture-based syndromes, as the DSM-IV recognizes (pp. 844–845), and they develop new idioms of distress in interaction with the host society (Rogler et al., 1994).

The hypothesis that culture plays a role in configuring symptoms, however, applies to more than culture-bound syndromes. It includes the more traditional DSM disorders. Once again, an epidemiological study in Puerto Rico is revealing. The researchers reported (Guarnaccia et al., 1992) how they coped with a critical problem: "The lay interview tended to over-diagnose schizophrenia relative to the clinician and to underdiagnose dysthymic disorder" (p. 102). The Puerto Rican psychiatrists made culturally informed additions to the DIS in symptom assessment (level 1 of the framework) and in the configuring of symptoms into disorders (level 2 of the framework). Specifically, features of Puerto Rican culture were taken into account—such as experiences with visions, presentiments, and the hearing of voices—and the prescribed algorithms were altered. The modifications were possible because "The addition of questions which asked people to describe their experiences, to provide their social context, and to assess the response of others to those experiences are major innovations by the Puerto Rican research team" (Guarnaccia et al., 1992. p. 107). Although these procedures were applied in a research project, they obey the intent of the subsequently published "Outline for Cultural Formulation" in the DSM-IV (pp. 843–844).

In the same study (Canino et al., 1987), prevalence rates for obsessive-compulsive disorder, psychosexual dysfunction, dysthymia, and cognitive impairment were computed in two ways: first, by using the standard National Institute of Mental Health Diagnostic Interview Schedule (DIS) mental health assessment procedures developed in the United States (Robins et al., 1981); second, by the previously reported expert cultural adaptations of the DIS procedures. There were substantial differences between the two rates of the four disorders. For example, the percentage change in the two rates, computed for a previous article (Rogler, 1993), indicated that the culturally adapted procedures produced lifetime prevalence rates for psychosexual dysfunction that were 81 percent lower than those produced by standard procedures; for dysthymia, the lifetime prevalence rates were 60 percent higher.

The marked change in prevalence rates in this study reflects the generality versus specificity dilemma of research definitions in cross-cultural epidemiology: generality in the epidemiological study in Puerto Rico stemmed from the conceptual meaning of the disorders given by the DSM-III and operationalized in the DIS; specificity involved modifications in the DIS made by the researchers sensitive to the cultural configuration of the disorders' symptoms in Puerto Rican society. Epidemiological rates, the study shows, are highly sensitive to the balance between generality and specificity in the research definitions of disorders. Thus, differences in the cultural grounding of research definitions within the same data set of the influential World Health Organization research program have produced marked differences in cross-cultural incidence rates of schizophrenia (Kleinman, 1987). Which definitions are "correct"? How do we know whether the appropriate kind and number of cultural modifications have been made? What is the appropriate balance between conceptual generality and cultural specificity?

These questions can be posed but cannot be satisfactorily answered because little is known about how culture helps to configure symptoms into mental disorders, and how such configurations relate to the DSM-IV criteria of disorders. Rather than imposing definitional fiats, I suggest one approach is to treat the dilemma as a problem for cultural research within the proposed framework. The task would be to study the effects of different research definitions of the disorder, starting with the DSM-IV standard criteria for disorders and then successively incorporating cultural modifications, including those proposed by the DSM-IV, to see which ones produce the best reliability and the most accurate criterion-related predictions. (Axis V in the DSM-IV provides some criteria for predictions oriented toward psychological, social, and occupational functioning.) After all, well-conducted cross-cultural studies *inevitably* incorporate such modifications. One study, which psychometrically evaluated alternative research definitions of schizophrenia but not with the cultural factor in mind, concluded: "Operational definitions are a step in the right direction and the studies reported in this paper allow rational choices to be made in favor of some rather than others" (Brockington et al., 1978, p. 395). The methodology enabling "rational choices" is applicable to this issue. The issue is to determine which cultural modifications improve the psychometric properties of research definitions of mental disorders.

So far, the discussion of culture's organizing role has focused only on symptoms in the culture-bound syndromes and in the more familiar disorders in the DSM-IV. Its organizing role, however, may extend beyond symptoms and single disorders to patterns of comorbidity of psychiatric disorders. A suggestion to this effect is evident in a recent demonstration of nationwide patterns of comorbidity. In a state-of-the-art epidemiological study of lifetime and twelve-month prevalence (Kessler et al., 1994), the comorbidity of psychiatric disorders emerges as a strong pattern. Of particular interest to our purpose, however, is that comorbidity is stronger among Hispanics than among non-Hispanics. This difference remains to be elaborated through statistical analyses, but it is not premature to suggest that comorbidity may be variable across cultural groups.

Moreover, differences between cultural groups also appear in technical studies attempting to predict thresholds of psychiatric disorder by means of scales measuring symptomatic dimensions. For example, Cho et al. (1993) undertook a concordance analysis between the Center for Epidemiological Studies Depression Scale (CES-D) (Radloff, 1977) and the DIS specification of major depression among stateside Puerto Ricans and Cubans. The CES-D is a psychometrically developed symptom scale; the DIS component operationalizes major depression as a DSM-III clinical syndrome. The concordance analysis sought to determine the cutoff point in the CES-D that most effectively predicted major depression. Although both groups form part of the Hispanic category, national cultural differences were evident: the most effective cutoff point in the CES-D for Puerto Ricans was substantially higher than for Cubans. The implications of this study, as well as the previous one on comorbidity, invite research on culture's multiple organizing role.

In sum, the attention the DSM-IV gives to culture-bound syndromes, as well as its formulation of such syndromes as not always instances of the traditional DSM disorders, implies, without making explicit, the hypothesis in the framework's second level of culture's configuring influence. Nor is the hypothesis of culture's configuring role stated explicitly in the DSM-IV discussion of those disorders not recognized as culture-bound syndromes, although here and there are glimpses of it, as in the case of anorexia nervosa. The hypothesis needs explicit research attention in cross-cultural studies of the traditional disorders. The psychometric scrutiny of culturally modified research definition of disorders forms part of such studies.

The Diagnostic Situation

Decisions about symptom assessment and about the configuring of symptoms into disorders do not exhaust the range of culture's relevance to psychiatric diagnosis. Whether such decisions are made with the aid of structured mental health instruments or in the course of fluid, open-ended assessments of the client's problem, whether they are made in clinical or research settings, they are always made in a social situation. The diagnostic situation itself, composed of the complex interactions between client and clinician, or between respondent and research interviewer, is subject to cultural influences likely to be consequential to diagnostic outcomes. This is the focus of the framework's third level.

The current volume of persons being transported by cross-national migration streams has increased the number of situations of cross-cultural pairing between diagnosticians and clients in mental health assessments. Transported, too, has been the situational organization of psychiatric diagnosis, away from its once notable tendency to be encapsulated as a professionally hidden sphere of dyadic interactions and toward settings providing opportunities for the open scrutiny of such interactions as objective researchable events.

The DSM-IV's "Outline for Cultural Formulation" (pp. 843–844), presented as a supplement to the manual's multiaxial diagnostic assessment, reflects such opportunities because it encompasses clinical, personality, and physical disorders as well as issues pertinent to the psychosocial environment and to the client's overall level of functioning. Confronting a cross-cultural diagnostic situation, the clinician is invited to provide narrative accounts of a variety of cultural components, such as the client's ethnicity and language, his or her culture's explanations of the distress, cultural interpretations of social stressors and level of functioning in the client's life, and the relevance of culture in the diagnostic interactions. The accounts are then synthesized into an "overall cultural assessment for diagnosis and care" (p. 844). The presence of such a statement in the DSM-IV acknowledges that cultural sensitivity in diagnosis requires much more than the clinician's personal sensitivity. It also requires research-based knowledge about culture's role in diagnosis.

Carefully constructed, the overall cultural assessment should buttress research that has recently begun to focus on the influence of culture on the diagnostic situation. Precedents for such clinical contributions to research can be found in the few studies on this topic that center mostly on the diagnostic experiences of Spanish-dominant Hispanics. In fact, the studies began with clinical observations about the relationship between the language of the diagnostic interview and the inference of psychopathology drawn by the clinician. The initial observation was that when such clients expressed their mental health problems in the unfamiliar language, which was English, they appeared less pathological (Del Castillo, 1970). The self-conscious discipline and the internal vigilance and control required when speaking an unfamiliar language were assumed to suppress the afflicted person's expression of mental health relevant emotions. In the familiar language, which was Spanish, such emotions were more openly expressed, thereby leading to inferences of greater psychopathology.

However, subsequent studies (Marcos et al., 1973a, 1973b), based upon more controlled observations varying the language of the diagnostic interview, arrived at the opposite conclusion: when the client speaks in the unfamiliar language "he creates problems both for himself and for the psychiatrist" because this "imposes an additional burden on the patient's already failing efforts to organize a fluid and chaotic subjective experience"; the result is "disturbances in fluency, organization, and integration" in the presentation of the problem (Marcos et al., 1973b, p. 658). Thus, the patient appears sicker when speaking the unfamiliar language.

Both the clinical and controlled observations, however, confound the language spoken during the psychiatric interview with the ethnicity of the diagnostician, which could account for the inconsistent inferences about psychopathology. Research has not yet resolved this inconsistency, but the inconsistency itself has given rise to the dominant hypothesis in the framework's third level: the cultural distance between the diagnostician and the client affects the degree of psychopathology inferred and affects, too, the type of disorder diagnosed. Cultural distance is rendered researchable with naturalistic studies or experimental designs that combine, on the one hand, similarities and differences between the ethnicity of the diagnostician and that of the client with, on the other hand, variations in the language of the diagnostic interview, that is, whether or not it is the client's dominant language.

The cultural distance hypothesis is an example of the need to frame hypotheses in the framework's third level in broad terms: in the absence of more definitive research, such hypotheses cannot yet specify the appropriate qualifiers designating how culturally relevant variations in symptom assessment and in the configuring of symptoms into disorders affect inferences of psychopathology in the diagnostic situation. Nor can they yet specify with testable precision how the less tangible but very real culture-laden nuances of interaction mediate the process of mental health assessment: eye contact, pacing and intonation of speech, physical posturing and behavioral accommodations of interpersonal distance, hand and body gestures, and other culturally patterned residual behaviors (Marcos, 1994).

Discussion

The application of the framework to the DSM-IV is designed to be helpful and not determinative of the specific research problems to be pursued. Its use is not restricted to the specific focus of the research projects discussed in this article, although the findings of each project invite replication and extension. Nor is it determinative of the order in which research on the three levels ought to proceed; each level contains diagnostic relevant hypotheses worthy of individual attention. However, when the levels are integrated into the framework, the cumulative character of cultural influences on psychiatric diagnosis can be appreciated.

Studies addressing such hypotheses included a striking variety of biomedical—and behavioral research—designs, from ethnographic documentations of indigenous patterns of distress, to epidemiological studies seeking to examine cultural processes in the configuring of symptoms, to experimental studies of the effects of cross-cultural pairings of diagnostician and client on diagnostic outcomes. However, since matters of research design are inevitably preeminent in the formulation of specific research projects, I would like to emphasize a general point: much can be learned from published studies that self-consciously report historical accounts of how culturally based modifications in concepts and procedures were made, why they were made, and in what way, if at all, they were consequential to the findings. Often, cultural modifications remain only in the researcher's memory, buried in the unwritten history of the project, as if they were perfunctory pretesting adjustments, even when they did or could have played a decisive role in shaping the research (Rogler, 1989). Knowledge needs to be based not only on research purposefully designed to examine cultural influences across the framework's levels, but based also on supplementary reports of the consequences of cross-cultural adaptations.

The application of the framework to the cultural insertions in the DSM-

IV makes clear that cultural influences on diagnosis are multifarious, not singular. The framework enables the situating of hypotheses about cultural influences on symptom assessment, the configuring of symptoms into disorders, and on the diagnostic situation, or on some interstitial area between or combining the three levels. It draws attention to the cumulative character of culture's effect on psychiatric diagnosis. The effects do not discretely appear then discretely disappear; they tend to increase from the first to the third level. Moving upward inductively, each level adds cultural increments to the mental health inferences of the previous level. Thus, the residues of cultural influences in the first phase—the assessment of symptoms—feed those of the second phase—the configuring of symptoms into disorders, which feed those in the third phase—the situation enmeshing diagnostician and client. The river of diagnostic decisions is fed by incoming tributaries, many of which are cultural. Culture suffuses even the most prosaic diagnostic inferences.

In less metaphorical terms, the second and third levels of the framework subsume the hypotheses of the previous level. Therefore, level-three hypotheses are markedly exploratory, not only because of the scarcity of research, but also because of their intrinsic complexity. Contextually, they are part of a broader unexamined matrix of other cultural variables likely to effect diagnosis. The diagnostic situation encompasses the terminal residues of cultural forces impinging on psychiatric diagnoses.

The views of Frances and his colleagues (1991) are appropriate here: "The highest purpose of the DSM-IV is that it encourage and facilitate the research that will render it obsolete" (p. 411). My purpose has been to encourage research on culture in psychiatric diagnosis to show how the cumulative process of cultural accretions intertwines with clinical inferences throughout the diagnostic process.

References

American Psychiatric Association. (1994). *Diagnostic and statistical manual of mental disorders*, 4th Edition. Washington, DC: American Psychiatric Association.

Angel, R., and Gronfein, W. (1988). The use of subjective information in statistical models. *American Sociological Review* 53:464–473.

Brockington, I. F., Kendell, R. E., and Leff, J. P. (1978). Definitions of schizophrenia: Concordance and predictions of outcome. *Psychological Medicine* 8:387–398.

Canino, G. J., Bird, H. R., Shrout, P. E., Rubio-Stipec, M., et al. (1987). The prevalence of specific psychiatric disorders in Puerto Rico. *Archives of General Psychiatry* 44:727–735.

Cho, M. J., Moscicki, E. K., Narrow, W. E., Rae, D. S., et al. (1993). Concordance between two measures of depression in the Hispanic health and nutrition examination survey. *Social Psychiatry Psychiatric Epidemiology* 28:156–163.

Del Castillo, J. C. (1970). The influence of language upon symptomatology in foreign-born patients. *American Journal of Psychiatry* 127:242–244.

Dohrenwend, B. (1966). Social status and psychological disorders: An issue of substance and an issue of method. *American Sociological Review* 31:14–34.

Egeland, J. A., Hostetter, A. M., and Eshleman, S. K. (1983). Amish study III: The impact of cultural factors on diagnosis of bipolar illness. *American Journal of Psychiatry* 140:67–71.

Frances, A. J., First, M. B., Widiger, T. A., Miele, G. M., et al. (1991). An A to Z guide to DSM-IV conundrums. *Journal of Abnormal Psychology* 100:407–412.

Gonzalez, C. A., Lewis-Fernandez, R., Griffith, E. E. H., Littlewood, R., and Castillo, R. (1994). The impact of culture on dissociation: On enhancing the cultural suitability of DSM-IV. In J. E. Mezzich, A. Kleinman, H. Fabrega, D. Parron, et al. (Eds.), *Cultural issues and DSM-IV: Support papers.* Submitted for the *DSM-IV Source Book* by the Steering Committee, NIMH Group on Culture and Diagnosis, January.

Guarnaccia, P. J. (1992). *Ataques de nervios* in Puerto Rico: Culture-bound syndrome or popular illness? *Medical Anthropology* 15:1–14.

Guarnaccia, P. J., Guevara-Ramos. L. M., Gonzales, G., Canino, G. J., and Bird, H. (1992). Cross-cultural aspects of psychotic symptoms in Puerto Rico. *Research Community Mental Health* 7:99–110.

Haberman, P. (1976). Psychiatric symptoms among Puerto Ricans in Puerto Rico and New York City. *Ethnicity* 3:133–144.

Hughes, C. C., Simons, R. C., and Wintrob, R. M. (1992). Selected glossary of "culture-bound" syndromes. In J. E. Mezzich, A. Kleinman, H. Fabrega, B. Good, et al. (Eds.), *Cultural proposals for DSM-IV.* Submitted to the DSM-IV task force by the Steering Committee, NIMH-Sponsored Group on Culture and Diagnosis.

Kessler, R. C., McGonagle, K. A., Zhao, S., Nelson, C. B., et al. (1994). Lifetime and 12-month prevalence of DSM-III-R psychiatric disorders in the United States. *Archives of General Psychiatry* 51:8–19.

Kleinman, A. (1987). Anthropology and psychiatry. *British Journal of Psychiatry* 151:447–454.

Kleinman, A. (1988). *Rethinking psychiatry: From cultural category to personal experience.* New York: Free Press.

Kleinman, A., and Good, B. (Eds.). (1985). *Culture and depression.* Berkeley: University of California Press.

Lin, K. M., Inui, T. S., Kleinman, A., and Womack, W. M. (1982). Sociocultural determinants of the help-seeking behavior of patients with mental illness. *Journal of Nervous and Mental Disease* 170:78–85.

Manson, S. M., Shore, J. H., and Bloom, J. D. (1985). The depressive experience in American Indian communities: A challenge for psychiatric theory and diagnosis. In A. Kleinman and B. Good (Eds.), *Culture and depression.* Berkeley: University of California Press.

Marcos, L. R. (1994). The psychiatric examination of Hispanics: Across the language barrier. In R. G. Malgady and O. Rodriguez (Eds.), *Theoretical and conceptual issues in Hispanic mental health.* Malabar, FL: Krieger Publishing.

Marcos, L. R., Alpert, M., Urcuyo, L., and Kesselman, M. (1973a). The effect of interview language on the evaluation of psychopathology in Spanish-American schizophrenic patients. *American Journal of Psychiatry* 130:549–553.

Marcos, L. R., Urcuyo, L., Kesselman, M., and Alpert, M. (1973b). The language barrier in evaluating Spanish-American patients. *Archives of General Psychiatry* 29:655–659.

Mechanic, D. (1968). *Medical sociology: A selective view.* New York: Free Press.

Mezzich, J. E., Kleinman, A., Fabrega, H., Parron, D., et al. (1994). *Cultural Issues and DSM-IV: Support Papers.* Submitted for the *DSM-IV Source Book* by the Steering Committee, NIMH Group on Culture and Diagnosis, January.

Radloff, L. S. (1977). The CES-D Scale: A self-report depression scale for research in the general population. *Applied Psychological Measures* 1:385–401.

Robins, L. N., Helzer, J. E., Croughan, J., Williams, J. B. W., and Spitzer, R. L. (1981). *National Institute of Mental Health: NIMH diagnostic interview schedule: Version III.* Developed for the NIMH Division of Biometry and Epidemiology.

Rogler, L. H. (1989). The meaning of culturally sensitive research in mental health. *American Journal of Psychiatry* 146:296–303.

Rogler, L. H., (1993). Culturally sensitizing psychiatric diagnosis: A framework for research. *Journal of Nervous and Mental Disease* 181:401–408.

Rogler, L. H., and Cortes, D. E. (1993). Help-seeking pathways: A unifying concept in mental health care. *American Journal of Psychiatry* 150:554–561.

Rogler, L. H., Cortes, D. E., and Malgady, R. G. (1994). The mental health relevance of idioms of distress: Anger and perceptions of injustice among New York City Puerto Ricans. *Journal of Nervous and Mental Disease* 182:327–330.

Rogler, L. H., and Hollingshead, A. B. (1985). *Trapped: Puerto Rican families and schizophrenia.* Maplewood, NJ: Waterfront Press.

Spitzer, R., Endicott, J., and Robins, E. (1977). *Research Diagnostic Criteria (RDC) for a selected group of functional disorders*, 3rd Edition. New York: New York State Psychiatric Institute.

Tylor, E. B. (1958). *The origins of culture.* New York: Harper.

Wilson, M. (1993). DSM-III and the transformation of American psychiatry: A history. *American Journal of Psychiatry* 150:399–410.

12

The Place of Culture in DSM-IV

Juan E. Mezzich, L. J. Kirmayer, A. Kleinman, Horacio Fabrega, D. L. Parron, Byron J. Good, K. M. Lin, S. M. Manson

Among the more innovative features of DSM-IV is the inclusion of explicit considerations of culture throughout the text (American Psychiatric Association, 1994). This effort was largely the result of an NIMH-sponsored Group on Culture and Diagnosis working collaboratively with, but outside the official framework of the DSM-IV Task Force and Workgroups. Many negotiations and editorial decisions took place in translating and incorporating some of the Culture and Diagnosis Group's suggestions into the text of DSM-IV. A close examination of this process reveals important tensions and contradictions in the effort to incorporate cultural knowledge and perspectives into the DSM. In this paper, we will review the process by which the cultural aspects for DSM-IV were developed and assess the successes and limitations of the final product. The results of this critical review have implications not only for understanding the place of culture in current and future nosologies and for the utility and potential limitations of DSM-IV as a clinical and research tool in multicultural settings, but also for understanding the sociopolitical process of constructing the DSM itself.

Interest in the cultural framework of illness, diagnosis, and care has been stimulated by increasing awareness of cultural diversity in U.S. society. The experiences of the latter half of the twentieth century have refuted the assumption that the "melting pot" of assimilation would level out major cultural differences or make them peripheral to individuals' everyday lives (Gor-

From *The Journal of Nervous and Mental Disease* 187, no. 8 (August 1999)

don, 1964; Weinfeld, 1994). Global migrations and telecommunications have increased the pace and extent of intercultural exchange at all levels and transformed clinical practice (Castles and Miller, 1993; Rogler, 1994). At the same time, there has been much progress in cross-cultural psychiatry and psychology and medical anthropology and sociology, the disciplines that study the interaction of culture and psychopathology (Fabrega, 1987; Kleinman, 1988a; Littlewood, 1990; Mezzich and Berganza, 1984). Together, these advances in research and the changing nature of patient populations and the social context of psychiatry have made careful consideration of culture in psychiatric diagnosis a clinical issue of compelling importance.

Culture is involved in psychiatric assessment and diagnosis in at least five ways (Mezzich et al., 2000; Rogler, 1993). First, culture shapes the phenomenology of symptoms themselves, their content, meaning, and configuration. Second, culture is manifested through ethnopsychiatric diagnostic rationales and practices of grouping symptoms together into patterns that include but are not limited to the familiar culture-bound syndromes found in various societies including our own Western culture. Third, culture provides the matrix for the interpersonal situation of the diagnostic interview. Fourth, because the clinical encounter is often intercultural, the dynamics of cross-cultural work are crucial for understanding and refining diagnostic categories and practices. Finally, culture informs the overall conceptualization of diagnostic systems, which are children of their time and circumstances.

History of the Culture and Diagnosis Group

In 1990, shortly after the American Psychiatric Association started preparing the fourth edition of its diagnostic manual, Juan E. Mezzich (also a member of the DSM-IV Task Force), Arthur Meirunan, Horacio Fabrega Jr., and Delores L. Parron began planning a process by which experts in cultural psychiatry could be brought together to prepare cultural proposals for DSM-IV. A conference on Culture and Diagnosis was held in Pittsburgh in April 1991 under the auspices of the National Institute of Mental Health and the American Psychiatric Association. Fifteen nosologists, who were members of the DSM-IV Task Force (chaired by Allen Frances), met with a multidisciplinary group of forty-five experts in cultural psychiatry, including cultural psychiatrists, psychologists, anthropologists, sociologists, and representatives of some prominent ethnic minorities.

At the outset, Allen Frances indicated that DSM-IV was intended to be a "conservative" revision and that there would be little chance of rearranging categories altering diagnostic criteria, or adding new diagnostic entities. Any such change would require a great deal of "hard" evidence, presumably from epidemiological studies. Cultural information was more likely to be incorporated into the text that accompanies each disorder.

The conference identified several places where cultural considerations could be readily introduced in the DSM: the introduction to the manual, in the various diagnostic categories and the multiaxial schema, and a glossary of culture-related syndromes. Meeting participants also emphasized the need to appraise the ethnic representativeness of the DSM-IV field trial samples and to develop research documentation and educational materials on cultural influences on psychiatric nosology and diagnosis (Mezzich et al., 1992, 1996).

The Pittsburgh conference led to the formation of a Culture and Diagnosis Group funded by the Office for Special Populations of the NIMH. This support was crucial because the DSM-IV leadership had declined to assign official work-group status to this network of persons. Although this lack of official endorsement may have limited direct access to the DSM-IV decision-making process, it also allowed for scholarly independence. The NIMH-sponsored group included fifty cultural experts, both clinicians and scholars, coordinated by a steering committee (J. E. Mezzich, A. Kleinman, H. Fabrega, D. L Parron, B. Good, K-M. Lin, and S. Manson, with G. Johnson-Powell participating during the initial phase of the project). To accomplish its self-assigned tasks, the steering committee designated a writing work-group and a primary reader and added advisors and consultants as needed to review the proposals. Comprehensive literature reviews were conducted for each major group of disorders and review papers with specific cultural proposals were circulated and revised from April 1992 to September 1993. Working documents with summary papers in support of the proposals were prepared in January 1993 and January 1994. The final versions of these brief review papers comprise the *DSM-IV Sourcebook* Cultural Issues section (Mezzich et al., 1997).

What Was Included in the Text?

In this section, we will summarize the major cultural contributions prepared for the DSM. After each brief synopsis, we present a brief discussion of what was actually included in the manual. We will highlight major changes or omissions that have a significant impact on the meaning of the text.

1. Introduction to the Manual

A statement was prepared for the introduction to alert the clinician to the challenge of using DSM-IV thoughtfully in a multicultural society. It outlined the concepts of culture and ethnicity and referred to the substantial anthropological research underlying the specific recommendations offered. It encouraged the clinician to become aware of his or her ethnocentric biases as well as attend to the personal and cultural perspectives of the patient being assessed. The statement also framed the entire DSM as a cultural document in that it inevitably reflects current implicit values and perspectives of certain segments of U.S. society (Fabrega, 1994, 1995).

A shortened version of the proposed text was included in the last two pages of the eleven-page introduction. Definitions of culture and ethnicity were deleted. This placement and the elimination of important distinctions had the effect of reducing the cultural perspective to an addendum to the core of the introduction. This core indicates that DSM is the "best and latest" and implies it represents universal, atheoretical, and, hence, "culture-free" categories.

2. Cultural Considerations for Specific Disorders

The most extensive contribution of the Culture and Diagnosis Workgroup involved detailed advice on modifications of diagnostic criteria, differential diagnosis, and accompanying text on cultural considerations. Most of the proposed text was targeted at specific disorders, but some important considerations applied to whole categories and their interconnections. Text was prepared for most disorders within all broad diagnostic classes, except Factitious Disorders. No cultural considerations were proposed for some individual diagnostic categories under Childhood Onset and Sexual Disorders. The cultural considerations summarized information on cultural variations in modes of describing distress, symptom patterns, dysfunctions, course, and sociodemographic correlates of the disorder. These remarks were intended to promote culturally sensitive application of the corresponding diagnostic criteria. At a minimum, cultural sensitivity in diagnosis implies that an examiner is able to take into account the social and cultural context of the person being examined in order to ascertain whether specific diagnostic criteria are applicable in the present case and generate an appropriate differential diagnosis.

In general, simplified versions of the proposed cultural comments on diagnostic criteria and accompanying text were incorporated into DSM-IV. Except for the Personality Disorders, cultural considerations proposed for the introductory sections of the broad classes were not included. A total of seventy-six individual diagnostic categories within all fifteen broad diagnostic classes have sections labeled "Culture, Age, and Gender Considerations." The degree of proposed text incorporated in DSM-IV varied markedly across its sections. There were some clear trends in the type of material included. For example, proposals involving cross-cultural variations in symptomatology or prevalence rates tended to be included whereas those presenting any challenge to the presumed universality of standard diagnostic categories and criteria tended to be ignored.

3. Cultural Annotations for the Multiaxial Schema

Text was proposed for each of the axes of the DSM-IV multiaxial schema drawing attention to the fact that application of the standardized axial typologies and scales requires careful attention to how cultural factors influence such assessments. This applies to the formulation of mental disorders in Axis I and, especially, Axis II, as well as to the general medical disorders in Axis III, which can be differentially distributed across social class and ethnic groups. As well, certain psychosocial stressors (Axis IV) are particularly frequent in minority, displaced, and economically disadvantaged populations. The accurate rating of levels of functioning (Axis V) can be enhanced by considering the collective experience of the individual's reference groups as well as demographic information.

The proposed cultural annotations for the Multiaxial Assessment are virtually absent from the published manual. Exceptions are the inclusion of one cultural example within Psychosocial Problems Related to Social Environment in Axis IV and a reference to the axes within the cultural statement in the general introduction and within the introduction to the Cultural Formulation.

4. Cultural Formulation Guidelines

This contribution emerged later than the other components of the cultural proposals for DSM-IV but was quickly recognized as a crucial innovation (Mezzich and Good, 1997). It supplements the nomothetic or standardized diagnostic ratings with an idiographic statement, emphasizing the patient's personal experience and the corresponding cultural reference group (Good and Good, 1986; Jones and Thorne, 1987; Kleinman, 1988b). A literature review found several broad dimensions relevant to a cultural formulation that were distilled into a brief set of guidelines with five elements: (1) the cultural identity of the patient, including reference group(s), language, spiritual/religious affiliation, and multicultural identity; (2) cultural explanations of the illness (i.e., idioms of distress, explanatory models, and popular and professional sources of care); (3) cultural factors related to the psychosocial environment and functioning (e.g., the meaning of social support and stigma); (4) cultural aspects of the relationship between patient and clinician (e.g., attitudes toward authority, dependency, and relevance to transference and countertransference); and (5) an overall formulation, synthesizing elements critical to diagnosis and care. Field trials of the guidelines with various ethnic groups (African American, American Indian, Asian American, and Latino) indicated their utility and yielded illustrative case formulations, four of which were included in the proposed text to clarify the application of the Cultural Formulation.

The introduction and five elements of the proposed Cultural Formulation outline were included almost completely. However, they are placed in the ninth appendix to the manual, not, as originally proposed, in the section immediately after the presentation of Multiaxial Assessment. The illustrative cases, which are important to facilitating clinicians' use of the novel contribution, were left out.

5. Glossary of Culture-Bound Syndromes (CBS) and Idioms of Distress

This collation of terms and their meanings was intended to provide definitions of some of the folk or popular psychiatric syndromes and idioms of distress—that is, culturally shaped constellations of symptoms and culturally prescribed ways of describing distress that may or may not have psychopathological significance and that are likely to be encountered in cross-cultural psychiatric work. It would provide a handy reference for terms used elsewhere in the DSM-IV text. By highlighting distinctive forms of illness experience and local approaches to describing, explaining, classifying, and responding to distress, the CBS glossary also illustrates the importance of an anthropological framework to understand any disorder. In many cases, folk terms do not refer to syndromes at all but to locally formulated descriptions and interpretations of illness and the proposed title reflected this diversity.

The glossary proposal began with a brief introduction and then presented twenty-five terms drawn from a much larger catalog (Simons and Hughes, 1985), focusing on those that have been most studied and that are widely recognized both in non-Western societies and in North America among African Americans (e.g., rootwork and falling out), American Indians and Alaska Natives (ghost sickness and *pibloktoq*), Asian Americans (*shenjing shuairuo* and *taijin kyofusho*), and Latinos (*susto* and *ataque de nervios*). Importantly, and in reference to DSM itself as a cultural document Western culture-related syndromes (e.g., anorexia nervosa and multiple personality disorder) were also identified and linked to special features of Western countries or highly Westernized statements of other societies.

The Glossary of Culture-Bound Syndromes is also the ninth appendix, and the title was shortened by eliminating the phrase "and Idioms of Distress." The section on Western culture-bound syndromes was excluded from the glossary. As well, many references to culture-specific terms in the cultural consideration sections of the text were cut, leaving the glossary virtually the only place where several of these terms are mentioned in the DSM. The divorce of the glossary from the body of the text and the exclusion of Western CBS has the effect of rendering the glossary "a museum of exotica."

Editorial Elisions and Transformations

The mere enumeration of what was included and left out in the editing of the DSM does not give an accurate picture of the presence of culture in DSM-IV. To appreciate this, we must look more closely at some examples of how the proposed text was translated and interpreted by the official workgroups and editors.

Cultural commentary on diagnostic categories was placed mostly within specific disorders and only minimally in the introductions to whole classes of disorders. Many cultural proposals, however, were intended to highlight salient cultural issues for a whole category of disorders. For example, the clinical assessment of Child Onset Disorders requires work with multiple informants including parents, extended family, school, and community. Cultural considerations are crucial both to engaging and interpreting the reports of informants and to evaluating the significance of social context. As an indication of the scope of this problem, we know that where a systematic attempt was made a few years ago to apply DSM-III criteria to a large community sample of children in Puerto Rico, without a culturally informed assessment of impairment in functioning, about half of the sample was rated as mentally ill (Bird et al., 1988).

Beyond this issue of generality, some of the most salient cultural considerations were most appropriate for the introduction to a section because they challenge a drastic separation of disorders at various hierarchical levels. For example, around the world, affective, anxiety, and somatoform disorders often overlap (contributing to the perception of comorbidity), and many patients present a variety of neurotic symptoms without fulfilling criteria for any single disorder (Guarnaccia and Kirmayer, 1997; Kirmayer and Weiss,

1997; Weiss et al., 1995). Eliminating cultural comments on the broad classes of DSM disorders deflected criticism of the major categories in the DSM. Although these are sometimes defended as atheoretical or purely phenomenological groupings, it can be argued (Fabrega, 1987; Kleinman, 1988a; Mezzich and Berganza, 1984) that they reflect implicit theories about (a) which disorders share common etiopathogenic mechanisms and (b) how psychopathological changes are shaped and experienced by individuals seeking care.

The text prepared for specific diagnostic categories fared better than that written for the introduction to sections. In many cases, however, specific examples were eliminated. As a result, the information presented in the cultural comments often is so sketchy it serves mainly to alert the clinician to the possibility of cultural variation. For example, the dissociative disorders section incorporated about half of the cultural proposals. Spurred on by the interest and receptivity of the DSM-IV Dissociative Disorders Workgroup, the initial proposals for Dissociative Disorders included alternative diagnostic criteria (Cardena, 1992). This receptiveness may have reflected the acknowledged plasticity of these disorders and an interest in enlarging the category to promote research and clinical services (Kirmayer, 1992). Nevertheless, although cross-cultural variation in the phenomenology of these disorders was readily accepted, the argument that there are cross-cultural differences in their basic nosology was rejected (Lewis-Fernandez, 1992). Trance and Possession Disorder—proposed as a new category to match that present in the Tenth Revision of the International Classification of Diseases (WHO, 1992)—was relegated to an appendix for further study.

Some of the major biases of DSM-IV concern ontological notions of what constitutes a real disease or disorder, epistemological ideas about what counts as scientific evidence, methodological commitments to how research should be conducted, and pragmatic considerations about the appropriate uses of the DSM. Contrary to its frequent portrayal as an atheoretical, purely descriptive nosology based on scientific evidence, the DSM is a historical document with a complicated pedigree and many theoretical notions expressed in its structure and content. Most of the disorders of the DSM are syndromes in search of underlying pathological mechanisms or course trajectories that would make them more bona fide diseases.

A second structuring principle in the DSM concerns distinctions among syndromes that have demonstrable implications for current therapeutics. Like the psychodynamic biases of older DSMs, much of the current DSM appears to have begun with criteria intended to promote psychopharmacological research and allow differential diagnosis in terms of effective pharmacotherapy (Wilson, 1993). However, because psychological and social mechanisms influenced by culture clearly play a role in both the pathogenesis and treatment of most, if not all, psychiatric disorders, it may be possible to construct alternative nosologies based on distinctions at the level of common psychological or social interactional mechanisms and corresponding differential therapeutics (Kirmayer, 1991).

A major architectural opportunity in DSM-III and DSM-IV to articulate more closely the reality of the patient is provided by the multiaxial diagnostic schema. However, this opportunity has not been fully realized as indicated by the diffidence and optionality with which the schema is presented. Furthermore, the proposals made to enhance the cultural suitability and sensitivity of the axes involved were minimally incorporated despite the obvious cultural anchorage of concepts such as adaptive functioning and psychosocial stressors and supports.

Context and Categories

Deference to established nosological categories that guide research and diagnostic practices may limit our ability to recognize situations when the data demand rethinking such categories. The tendency to reproduce uncrititically preexisting constructs has been termed the "category fallacy" (Kleinman, 1977).

The clinical experience encoded in the diagnostic criteria of DSM III and subsequent revisions were largely based on relatively homogeneous clinical populations of patients at university clinics, initially in the Midwest and East Coast of the United States. There has been strikingly little effort to appraise the clinical and predictive utility of DSM categories, criteria, and axes on culturally diverse populations within the United States.

In contrast to a biomedically reductionistic approach, a culturally informed clinical psychiatry links knowledge of human biology and a person-centered view of predicaments (Corin, 1990; Strauss, 1992) with social science perspectives relevant to understanding all human experience, including psychiatric disorders (Fabrega and Nguyen, 1992; Gaines, 1992; Hughes, 1993; Kleinman, 1988a). This type of formulation is more than an academic exercise; the experience of family and other systemically oriented therapists shows how it can lead to ways of construing problems that generate effective solutions (Ho, 1993; Phillips et al., 1994).

The DSM has traditionally concentrated on pathology conceptualized as rooted and fixed in the biological individual. This ignores the way in which many psychiatric problems are not only substantially more prevalent among individuals facing social disadvantage but, in important ways, constituted by those same economic, family, social, and cultural predicaments (Desjarlais, et al., 1995; Kirmayer, 1989; Littlewood, 1993). It is instructive in this regard to read in the introduction to the WHO's 1995 World Health Report (WHO, 1995) that poverty is the chief cause of mortality and morbidity in the world. To the extent that individuals' problems are manifestations of larger social problems, a diagnostic process exclusively centered on individual pathology may work against a clinically accurate—and a professionally and morally adequate—response.

Discussion and Future Tasks

The process of developing cultural proposals has provided a fascinating case study in the sociology of science. It involved an exchange between nosologists and cultural experts in which there were two channels or levels of communication: a normal channel in which each tried to speak the same language of empiricism (e.g., biological and epidemiological psychiatry) and a second level or back channel in which the cultural experts were engaged in understanding the whole nosological enterprise as a socially mediated activity. Although the cultural perspective is primarily concerned with understanding human problems, illness, and suffering contextually, the biomedical nosological enterprise is traditionally committed to abstracting the assumed "basic" patterns of distress in a way that allows disorders to be studied in and of themselves, divorced from context. To the extent that the cultural experts adopted the language of discrete disorders separated from the particulars of human lives and social situations, they risked losing what is most distinctive about their perspective. To the extent the nosologists engaged the cultural critique of their categories as situated, socially constructed, and limited by various sorts of blinders, they were in danger of losing the conviction that the diagnostic categories in DSM mirror the natural categories of disease in the world ("carving nature at its joints").

We note also that there were several failures in the effort to incorporate culture into the DSM for which the Culture and Diagnosis Group itself must take primary responsibility. Although a meaning-centered anthropological approach directly or indirectly informed our analyses, it should be recognized that cultural psychiatry involves an amalgam of principles and generalizations drawn from several social sciences and a broadly based clinical psychiatry. There was too little attention to social factors in the cultural considerations. For example, quite aside from the pervasive importance of the cultural programming of behavior, social class status is the best predictor of health status (Evans et al., 1994). In North American cultural psychiatry, not unlike cultural anthropology, there has been a tendency to use culture as a proxy for harder issues of class, economic disadvantage, racism, and power (Comas-Diaz and Griffith, 1987; Littlewood, 1993; Pinderhughes, 1989).

The complex issue of intracultural heterogeneity was also not adequately addressed. For example, gender issues were treated superficially in terms of sex ratio, and there was little attention to how gender and culture interact.

Looking ahead to future revisions of diagnostic systems, the following recommendations on strengthening their academic base, developmental process, and actual content appear to be in order:

1. Further research on the cultural framework for diagnosis and care is essential. This research should be organized programmatically and longitudinally and cover pathways, the diagnostic process, the predictive power of alternative categories, criteria and axes, and help-seeking pathways (Guarnaccia et al., 1993; Rogler, 1992).
2. There is a need for alternative assessment tools that promote the process of interviewing, field observation, community participation, and interdisciplinary collaboration required for culturally responsive diagnosis. Such tools should improve on current structured interviews, which tend to focus on reliability with little concern for comprehensive diagnostic validity.
3. Educational aids are needed to facilitate the appropriate use of the Cultural Formulation Outline and the other cultural contributions in DSM-IV. The NIMH Group on Culture, Diagnosis, and Care is preparing an introductory booklet with practical guidelines and illustrations for the Cultural Formulation.
4. Empirical research is needed to evaluate the impact of the DSM-IV Cultural Formulation on the quality of diagnosis and care. This question takes a special urgency in the emerging world of managed care, where cost-effectiveness is the great leveler of quality of care.
5. There ought to be cultural expertise in the leadership of the diagnostic system developmental task force so that sociocultural issues (along with other key perspectives) are central considerations from the start of the process.
6. The workgroup in charge of preparing cultural proposals should more effectively interact with other components of the diagnostic system enterprise in order to facilitate cross-fertilization of perspectives and the introduction and refinement of relevant materials.
7. There must be a more explicit process of accountability and feedback to the various groups and individuals contributing expertise to the construction of the diagnostic system.
8. A future diagnostic manual, from the beginning of its introduction,

should articulate a truly comprehensive framework based on a historically and culturally informed human biology that is responsive to the complexity of health problems in their social context.

9. Diagnosis in a future manual should not be limited to the identification of individual syndromes or disorders but should provide a fuller assessment of the patient's whole clinical condition. This may be accomplished by emphasizing a multiaxial diagnostic formulation, as recommended by the Psychiatric Evaluation Task Force of the American Psychiatric Association (1995) and by considering a more comprehensive diagnostic model, integrating a standardized statement with an idiographic formulation (that articulates the perspectives of the patient and his/her cultural reference group), such as that currently under development by the World Psychiatric Association (Mezzich et al., 2000).
10. Specific cultural elements of a diagnostic system, such as cultural considerations on diagnostic categories and criteria, culture-related syndromes and idioms of distress, and a cultural formulation, should be better integrated with other diagnostic components and more appropriately placed within the manual.

Although much more work is needed, it is clear that the door has been opened and, given the compelling reality of multicultural societies and globalization, it is certain not to close until culture has been thoroughly integrated into the essential framework of diagnostic systems.

References

American Psychiatric Association. (1994). *Diagnostic and statistical manual of mental disorders*, 4th Edition. Washington, DC: American Psychiatric Association.

American Psychiatric Association. (1995). Practice guidelines for psychiatric evaluation of adults. *Am J Psychiatry* 162(Nov Suppl): 65–80.

Bird, H. R., Camino, G., Rubio-Stipec, M., Gould, M. S., Ribera, J., Sesman, M., Woodbury, M., Huertas-Goldman, S., Pagan, A., Sanchez Lacey, A., and Moscoso, M. (1988). Estimates of the prevalence of childhood maladjustment in a community survey in Puerto Rico. *Arch Gen Psychiatry* 45:1120–1126.

Cardena, E. (1992). Trance and possession as dissociative disorders. *Transcult Psychiatr Res Rev* 29:287–300.

Castles, S., and Miller, M. J. (1993). *The age of migration: International population movements in the modem world.* New York: Guilford.

Comas-Diaz, L., and Griffith, E. E. H. (1987). *Clinical guidelines in cross-cultural mental health.* New York: Wiley.

Corin, E. (1990). Facts and meaning in psychiatry: An anthropological approach to the life world of schizophrenics. *Cult Med Psychiatry* 14:153–188.

Desjarlais, R., Eisenberg, L., Good, B., and Kleinman, A. (1995). *World mental health: Problems and priorities in low-income countries.* New York: Oxford University Press.

Evans, R. G., Barer, M. L., and Marmor, T. L. (Eds.). (1994). *Why are some people healthy and others not? The determination of health of populations.* New York: W. de Gruyter.

Fabrega, H. (1987). Psychiatric diagnosis: A cultural perspective. *J Nerv Ment Dis* 175:383–394.

Fabrega, H. (1994). International systems of diagnosis in psychiatry. *J Nem Ment Di* 182:256–263.

Fabirega, H. (1995). Cultural challenges to the psychiatric enterprise. *Compr Psychiatry* 36:377–383.

Fabrega, H. Jr., and Nguyen, H. (1992). Culture, social structure, and quandaries of psychiatric diagnosis: A Vietnamese case study. *Psychiatry* 55:230–249.

Gaines, A. D. (1992). From DSM-1 to III-R: Voices of self, mastery and the other. A cultural constructive reading of U.S. psychiatric classification. *Soc Sci Med* 35:3–24.

Guaniaccia, P. J., Canino, G., Rubio-Stipec, M., and Bravo, M. (1993). The prevalence of *ataques de nervios* in the Puerto Rico disaster study: The role of culture in psychiatric epidemiology. *J Nerv Ment Dis* 181:157–165.

Guarnaccia, P., and Kirmayer, L. J. (1997). Cultural considerations on anxiety disorders. In T. A. Widiger, et al. (Eds.), *DSM-IV sourcebook*, Vol. 3. Washington, DC: American Psychiatric Press.

Good, B., and Good, M-J. D. (1986). The cultural context of diagnosis and therapy: A view from medical anthropology. In M. R. Miranda, H. H. L. Kitano (Eds.), *Mental health research and practice in minority communities.* U.S. Department of Health and Human Services Publication No. ADM 86–1466. Washington, DC: Government Printing Services.

Gordon, M. M. (1964). *Assimilation in American life.* New York: Oxford University Press.

Ho, M. K. (1993). *Family therapy with ethnic minorities.* Newbury Park, CA: Sage Publications.

Hughes, C. C. (1993). Culture in clinical psychiatry. In: A. C. Gaw (Ed.), *Culture, ethnicity and mental illness*, pp. 3–41. Washington, DC: American Psychiatric Press.

Jones, E. E., and Thorne, A. (1987). Rediscovery of the subject: Intercultural approaches to clinical assessment. *J Consult Clin Psychol* 55: 488–496.

Kirmayer, L. J. (1989). Cultural variations in the response to psychiatric disorders and emotional distress. *Soc Sci Med* 29:327–339.

Kirmayer, L. J. (1991). The place of culture in psychiatric nosology: Taijin kyofusho and DSM-III-R. *J Nerv Ment Dis* 179:19–28.

Kirmayer, L. J. (1992). (Editorial) Taking possession of trance. *Transcult Psychiatr Res Rev* 29:283–286.

Kirmayer, L. J., and Weiss, M. G. (1997). Cultural considerations on somatoform disorders. In T. A. Widiger, et al. Eds., *DSM-IV sourcebook*, Vol. 3. Washington, DC: American Psychiatric Press.

Kleinman, A. M. (1977). Depression, somatization and the "new cross-cultural psychiatry." *Soc Sci Med* 11:3–10.

Kleinman, A. (1987). Anthropology and psychiatry: The role of culture in cross-cultural research on illness. *Br J Psychiatry* 151: 447–454.

Kleinman, A. (1988a). *Rethinking psychiatry.* New York: Free Press.

Kleinman, A. (1988b). *The illness narratives.* New York: Basic Books.

Lewis-Fernández, R. (1992). The proposed DSM-IV trance and possession disorder category: Potential benefits and risks. *Transcult Psychiatr Res Rev* 29:301–318.

Littlewood, R. (1990). From categories to contexts: A decade of the "new cross-cultural psychiatry." *Br J Psychiatry* 156:308–327.

Littlewood, R. (1993). Ideology, camouflage or contingency? Racism in British psychiatry. *Transcult Psychiair Res Rev* 30:243–229.

Mezzich, J. E., Berganza, C. E. (1984). *Culture and psychopathology.* New York: Columbia University Press.

Mezzich, J. E., Fabrega, H., and Kleinman, A. (1992). Cultural validity and DSM-IV. *J Nerv Ment Dis* 180:4.

Mezzich, J. E., and Good, B. J. (1997). On culturally enhancing the DSM-TV multiaxial formulation. In T. Widiger, A. Frances, H. A. Pincus, et al. (Eds.), *DSM-IV sourcebook*, Vol. 3. Washington, DC: American Psychiatric Press.

Mezzich, J. E., Kleinman, A., Fabrega, H., and Parron, D. L. (1996). *Culture and psychiatric diagnosis.* Washington, DC: American Psychiatric Press.

Mezzich, J. E., Kleinman, A., Fabrega, H., Parron, D. L., Good, B. J., Lin, K., and Manson, S. M. (1997). Introduction to cultural issues section. In T. Widiger, A. Frances, H. A. Pincus, et al. (Eds.), *DSM-IV sourcebook,* Vol. 3. Washington, DC: American Psychiatric Press.

Mezzich, J. E., Otero, A. A., and Lee, S. (2000). International psychiatric diagnosis. In H. I. Kaplan, and B. J. Sadock (Eds.), *Comprehensive textbook of psychiatry*, 7th Edition. Baltimore: Williams & Wilkins.

Phillips, M. R., Pearson, V., and Wang, R. (1994). Psychiatric rehabilitation in China: Models for change in a changing society. *Br J Psychiatry* 165 (Suppl 24):1–142.

Pinderhughes, E. (1989). *Understanding race, ethnicity, and power: The key to clinical efficacy.* New York: Free Press.

Rogler, L. H. (1992). The role of culture in mental health diagnosis: The need for programmatic research. *J Nerv Ment Dis* 180: 745–747.

Rogler, L. H. (1993). Culture in psychiatric diagnosis: An issue of scientific accuracy. *Psychiatry* 56:324–327.

Rogler, L. H. (1994). International migrations: A framework for directing research. *Am Psychologist* 49:701–708.

Simons, R. C., and Hughes, C. C. (1986). *The Culture-bound syndromes: Folk illnesses of psychiatric and anthropological interest.* Dordrecht: D. Reidel.

Strauss, J. S. (1992). The person-key to understanding mental illness: Towards a new dynamic psychiatry, III. *Br J Psychiatry* 161:19–26.

Weinfeld, M. (1994). Ethnic assimilation and the retention of ethnic cultures. In J. W. Berry, J. A. Laponce (Eds.), *Ethnicity and cultures in Canada*, pp. 238–266. Toronto: University of Toronto Press.

Weiss, M. G., Raguram, R., and Channabasavanna, S. M. (1995). Cultural dimensions of psychiatric diagnosis: A comparison of DSM-III-R an illness explanatory models in South India. *Br J Psychiatry* 1 353–359.

Wilson, M. (1993). DSM-III and the transformation of American psychiatry: A history. *Am J Psychiatry* 150:399–410.

World Health Organization. (1992). The ICD-10 *Classification of mental and behavioral disorders: Clinical descriptions and diagnostic guidelines.* Geneva: World Health Organization.

World Health Organization. (1995). *World health report.* Geneva: World Health Organization.

13

Using DSM-IV Cultural Formulation to Enhance Psychodynamic Understanding

Giovanni Caracci

THE FUNDAMENTAL ROLE cultural factors play in the recognition and treatment of mental illness has received widespread attention in the past decade (1–4). Culture permeates the patient-physician encounter at several levels. The patient's map of belief systems derived from his cultural background affects the expression of symptoms, whether they are viewed as normal, how a physician and treatment are perceived, the family's response to mental illness, compliance with treatment, and communication of emotional suffering. One of the main advances in our cultural understanding of psychiatric illness has been the development of the DSM-IV Cultural Formulation Outline, which was the result of years of research and discussion within the DSM-IV Task Force and the National Institute of Mental Health (NIMH) (5). The outline is meant to supplement the multiaxial diagnostic assessment and to address difficulties that may be encountered in applying DSM-IV criteria in a multicultural environment. Five elements of the formulation are listed: cultural identity of the individual, the cultural explanation of the individual's illness, cultural factors related to the psychosocial environment and level of functioning, cultural elements of the relationship between the individual and the clinician, and overall cultural assessment for diagnosis and care (6).

Over the last few years some authors have advocated supplementing the descriptive diagnosis that is based on the observation of the presenting symp-

From *Dynamic Psychiatry* 33 (2000)

toms with a comprehensive evaluation of the human being behind the symptoms, emphasizing the patients subjective experience, his unique form of suffering, and the idiosyncratic expression of psychopathology in his interpersonal world as well as within the therapeutic relationship. The two views have also been called nomothetic and idiographic (5). By acquiring information close to the essence of the patient, the idiographic view of psychopathology greatly enriches our understanding of the patient as a whole. The process of obtaining information to arrive at an idiographic formulation shares some similarities with an interview with a focus on psychodynamic formulation. To mention a few similarities: In both approaches the subjective experience of the patient is seen as unique rather than similar to other patients. Both use an empathic listening mode, where the patient is encouraged to verbalize his perspective on his mental anguish. In both the goal is to achieve an understanding of the patient's psychosocial and intrapsychic strengths as well as weaknesses. Moreover, in both formulations transferential and countertransferential considerations are useful to grasp the patient's inner experience and his interaction with the external reality.

Cultural formulation is uniquely positioned as an invaluable bridge between the nomothetic and the idiographic/psychodynamic domains. By exploring the multiple layers of interaction between patient and cultural environment it provides the clinician with a different prism through which he can view the patient's symptoms, his psychosocial functioning, and his interpersonal relations (7). In the process, maladaptive behaviors and thoughts can be uncovered and recorded.

One clarification worth addressing is the meaning of the word *psychodynamic*. While this word has often been equated with *psychoanalytic* we prefer to use it in a wider context, reflecting theoretical underpinnings from different schools of thought. Thus, we adopted the following definition: psychodynamic psychiatry is an approach to diagnosis and treatment characterized by a way of thinking about the patient and clinician that includes unconscious conflicts, deficit and distortions of intrapsychic structure, and internal relations (8). The main theoretical guiding concepts derive from the schools of ego psychology, self psychology, and object relations. In addition, we supplemented these three models with principles from a cognitive model. The theory postulates that the adverse experiences producing psychopathology are represented as beliefs linked to expectations of injury. Moreover it states that many of these beliefs, when carried unchanged into the adult life, become irrational, determine inappropriate affects and the maladaptive attitudes and behaviors that constitute adult psychopathology (9). These are theoretical constructs that explain psychological conflicts and mental functioning. Their concepts greatly overlap and some of them are better suited for some types of disorders, for example, object relations for borderline personality and self-psychology for narcissistic disorders. In line with the eclectic nature of our exploration, a blend of these three approaches was used for this work.

This article illustrates how cultural formulation can help residents enhance their psychodynamic understanding of patients. It is the product of a year-long seminar taught to graduate and postgraduate students at our institution. The initial objective of the seminar was learning to formulate patients according to the outline and to understand the interface between the multi-axial system and the five elements of cultural formulation. However the focus of the seminar gradually shifted as it became increasingly evident that the outline was allowing the students to sharpen their understanding of patients' personality traits and psychodynamic world. The challenge soon became to understand how cultural factors and psychodynamic ones interplay in a unique way for each patient. It is interesting that while at the beginning of the seminar residents saw cultural and psychodynamic factors as separate, mostly due to their tendency to compartmentalize domains, this was no longer the case toward the end of the seminar, when cultural and intrapsychic factors were seen as intricately intertwined. Although these were PGY 1 and 2 residents, they followed their patients beyond their inpatient stay in the day hospital and outpatient and took notes which they regularly brought to the seminar. Therefore, over time the seminar became a cultural/psychodynamic formulation continuous case seminar with regular updates.

The cultural identity of the individual is divided into cultural reference group, language, involvement with the culture of origin, and involvement with the host culture. The cultural reference group is on the surface a given one. But in the present multiethnic society it is not so simple a matter. A patient told a resident "I am one-quarter Indian, one-quarter Spanish and the rest is German, and I came here when I was five; therefore I am an American. What does that make me? I don't know." Further exploration of the case showed a strong identification with the Spanish heritage mostly traceable to her being brought up by their Hispanic grandmother, who was the only stable presence in a very chaotic family environment.

Language on the other hand is a complex function that can reveal important nuances of the person's psychodynamics. Especially in immigrants, whether the language of the host culture is spoken or not, the patient's relationship with the language of origin as well as with the acquired language offers a view into the characteristics of the ego, quality of object relations, and characteristics of the self.

A thirty-year-old Dominican female with panic disorder and agoraphobia in the United States for thirteen years did not speak English, nor did she express any desire to learn it. An in-depth interview revealed that the patient viewed learning the new language as a threat to her dependency needs and fear of abandonment by her family (i.e., acculturation equaled independence and losing the loved ones). Her fears were defensively displaced onto her phobias.

The cultural factors in development: This is an area which can greatly contribute to understanding the patient's self-objects, family relations, defense mechanisms, superego issues, and irrational belief systems.

An Eastern European patient with a history of dysthymia, multiple somatic complaints, and borderline traits described his migration to the United States at the age of seven as traumatic. He verbalized his resentment at being uprooted. His family confirmed that around that age he had changed from an extroverted child to a brooding one. His massive denial of unacceptable angry feelings was turned inward with ensuing depression as well as hypochondriacal somatizations. His parents spoke their native language and constantly romanticized their country of origin, overtly expressing regret about their decision to move. Over time he had developed a maladaptive belief of not belonging and that there was a place out there where he could be happy and fulfilled. This idea greatly restricted his social and romantic life and needed to be addressed in psychotherapy.

Information about involvement with the culture of origin is very useful in uncovering conflictual and ambivalent feelings toward parental figures and siblings. This is the area where primitive defenses such as splitting and projective identification are more often identified. The culture of origin may become an idealized parental imago while the host culture may be devalued as the bad self-object.

An Indian patient with borderline personality disorder and intermittent psychotic episodes secondary to psychosocial stressors was a devout follower of an Indian guru in the United States, at various points living in his commune. She was completely consumed with following the traditions of her native India and derided the American culture as degrading. When psychotic, she heard the voice of the guru telling her she was the chosen one to save this country from moral decay. Further exploration revealed an ambivalent relationship with a rigid and distant father and a yearning for his affection. The guru had become the idealized parental image while the entire host culture was split off as the bad self-object.

The involvement with the host culture also provides valuable information about, for example, ego strengths or weaknesses, characteristics of the self such as self-esteem and continuity of the self. A Chinese patient hospitalized for major depression and a suicide attempt at first refused to talk about his origins; than he gradually spoke about his not wanting to identify himself as a Chinese, which eventually led to his changing both his first and last name to an American one. This was secondary to a poor sense of self and ambivalence about his culture of origin. Within an object relations theory, he had idealized the host culture and devalued the culture of origin (representing the rigid, distant, and bad parents), within the self-psychology framework he was reacting to the empathic failures of his family by assigning perfection to an idealized parental imago, in the process protecting a defective self prone to fragmentation. From a cognitive viewpoint he harbored an irrational belief that to be successful he had to totally renounce his ethnicity.

The cultural explanation of the individual's illness provides several points of entry into the patient's psychological world. These include the predominant idioms of distress, the meaning and perceived severity of the individual's symptoms in relation to norms of the culture reference group, the perceived causes and explanatory models of the illness, and help experiences and plans. The predominant idioms of distress through which symptoms are communicated convey a meaning that can be clinically useful.

A twenty-seven-year-old African American woman with a diagnosis of depressive psychosis experienced auditory hallucinations telling her that she will never be forgiven. When she was brought to the ER, her father related that she had been "speaking in tongues," an expression used by followers of the Pentecostal faith to describe a trancelike phenomenon during which communication with the Holy Spirit is established. Since within her religious group the phenomenon was seen as normal, she did not come to the attention of a mental health professional until a few months later. The voice of God was a culturally acceptable manifestation of her emotional distress. Further exploration into these idioms of distress revealed a conflictual relationship with a highly controlling father on whom she was very dependent. Unable to accept her rage at her overbearing father, she had incorporated him into her delusions as the unforgiving God. Her core belief was that since she had disrespected her father by cursing at him she was never going to be forgiven and she would be condemned to being eternally punished by him.

Closely related to the idea of distress is that of the meaning and perceived severity of the individual's symptoms in relation to norms of the culture reference group. A fifty-four-year-old Burmese male with depression and multiple somatic complaints thought that his malaise was secondary to gardening, an activity he had engaged in for five months after he had been laid off from his job. He only acknowledged the somatic manifestations and strongly denied being depressed. This view was also shared by some of his family members. Other members of the patient's family had different interpretations as to what had happened. These discrepancies revealed some insights into the patient's family dynamics, which were useful in the treatment. In sum, after years of hard work as an immigrant, being the breadwinner in the household, he had found himself unemployed and no longer indispensable. This loss led him to becoming increasingly despondent and withdrawn. His sons had decided that he could spend his time gardening when "all of a sudden, while in the garden" he began complaining of headaches and other somatic symptoms. From that moment on he assumed the sick role, as he and the entire family perceived the illness to be very serious as well as incapacitating. The somatization of his depression was interpreted as normal within the Burmese perception of mental illness as unacceptable or flatly denied.

Similarly, the perceived causes and explanatory models offer invaluable information about the patient's awareness of his illness as well as of the issue of attribution of symptoms. This is an interesting interface between the cultural domain and the psychodynamic one. Insight into the illness is usually assessed early on by the clinician, as it will guide assessment of prognosis as well as approach to treatment. Understanding the dynamics behind some of the irrational beliefs about what causes our patients' problems can considerably illuminate the therapeutic journey. It is important however to underscore that lack of insight is indeed a symptom in some psychopathological entities such as schizophrenia.

A forty-year-old Italian American with bipolar affective disorder was hospitalized for a severe depressive disorder. She believed that her illness was due to "malocchio," literally, evil eye from her husband's family. "Malocchio" is a pervasive belief among Mediterranean and Hispanic cultures and it is rooted in the idea that a malevolent person can bring on misfortunes and illness. An exploration into the family dynamics revealed that for years she had made unrealistic demands on his family, whom she perceived as a threat to her marriage. She constantly questioned her husband's love, blaming his excessive attachment to his family for his lack of love toward her. Her paranoid reactions served the purpose of protecting her from self-blame and a sense of unworthiness, while at the same time denying her own involvement in her marital difficulties. Eventually, we were able to trace her reaction to growing up in an environment perceived as ambivalent and hostile, especially on her mother's family side.

Help-seeking experiences and plans: All the cases mentioned above resorted to culturally related forms of healing that were outside of the psychiatric realm. This is usually due to culturally sanctioned stigma surrounding psychiatry, and these patients feel more comfortable with culturally accepted means of delivering mental health. The patient's first approach to dealing with his emotional suffering often offers the clinician helpful insights. In each individual case different variables play a role in this first step, including whether the patient himself or a family member sought help, availability of means for treating mental illness, religious affiliation, socioeconomic status, and level of education. Much can be learned from this process, especially from transferential reactions patients develop toward folk healers and from the validation the healer gives to the patient's symptoms.

A thirty-five-year-old Puerto Rican woman who suffered from dizziness, weakness, anxiety, and a host of somatic complaints presented with unresolved sexual conflicts centering around a core idea that a family member had sexually molested her when she was a child. At first she had resorted to a "curandero" to heal her symptoms. The healer used several local techniques, which resulted in partial improvement of her symptoms. However, in the process she developed a strong erotic transference toward him, which eventually led to the worsening of her anxiety and ultimately to her hospitalization. Underlying her anxiety were ideas of sex as dirty and unacceptable based on prominent oedipal conflicts that were explored in psychotherapy.

Cultural factors related to psychosocial environment and levels of functioning: Attaining an understanding of the significance of psychosocial stressors and how they are perceived by the patient is a crucial step in every psychodynamic formulation. Here the emphasis on the cultural element facilitates a view into the patient's fears, beliefs, adaptations, and defense mechanisms.

A thirty-year-old Korean physician was hospitalized with a major depressive episode following his being denied renewal of his contract in the second year of residency because of poor performance on the job. He had become suicidal with clear plans to carry it out. An exploration of his perception of the stressor revealed that he had experienced the job loss as catastrophic and final. He then proceeded to describe what he called "Korean values" regarding education, describing an all-or-nothing belief that a person without a completed education is unworthy and considered a social outcast. His perception of his cultural norm was that anything short of completing education was to be considered a failure. Exploring the patient's family dynamics showed that his father, himself a successful physician, had chosen him to continue his legacy. In the process he had shown parental preference over a troubled younger sibling who had dropped out of medical school. The patient's grandiosity masked inferiority feelings and guilt toward his brother. His anxiety over becoming a successful doctor was based on the idea of depriving the unfavored brother of parental affection, to which he adapted masochistically by making an astonishingly naive series of mistakes at work.

Social Supports: In this subset we can assess the resources available to the patient and how they are used. A patient with a variety of support systems may hardly utilize them while another with limited resources may maximize their usefulness. In this context, important dynamics may be uncovered within the patient's relationship with family, mental health providers, and social structure. An elderly Russian woman evaluated for depression on our medical unit verbalized feelings of being a burden to her family and suicidal ideation. A family meeting showed that the patient's family was very supportive but after the loss of a sister in Russia she had gradually withdrawn from her family, refused help, and stopped socializing with her peers. Her close relationship with her sister had been seriously strained at the time the patient had made the decision to emigrate. Eventually her sister had decided to remain in Russia, and the two were estranged for one year. Addressing the patient's irrational conviction that she had caused her sister's death by her decision and her consequent guilt feelings was crucial for her to rely on her family again.

Level of Functioning and Disability: This is an area of inquiry that affords many insights into the interaction between cultural values and psychodynamics. For example, how does a commonly held Chinese belief that in life one "is supposed to eat bitter" influence a patient's difficulty to work due to depression? A frequently seen compromise is the manifestation of somatic symptoms, which in many cultures are better accepted than psychiatric ones. In some cultures the expectation to function in the work, social, or romantic domain is imposed on the mildly or moderately ill patient, while it is waived in the more severely mentally ill. Gender factors also account for much variance. DSM-IV Axis V scoring clearly needs adjustment in non-Western societies where expectations may be different, as are social reactions to disability. A twenty-four-year-old Greek American attempted suicide on the eve of his college graduation. His father, a prominent Greek American business man, embraced the prevailing cultural idea from his background that successful men are self-made and success only comes to the ones who try hard enough. His larger-than-life figure was supported by an actually very insecure core, which led him to be overly critical of his son in whom he saw his inadequate self. The patient was convinced that no matter how hard he tried he would be unable to measure up to his father. Consequently, he had developed a defensive need to be nearly perfect, but his unrealistic demands on himself made him vulnerable to failure, work inhibition, and masochistic defenses such as inability to finish college. This in turn prevented him from the very anxiety-provoking possibility of "being like my father" or even "beating my father at his own game."

Clinician/Patient relationship: The exploration of this domain can potentially yield information crucial to successful treatment. Whether the patient shares the same cultural background of the therapist or is culturally from a world apart, he develops transferential reactions which need to be identified. Equally important is the understanding of the doctor's countertransference toward the patients and how cultural factors may play a role. Much of our residents' understanding about cultural bias and cultural "blind spots" have come from this section. In another seminar that is entirely devoted to identification and handling of counter transference, cultural factors constantly emerge as a fundamental for shedding light on the patient/clinician interaction. A thirty-year-old Polish patient admitted to the inpatient with depression and obsessive compulsive disorder was assigned to a Polish resident. She rapidly developed a strong positive transference toward the resident, who was seen as being from the same background and language. Her compliance and response to treatment were both excellent and when she was discharged she continued to be followed by the resident on an outpatient basis. After one month in the outpatient the patient became noncompliant with treatment, stopped taking her medications, and began to ventilate anger and hostility at the resident. An analysis of the process as well as the patient-resident relationship uncovered that the initial glowing transferential reaction had been replaced by a highly defensive negative one, which could be traced to her ambivalent relationship with an older sister whom she perceived as preferred by her mother. The patient had developed toward the resident the same feelings of inferiority, hostility, envy, and competitiveness she had experienced with her sister. Identifying and containing the resident's opposing countertransferential reactions was challenging but instrumental for the continuation of treatment.

Overall Cultural Formulation: This is a summary of the most relevant findings that may help highlight the most prominent dynamics of the case.

A thirty-seven-year-old African American from North Carolina was admitted with a diagnosis of alcohol dependence and major depression. Upon admission he identified himself as being a Southern Baptist, a faith that stresses profound family ties, strong work ethics, stoicism in the face of adversities, high moral values, and a strong belief in sin. Both patient and his family believed that by drinking excessively he had "turned from God." His family also expressed disdain about the patient's life choices, that is, moving to New York, studying Russian and Spanish and marrying a "white Russian" immigrant. His illness was perceived by the family as incurable, unresponsive to conventional medical treatment. His only hope for recovery from "walking off from Jesus" was "spiritualist" healing by a reverend at his congregation. The event that precipitated his depression and relapse into alcoholism was the death of his mother by breast cancer sixty days prior to his hospitalization. The patient had not visited his mother before she died or during her illness although he was distinguished in the family as being her "favorite son." While he had claimed to have no social support, he was visited by a large number of family members with whom he seemed to assume a "sick role." The patient had a good rapport with the resident although he expressed some doubts that she would understand his culture of origin. The resident verbalized some puzzlement at the dogmatic rigidity of his faith but overall empathized by feeling sorry about his depression and self-destructive behavior. Clearly he had ambivalent feelings about his cultural background. Although he had identified himself as Southern Baptist he broke away from its norms in several ways. On the surface he had rejected his culture, but he remained heavily influenced by it with his pervasive guilt about sinning and feelings of unworthiness. Seeking an identity of his own, he had embraced other cultures and other languages but his "cultural conscience" continued to haunt him after his mother died, ravaged by guilt about having abandoned her as well his family. This patient's apparent rejection of his cultural norms masked deep psychological conflicts which originated in his family dynamics. Uncomfortable with the idea of being the mother's favorite he developed defense mechanisms to deal with his anxiety, such as excessive drinking and masochistic acting out at work. Interestingly, over the years he had come to embrace those concepts he had rejected, that he was unworthy, because mentally ill, that he had sinned and beyond help and that his life had been a useless and unproductive waste.

The resident was instructed to elicit core belief systems related to his anxiety about being her mother's favorite and how, within the family dynamics this idea explained his ambivalence toward his culture of origin.

In conclusion, cultural formulation outline can be used as a road into the exploration of patients' dynamics. This is mostly due to the outline's versatility of its elements, as they allow the clinician to reach into domains of psychodynamic interest with considerable overlap between the two. From a purely academic viewpoint this juxtaposition allows for teaching layers of complexity a student might otherwise not be able to grasp. It also gives the teacher the possibility of reframing the meaning of the words *culture* and *cultural*, which at times are used as meaningless clichés that interfere with deeper understanding. For the educator, the challenge remains to continuously refine creative ways to teach how to understand the patient's biopsychocultural core without overlooking important nuances and most of all without losing sight of his human side.

References

1. Mezzich, J. E. (1996). *Culture and psychiatric diagnosis: A DSM-IV perspective.* Washington, DC: American Psychiatric Press.

2. Alarcon, R. D. (1995). Culture and psychiatric diagnosis: Impact on DSM-IV and ICD-10. *Psychiatric Clinics of North America*, 18, 449–455.

3. Kleinman, A. (1988). *Rethinking psychiatry.* New York: Free Press.

4. Good, B. J. and Good, M-J. D. (1986). The cultural context of diagnosis and therapy: A view, from medical anthropology. In M. R. Miranda and H. H. L. Kitano (Eds.) *Mental health research and practice in minority communities.* U.S. Department of Health and Human services, Publication No. (DDM) 96-1466). Washington, DC: Government Printing Office.

5. Mezzich, J. E. (1995). Cultural formulation and comprehensive diagnosis: Clinical and research perspectives. *Psychiatric Clinics of North America* 18, 649–658.

6. American Psychiatric Association. (1994). *Diagnostic and statistical manual of mental disorders,* 4th Edition (DSM-IV) Washington, DC: American Psychiatric Association.

7. Alarcon, R. D.; Foulks, E. F.; Vakkur, M. (1988). *Personality disorders and culture.* New York: John Wiley and Son.

8. Gabbard, G. O. (1994). *Psychodynamic psychiatry in clinical practice.* American Psychiatric Association.

9. Bieber, I. (1980). *Cognitive psychoanalysis.* Lanham, MD: Jason Aronson.

14

Introducing the Cultural Formulation to Mental Health Care in Stockholm, Sweden

Sofie Bäärnhielm

I WOULD LIKE TO TALK ABOUT my experiences of introducing the Cultural Formulation (CF) to Mental Health Care in Stockholm, Sweden. These experiences come from the training of clinicians and from beginning to apply the CF in a clinical context.

I am a psychiatrist and the head of the Transcultural Centre in Stockholm, which is a knowledge center for transcultural psychiatry and asylum and refugee care in the county of Stockholm. Before discussing my experiences with the CF in Sweden it might be helpful if I say a few words about the Swedish context.

First, a very rough view of cultural diversity in Sweden, the official Swedish policy toward cultural diversity, the organizational model of providing mental health care, and how mental health care in Sweden has responded to cultural diversity. I shall also say something about my views regarding needs for future development. Much of this first part is included in a paper written for the journal *Transcultural Psychiatry.* After a condensed presentation of the Swedish context I shall talk about psychiatric assessment and experiences of introducing the CF in Stockholm. My final point consists of reflections on the future development of the Cultural Formulation.

The Swedish Context

Cultural Diversity and Official Policy

Sweden has become a multicultural society mainly through immigration. Sweden is a country that has experience of mass emigration. It is estimated

Presented at the symposium "The Cultural Formulation: International Perspectives" World Psychiatric Association Conference on Psychiatry and Its Contemporary Context, New York, April 30, 2004

that more then 25 percent of the population once emigrated, mainly to the United States. People emigrated for economic, religious, and political reasons.

Immigration to Sweden has taken place mainly since World War II. We have almost 9 million inhabitants and almost 12 percent were born outside Sweden (see table 14.1 for population statistics). Until the mid-1970s, immigration was primarily labor-force-related, mostly from Europe. There were, however, small groups of refugees from Eastern Europe. At that time, the manufacturing sector in Sweden was able to expand with the help of an immigrant labor force.

Immigration of labor was basically stopped in 1972 for people born out-

TABLE 14.1
Swedish Statistics

Population	2002 8,940,788			
Foreign-born	1970 537,585	1980 626,953	1990 790,445	2002 1,053,463
Foreign-born: % of total population	6.7	7.8	9.2	11.8

	Population by Country of Birth 2002
Sweden	7,887,325
Foreign-born	1,053,463
The Nordic Countries	279,570
(1. Finland 2. Norway 3. Denmark)	
Europe other than Nordic Countries	343,782
(1. former Yugoslavia, 2. Bosnia-Herzegovina, 3. Germany)	
Africa	59,507
(1. Somalia 2. Ethiopia 3. Morocco).	
North America	
(1. USA)	25,450
South America	
(1. Chile, 2. Argentina 3. Bolivia)	53,638
Asia	
(1. Iran 2. Turkey 3. Lebanon)	280,916
Former USSR	7,285
Oceania	3,285
Unknown country	353

Statistics Sweden, *Statistical Year Book* (Stockholm: Nordstedts, 2004).

side the Nordic countries. The same year, a door was opened to refugees and asylum seekers. As a consequence, immigration to Sweden during the past thirty years has mainly been through people who seek asylum and family reunions. Since the 1970s, the cultural background of the immigrant population has shifted from being mainly Nordic and European to more non-European.

The official Swedish model includes an acceptance of cultural diversity and of equal rights for minorities. Immigrant policy is based on ideas of equality, freedom of choice, and partnership. However, there is a gap between official policy and reality. Since the beginning of the 1980s, immigrants have found it difficult to get jobs, especially immigrants born outside Europe. Many immigrants, and especially newly arrived refugees, have settled in poor and exposed suburbs of the major cities in Sweden. There is an increasing segregation in Swedish society.

Mental Health Care in Sweden

The health care system in Sweden is based on everyone's equal right to health care and is state funded. Development of mental health care in Sweden during the past century shares many similarities with other Western nations and has included a shift toward community-based care. Today, mental health care is organized in sectors with responsibility for the population in geographically defined catchment areas.

Responding to Cultural Diversity

I consider the response to immigration and cultural diversity in mental health care in Sweden to have included three waves: first, responses to language, then responses to trauma and the stress of immigration, and lately also an interest in responding to cultural and ethnic diversity.

The interest in cultural psychiatry in Sweden grew at the end of the 1990s in psychiatric clinics encountering the new multicultural population in the segregated suburban areas. The interest in culture started out in the margin of the mental health care system and is still mainly in the margin.

However, I perceive a growing awareness also within mainstream psychiatry for the importance of responding to cultural diversity. I think that today in Sweden, mental health care is at the crossroads of choosing its future direction: either it takes up the challenge raised by immigration of an increasing cultural diversity or it satisfies itself with rhetoric, thus leaving reality in the margin.

Psychiatric Assessment and Experiences of Using the Cultural Formulation

Psychiatric Assessment

I consider understanding and evaluating the impact of culture in psychiatric assessment and diagnosis to be a pivotal concern for mental health care in Sweden. Addressing this issue is important with regard to both the individual patient and the development of mental health service delivery.

In the way mental health care is organized today in Sweden, psychiatric diagnosis is central for understanding and helping the patient. Diagnoses are also the core of the system regarding statistics, registrations, evaluations of treatment outcomes, and so forth, thus affecting future development of mental care and research.

Experiences of Using the Cultural Formulation

In Sweden the ICD-10 and DSM-IV are used. ICD-10 is used in patient care and DSM-IV in outpatient care and research. DSM-IV has had a great impact and is widely accepted within psychiatry. The quick reference to DSM-IV has been translated into Swedish but not the entire manual. The Cultural Formulation has not been translated and is not well-known among clinicians. I first learned of its existence from Professor Laurence Kirmayer of McGill University. He has been lecturing in cultural psychiatry at an annual one-week course in Stockholm and has presented the CF.

My view of the importance of understanding and evaluating the impact of culture in psychiatric assessment and diagnosis originates from three sources. The first is many years of clinical practice in a very multicultural and segregated suburban area of Stockholm. The second is my PhD work in which I explored meaning and restructuring of meaning among a group of Turkish- and Swedish-born female patients assessed as somatizing. I have also explored the views of their caregivers. The third source is my current work at the Transcultural Centre in Stockholm. The Centre provides, among other things, training, networking, and consultations to clinicians in psychiatry for the whole Stockholm area. Through this work I have come into contact with other clinicians' experiences. A central problem area brought up by clinicians in their consultations at the Centre has been their difficulties with cross-cultural psychiatric assessments and their experiences of having insufficient tools to evaluate the impact of culture in individual clinical cases.

When it comes to research about mental health care and cultural diversity in Sweden, this has until now focused on immigrants' health situation and on trauma. Few studies in Sweden have focused on the interaction between mental health care and cultural groups. There are some indications that there may be an underutilization of mental health care among some immigrant groups.

There is also some evidence pointing to problems with cross-cultural psychiatric assessment. In a doctoral thesis, Al Saffar (2003) looked at the distribution of different patient groups in the multicultural area of Stockholm where I worked previously. She used statistics from 1993 and found differences in psychiatric diagnoses for ethnic groups. Africans ran a higher risk than others of receiving a diagnosis of psychotic disorder—except schizophrenia. Greek patients were more likely to receive a diagnosis of somatoform disorder, and native Swedes to receive a diagnosis of personality disorder. Al Saffar does not offer any explanation as to the differences. It might be that the figures correspond to some form of reality. They can also be related to differences in help-seeking patterns and difficulties with cross-cultural psychiatric assessment.

Current statistics from the same multicultural area show some differences with other less multicultural areas in the same part of Stockholm. For example, there is a lower frequency of bipolar disorder and a higher frequency of nonspecific psychosis in the multicultural area compared with neighboring areas. The differences may be linked to differences in expressions of distress among patients, to help-seeking patterns, and also to difficulties with cross-cultural assessments.

Clinicians failing to understand the patient's expressions of distress and misdiagnosing mental illness affect each individual patient but also the future development of services and care. Just to give an example: work is currently being carried out in Swedish psychiatry to create national registers of treatment and treatment outcome for bipolar disorder and first episode schizophrenia. Clinical problems in identifying bipolar disorders and correctly diagnosing schizophrenia among patients in multicultural areas may have an effect on the future development of care.

Using the Cultural Formulation

Experiences of Using the Cultural Formulation

And now a few words about my experience of using the CF (Bäärnhielm 2000, 2003). At the Transcultural Centre where I work we have started to introduce the CF to clinicians and residents in training. I have also started to introduce it into clinical practice at the outpatient clinic in the multicultural area where I worked earlier. My experience of the CF is limited, and I can therefore only give you my first impressions.

My overall impression is that it is very important that the CF is included in DSM-IV. I also find very important the fact that it is suggested in the introduction to DSM-IV that the symptoms and course of a number of disorders are influenced by cultural and ethnic factors. The introduction also points to the importance of ethnic and cultural considerations. In my particular work context, this gives the issue of culture and diagnosing a degree of social acceptance.

Another important aspect with the CF is that it is formulated to promote a narrative approach, which I believe promotes a reflective stance and counteracts ethnical stereotyping and presumptions.

Future Development

After having used the Cultural Formulation, my impression is that there is a need for increased concern about the consequences of immigration, of patients being uprooted, dislocated, and relocated.

The CF points to the importance of referring to the patient's reference group. I found this to be problematic, as many of the patients in our multicultural areas in Sweden are refugees with a restricted affiliation to a clear reference group in their new host society.

One of the categories in the CF is the "Cultural explanations of the individual's illness." The text points to predominant idioms of distress and perceived causes of explanatory models that the individual and the reference group use to explain the illness. I think that the CF tries to grasp something important here, but I would like to suggest that there might be a problem with focusing on causality and explanatory models.

I shall explain how I arrived at my standpoint. As I mentioned earlier, I interviewed a group of Turkish- and Swedish-born women assessed as somatizing, and I asked them how they gave meaning to their illness. This was done in qualitative interview studies. I was initially inspired by the explanatory model perspective. I found that for the Swedish-born patients causal explanation was important and they often had several noncompeting explanations. This was not the case with the Turkish-born patients. For them causal explanation was seldom a core issue. When I asked them to explain I received answers like, "You should know, you are the physician." Sometimes direct interview questions about causal explanations even created confusion. Their attribution pattern was characterized by verbalizing links of coherence between health and aspects of life.

The findings in these studies have left me with the impression that it might be that we need to explore the important issue of patients' perspective of understanding their distress in a broader frame than causal explanations and explanatory models, especially if the patient lacks an alternative medical system to refer to. It has often been the patient's own formulation of his or her problem that has given me access to the patient's meaning.

In order to continue with the work of introducing the CF in Sweden we need to translate it, implement it in training, write guidelines about how to use it, and start clinical research on its application. One aspect of concern with regard to introducing the CF is its meaningfulness for the patient.

The CF is designed to assist the clinician in reporting the impact of the individual's cultural context. I think that we also need to look at the interaction in terms of how the patient perceives the clinician. We need to know whether the CF assists the patient in making psychiatric assessments and categorizations meaningful.

To summarize, in mental health care in Sweden we need to improve our capacity to respond to the increasing cultural diversity of the population. A central issue in this process is that of including the heterogeneity and complexity of the population in psychiatric assessment. To make this a part of the everyday clinical reality we need structured tools like the CF to assist the clinicians.

Finally, I want to thank you for this opportunity to share my still limited experiences of using the CF in Sweden, in this international context.

References

Al Saffar, S. (2003). *Trauma, ethnicity and posttraumatic stress disorder in outpatient psychiatry.* Dissertation, Psychiatry section, Department of Neurotec, Karolinska Institutet, Stockholm, Sweden.

Bäärnhielm, S. (2000). Making sense of suffering. Illness meaning among somatizing Swedish women in contact with local health care services. *Nordic Journal of Psychiatry* 54(6):423–430.

Bäärnhielm, S. (2003). *Clinical encounters with different illness realities: Qualitative studies of illness meaning and restructuring of illness meaning among two cultural groups of female patients in a multiracial area of Stockholm.* Dissertation, Division of Psychiatry, Neurotec Department, Karolinska Institutet, Stockholm, Sweden.

Bäärnhielm, S., and Ekblad, S. (2000). Turkish migrant women encountering health care in Stockholm: A qualitative study of somatization and illness meaning. *Culture, Medicine, and Psychiatry* 24(4):431–452.

Bäärnhielm, S., Ekblad, S., Ekberg, J., and Ginsburg, B. E. (2005). Historical reflections on mental health care in Sweden: The welfare state and cultural diversity, *Transcultural Psychiatry* 42(3):394–419.

15

The Cultural Interview in the Netherlands

The Cultural Formulation in Your Pocket

Hans Rohlof

THE NETHERLANDS is a small and densely populated country in the North East of Europe. In a country of about 200 miles from north to south and 150 miles from east to west, 16 million people are living. In the four large cities Amsterdam, Rotterdam, The Hague, and Utrecht, with their suburbs, around 8 million people are living. This is called "the city of Holland." The Netherlands has been a member of the European community for a long time. It is a kingdom, but the kings submit to the constitution and the parliament has the law-making power. The country is wealthy and prosperous, mainly because of the presence of international companies, a strong and intensified agriculture, the traditional trade firms, the harbor in Rotterdam and the airport in Amsterdam, and the exploitation of natural gas. Since the Second World War there have been no conflicts with other countries or tensions between population groups.

Because of the prosperity the attraction of the Netherlands as a country to work in has been great in the recent past. And because of the peaceful atmosphere a lot of refugees from war-stricken parts of the world sought asylum.

In the Netherlands the number of people who were born outside the country is therefore growing. Of the population of almost 16 million people the number of people who were born outside the country was 1.2 million in 1995, but 1.5 million in 2002. The number of children with at least one of

Presented at the World Psychiatric Association Conference on Psychiatry and Its Contemporary Context, New York, April 30–May 2, 2004

the parents born outside the country was 1.2 in 1995, and 1.4 in 2002 (Centraal Bureau voor de Statistiek, 2002). Responsible for this growth was the large influx of non-Western immigrants and refugees. The number of people who were born in a Western country stayed stable at around half a million, and 800,000 for the second generation. Included in these last numbers were those born in Indonesia, since they were mostly people of Dutch origin living in a former colony (see table 15.1).

The four largest groups of non-Western immigrants were Turks, Moroccans, and people from the former colonies Surinam and the Netherlands Antilles. The last country, a group of islands in the Caribbean, is still a part of the kingdom of the Netherlands, but has its own government. In table 15.2 there is a view of the four largest groups in 2002.

The number of people with a refugee background is also growing. In 2002 there were 56,000 people who were born in former Yugoslavia; 36,000 people from Iraq; 23,000 from Iran; 28,000 from Afghanistan; 21,000 from Somalia; and 11,000 from Vietnam. These numbers are only about the legal inhabitants, and do not take into account the number of asylum seekers and illegal immigrants.

Because of these growing numbers we see also more patients from non-Western origin in our mental health care institutions. In 1994 Centrum '45, which is an institution for treatment for people with traumatic experiences from the Second World War (1940–1945), decided to build a branch for the treatment of traumatized refugees. In that year the Bosnian War (1992–1995) was at its height, so many refugees from Bosnia came to Western Europe.

The department for the treatment of traumatized refugees is called *de*

TABLE 15.1
Immigrants in the Netherlands in 2002, in Thousands

	1st generation	2nd generation
Western	575	831
Non-Western	972	587

TABLE 15.2
Largest Non-Western Population Groups in 2002, in Thousands

	Surinam	Turkey	Morocco	Netherlands Antilles
1st generation	186	186	160	82
2nd generation	129	145	125	43

Vonk, which means "the sparkle," which was the original name of its main building, constructed in 1923 for factory girls by a liberal spouse of a factory owner.

In the center there are twenty-seven clinical beds for refugees and also for their children when they cannot be abandoned, with a maximum of five children. There is also a day clinic with five different groups, whose participants come for one day in the week. This puts the number of day clinical chairs at forty. The outpatient units in Amsterdam and Noordwijkerhout give ambulant treatment to 400 new patients every year, with a total number of 5,900 ambulant visits.

The patients in the center come from more then fifty different countries. The largest numbers of patients are from Bosnia, the Middle East, the former Soviet Union republics, and West Africa. Surprisingly, people from Vietnam and Somalia are rarely seen in the clinic.

The Cultural Interview

In the "de Vonk" center the patients show all kind of symptoms that can be described as post-traumatic. They have experienced all kinds of traumatic situations, such as war, imprisonment, persecution, violence and torture, and loss of family members and belongings. The symptoms they show are part of the post-traumatic stress disorder as described in DSM-IV, but are also of a different nature. Patients show delusions and hallucinations that can be ascribed to former traumatic events. Also, they very often have somatic complaints that could be explained by psychological problems and traumatic experiences. These clinical impressions about the patients were confirmed by a research project in which a larger number of post-traumatic complaints were found that the DSM-IV describes (Ghane, 2003). In addition, clinicians in the center often have problems with communication about symptoms and about treatment options. About half of the patients are not able to communicate in a Western language such as English, French, German, or Dutch—languages most clinicians in the Netherlands are able to speak. So the use of interpreters in the center is needed. But even with interpreters, miscommunication about information and about expectations in treatment are not rare.

More cultural information was also needed. The Cultural Formulation of DSM-IV (American Psychiatric Association, 2000) seemed to be a good format to obtain more information about cultural identity, cultural illness explanations and treatment expectations, and cultural factors in support seeking and stress. This Cultural Formulation, as described in the case report in the journal *Culture, Medicine, and Psychiatry* seemed to be an instrument that could be used at the end of a treatment. Wanted was an instrument that could implement the Cultural Formulation during the assessment procedure.

Therefore the so-called Cultural Interview was constructed (Rohlof et al., 2002). This is a structured interview of about forty questions (see appendix). With the completion of the interview, one could make a cultural formulation of a given patient during the assessment procedure. A disadvantage could be that after completing the interview the clinician may have the tendency to forget about the cultural aspects of the treatment. The Cultural Formulation begins with the Cultural Interview, but it does not end with it.

Experiences

After the construction of the interview, thirty patients were interviewed. The experiences with the interviews were presented elsewhere (Loevy et al., 2000). The interview turned out to be feasible, taking about one and a half hours, depending on the patient, the interviewer, and the presence of an interpreter. The interview was even considered as pleasant by most patients, since they were able to talk about good things in their past, and not about the bad experiences or their symptoms. The interview asked about events, behaviors, and attitudes in the culture of origin, and thus denied in a way the reality that the patients lived in a new culture: the immigrant culture in the Netherlands. However, that aspect seemed to be less important.

With the interview it was possible to gather much information from the cultural background of the patient. It was enough to make a cultural formulation of the patient. Several findings were:

1. Beginning therapists tend to take the interview as a more rigid structure than experienced therapists. The latter tend to ask their own questions, which leads in some cases to the gathering of less relevant data.
2. The structure of the interview with the beginning asking about cultural identity (as in the Cultural Formulation) makes the interviewee feel at ease. The questions about the cultural backgrounds of the complaints were more difficult and less pleasant to answer.
3. It is helpful to give the patient examples from Dutch culture, for example, asking about the most important thing in life can be illustrated by telling about the practice of having a wall plate with the family maxim by the fireplace.
4. In the interview, questions about conflicts with cultural things were avoided. This is something to keep in mind. Sometimes patients can have conflicts with, for instance, their Muslim background.

5. The interview proved to be important in the process of building a better image of the patient. For clinicians it is common to make stereotypical assumptions about a patient from the first look. The interview can help to create a more detailed image.
6. The interview is better taken by a third person, rather than the patient's own therapist. This improves the objectivity of the interview (Rohlof and Ghane, 2003).

In the meantime, the third improved edition of the Cultural Interview in Dutch has been made. Translations into English and German are complete, and a translation into Spanish is in preparation. The interview is used in mental health care, in general health care, and in research. Although the interview needs more scientific elaboration, such as the clustering of questions, and perhaps also a more quantitative approach, it has been instrumental in increasing the interest in the Cultural Formulation in the Netherlands.

Culture, Classification, and Diagnosis

In 2000, Ria Borra, Rob van Dijk, and Hans Rohlof decided to publish a book on transcultural diagnostics using the Cultural Formulation and the cultural interview and asked other authors to write case histories according to the Cultural Formulation. This resulted in a book (Borra et al., 2002) with three theoretical chapters, seventeen case histories, a concluding chapter, and the text of the cultural interview. The book, *Culture, Classification, and Diagnosis* illustrates that a classification according DSM-IV is far from a real diagnosis and that culture is a missing link in the practice of classification. In the Netherlands the book was greeted as a welcome guidebook for transcultural cases.

The concluding chapter of the book recorded some comments on the Cultural Formulation. Gaps in the Cultural Formulation were described, such as the failure to mention aspects of communicating in different languages and the use and role of interpreters. In addition, there is not much attention to the culture of mental health care itself: what does the patient think about talking and insight-oriented therapies, for example. Also, the interest of subcultures in the culture of origin should be stressed more. Culture is not static, but dynamic, especially for recent migrants, who tend to take cultural behavior and attitudes from the host country or from the migrant culture in the host country very quickly. Finally, there should not be any overemphasis on culture. Culture does not account for all differences between population groups. Social and economic factors are also important. There are also differences in power and in accessibility to health care systems. Stigmatization plays also a big role.

In 2003, a conference took place to introduce the book into Dutch mental health care. From the lectures of this conference a new book was published (van Dijk et al., 2003). The discussion about cultural factors in mental health care has not ended. New plans arise. The section on Transcultural Psychiatry of the Netherlands Psychiatric Association, which was founded in 2003, sees it as an important task to comment on the basic concepts in psychiatry, in assessment, therapy, and research. One of its activities in 2003 was to comment on the new protocol for the assessment procedure published by the Netherlands Psychiatric Association. At the moment a small working group is busy constructing a new format for assessment in psychiatry, with attention to cultural data. Work in this field proceeds. To be continued.

References

Borra, R., van Dijk, R., and Rohlof, H. (Eds.). (2002). *Cultuur, classificatie en diagnose.* Houten: Bohn, Stafleu van Loghum.

Centraal Bureau voor de Statistiek. (2002). *Allochtonen in Nederland.* Voorburg/Heerlen: CBS.

Ghane, S. (2003). *An exploration of posttraumatic reactions among treatment-seeking refugees.* Amsterdam: University of Amsterdam.

Loevy, N., Rohlof, H., and Sassesn, L. (2000). *Een gestructureerd interview voor de culturele formulering van de DSM-IV bij vluchtelingen.* Lecture presented at the conference Cultuur en Gezondheid, Amsterdam.

Rohlot, H., Loevy, N., Sassen, L., and Hehnich, S. (2002). The cultural interview. In R. Borra, R. van Dijk,and H. Rohlof (Eds.), *Cultuur, classificatie en diagnose.* Houten: Bohn, Stafleu van Loghuin.

Rohlof, H. and Ghane, S. (2003). Het culturele interview. In R. Van Dijk and N. Sönmez, (Eds.), *Cultuursensitief werken met DSM-IV.* Rotterdam: Mikado.

Van Dijk, R. and Sönmez, N. (Eds.). (2003). *Cultuursensitief werken met DSM-IV.* Rotterdam: Mikado.

Internet:
www.rohlof.nl
www.centrum45.nl
www.mikado-ggz-nl

Appendix:
The Cultural Formulation Interview

English version
Hans Rohlof, Noa Loevy, Lineke Sassen, and Stephanie Helmich

Summary and Case History

Filled in using the dossier before the interview.

1. Biography (personal and social details)
2. History of current symptoms
3. Earlier treatments
4. Psychiatric illness within the family
5. Course of illness

Introduction

Aim: explaining the interview and setting the tone.

"People from all over the world come to our clinic. Every country and every culture has its own way of life. You only really notice when you leave your own country and go to live in a foreign country. People look different, speak another language, behave and express themselves in different ways. We can sometimes get the feeling that we are not understood. Have you ever had that feeling? (If yes, listen briefly to explanation—'we will deal with this later on in the interview.' If no, 'Maybe you will understand what I mean when we discuss it later.')

"Problems in communication are sometimes partly the result of a lack of knowledge of cultural differences. Since we would like to help you as best we can, it is important for us to understand something of your country and your culture. By this we mean your way of life, which days you celebrate, what it means for you to be ill, and so on.

"I will now ask you a few questions about your culture and your symptoms."

A. Cultural Identity of the Individual

What is your native language?

What language do you speak at home/ with your friends/ in your dreams?

What other language(s) do you speak?

How well do you speak Dutch? How does it feel to always have to speak Dutch? Does it sometimes cause problems?

To which ethnic group do you officially belong? Do you feel that you do belong to this ethnic group, or to another one? Does this ever change? (e.g., do you always feel that you are ____ or sometimes something else?)

Do you miss other people having the same cultural background as yourself. (If yes:) Explain/ Why?

What aspects of your culture are most important to you. (e.g., family structures, norms and values, feast days, faith . . .)

Do you have children?

(If they have children:) Do you bring up your children in the same way that you were brought up? Explain.

(If no children:) Would you bring up your children in the same way? Explain.

To what extent can you follow your culture's way of life here in the Netherlands? Are their aspects of your culture that bother you or that you find less attractive?

Do you feel involved with Dutch culture (E.g., do you interact much with Dutch people, do you go to Dutch social events, do you read Dutch literature, are you interested in how things work in Dutch society, are there things in the Dutch culture which you are adopting . . .) ?

If so, what aspects of Dutch culture do you like, and what aspects bother you?

B. Cultural Explanations of the Individual's Illness

(Record explanation in individual's native language)

Now, about your symptoms,

What are your worst symptoms? What do you call them in your own language?

How do you think your symptoms started? (If only single answer: do you think that there are alternative/more explanations for your symptoms?)

How do your friends, family, and those around you explain your symptoms? How would people of your culture explain your symptoms?

Do you feel understood by your friends, family, and those around you?

Have you felt up to now that the staff here understand you? Would you expect them to?

If someone in your home community was sick, or had roughly the same symptoms as you, how would those around them try to help (e.g., pray for them, leave them to rest, care for them)?

Are you being cared for in that way now?

Do people where you come from sometimes make use of alternative, native, or faith healers, or do people go to a normal doctor or hospital?

What kind of help have you had up to now for your symptoms (both normal and alternative)? What helped most?

What kind of treatment would you like to receive now? What would you personally prefer?

(Examples: Talking about events in the past, adapting to the present, make plans for the future, talking about your emotions, receive advice, exercises, medicines . . .)

C. Cultural Factors in Psychosocial Surroundings and in Functioning

Now, let's discuss your daily life here rather than your daily life in your native country.

What is your current situation—are you married, do you have a family here?

What is your position in you family? Is this different to the situation in your country of origin? Explain.

Is there someone in your family who people go to for advice?

(If married:) How is your relationship with your spouse? Is this different to what it was in your country of origin? Explain.

(If has a family:) How is your relationship with your family? Is this different to what it was in your country of origin? Explain.

Have there been important changes in your social position in recent years? If yes: what does this mean for you?

If you have a practical problem, such as something you do not understand (e.g., train journeys, the immigration service, a letter from your lawyer), whom would you ask about it? From whom would you get the information?

If you had (emotional) difficulties in your own country, what did you do? To whom did you go?

Is there someone in the Netherlands from whom you receive (emotional) support (e.g., when you are sad)? Is this person family of yours? How often do you make use of this opportunity?

Is there someone in the Netherlands with whom you talk about your symptoms and traumatic experiences? (If yes:) Why him/her? Is there someone you would like to talk to? Explain. Some people are greatly strengthened by their faith. Are you religious?

Do you pray? How often?

Do you feel that prayer helps you? In what way?

Has your faith changed since the experiences you had? Do you still pray as often as you did?

Do your prayers help you as much as they did?

Do you go to a place of worship (church, mosque, etc.) in the Netherlands? Do you always go to the same one? How often do you go? Do you know the people there?

Do those people help you? Is there someone in particular who helps you? In what way do they do that?

D. Cultural Elements in the Relationship between the Individual and the Career

To which social class did you belong in your country of origin? Did you live in a town or in the countryside? What education have you had?

Some people consider clinical staff to be their equals, sometimes even their friends. Others feel that the staff are above them, or beneath them. How do you see this? Do you feel that the medical staff and social workers are equal to you, beneath you, or above you? When they advise something or prescribe medicines do you feel that you must take the advice or use the medicines?

If you had a free choice in selecting the personnel treating you, would you prefer male or female personnel? (As a choice:) Why? (trust, shame, more likely to understand, easier to express yourself . . .)

If you had a free choice in selecting the personnel treating you, would you prefer personnel with a similar cultural background to yourself, or do you not think that this matters? (As a choice:) Why? (trust, shame, more likely to understand, easier to express yourself . . .)

How do you feel about the fact that you don't receive therapy in your own language? Would you like to be given therapy in your own language? Would it help you feel that you were being understood properly?

(If an interpreter is being used:) How does it feel to work with an interpreter? If you could choose would you prefer a male or a female interpreter?

This is the end of the interview. Thank you very much indeed. I personally found it very interesting to learn about how these things work outside the Netherlands, and I hope that we can use what you have told me to understand and help you better.

Is there anything else that has not been mentioned in this discussion and that you would like to tell me about?

To be completed by interviewer after interview (optional, some matters will only become clear during the course of the treatment):

Communication problems experienced within the patient's own language (use of terms/concepts and motivation/interest)
Extent to which symptoms have a cultural meaning for the patient
To what extent is the patient prepared to engage in a working relationship with the therapist?
Degree of closeness (personal contact)
Pathology or otherwise of behavior.

E. Observations during the Interview

What was the contact with the client like? What kind of impression did he/she make? Record other notable issues from the conversation.

F. Summary

Summary of the most important issues raised during the interview.

G. Advice for Further Treatment

Possible problems in the area of cultures that could be an obstacle communicating with patient and specifying the diagnosis and the treatment. At the same time, things can be noted that can be looked at in treatment.

Part IV

Clinical Case Illustrations on the Cultural Formulation

AMONG THE MANY PUBLISHED CASES prepared following the DSM-IV Cultural Formulation Outline, we selected the following five because of their clinical interest and their value in illustrating cultural influences on diagnosis and care.

Lim and Lin's (1996) account of psychosis in a Chinese immigrant who practiced Qigong shows how a particular traditional exercise may contribute to the emergence of serious psychopathology. It also illustrates the nuances of illness presentation in China, including the frequent somatic expressions of psychiatric disorder.

Lewis-Fernandez's (1996) case illustrates diagnosis and treatment of *nervios* and *ataques* in a female Puerto Rican migrant. The author documents how the erroneous interpretation of culturally mediated idioms of distress may lead to inappropriate treatment choices and deleterious consequences for the patient.

Oquendo and Graver (1997) present a cultural formulation for an Indian woman with major depression cared for by a Latina therapist. It discusses the conflicts generated in a patient by the struggle between family cultural values and recently acquired Western values as seen by a therapist of a different ethnic and cultural background.

Yilmaz and Weiss (2000) offer a cultural formulation of a young male Turkish immigrant in Basel, Switzerland, who experiences depression and back pain. They illustrate how the Cultural Formulation Outline enriches understanding of various aspects of clinical problems and can be helpful for treatment planning.

Browne (2001) presents the case of a twenty-nine-year-old Javanese woman with a complex psychopathological picture experienced as a disturbance of mental and spiritual balance. The relevance of the cultural framework to understand the clinical case and design a treatment plan is indeed compelling.

16

Psychosis Following Qi-Gong in a Chinese Immigrant

Russell F. Lim and Keh-Ming Lin

Clinical History

PATIENT IDENTIFICATION. Mr. A is a fifty-seven-year-old married Chinese-American man with no previous psychiatric history who presented at the psychiatrist's office in 1989 with a three-week history of auditory hallucinations and delusions.

History of present illness. The patient was in his normal state of good health until two years prior to presentation, when he stared developing intermittent acute backaches. He went to his physician and was told that he had kidney stones. Conventional medical treatment did not provide much alleviation of his symptoms, and Mr. A gradually lost confidence in his Western-trained physician. Mr. A's back pain continued to flare up intermittently. After almost two years of treatment failures, Mr. A was willing to try treatments from China. Three weeks prior to evaluation, he started practicing Qi-gong, a Chinese folk health-enhancing practice similar to Tai Chi, which consists of controlled, synchronized breathing and body movements, and is expected to have curative effects on physical illnesses. His practice of Qi-gong was intensive. Several days after starting these practices, he developed delusional and hallucinatory experiences, which he had never experienced before. These conditions persisted and intensified, interfering with his concentration, and prevented him from working as an engineer. His auditory hallucinations

From *Culture, Medicine, and Psychiatry* 20, no. 3, 369–78 (September 1996) with kind permission from Springer Science and Business Media

consisted of voices of supernatural beings communicating with him regarding how he should practice Qi-gong and delusions that he was contacting beings from another dimension. He returned to the Qi-gong masters for help, but they were unable to provide any relief. His wife, who was a registered nurse, became increasingly concerned over his inability to work. She consulted with a Caucasian psychiatrist co-worker from their health maintenance organization (HMO) who referred her husband to a Chinese-American psychiatrist in private practice. On presentation, the patient denied depressed mood, suicidal ideation, racing thoughts, spending sprees, insomnia, anxiety, substance abuse, appetite or weight changes, and showed no pressured speech.

Psychiatric history and previous treatment. None.

Social and development history. Mr. A was born in Fukien Province, China. He is the oldest of four children with a younger brother and two younger sisters. His parents owned their own import/export company and passed away in Taiwan several years ago. He had an uneventful childhood and moved with his parents and siblings at age eighteen to Taiwan in 1949, after the Communist takeover of mainland China. He completed college in Taiwan and earned a bachelor's degree, and migrated to the United States to obtain a doctorate in engineering. He met and married his wife while he was in graduate school, and he has been married for thirty years. The couple has two children, a son, age twenty-five, and a daughter, age twenty-three. Mr. A has worked as an engineer for over thirty years. He lives with his wife; his two children are married, have families of their own, and have moved out of the area.

Family history. Family psychiatric history was denied. This does not rule out the possibility that he may have been concealing some family secrets, as many Chinese patients are unlikely to discuss mental illness in the family with strangers or health professionals because having a mentally ill relative could subject the family to subsequent discrimination that could preclude marriage opportunities and undermine social connections. However, the examining psychiatrist felt that Mr. A was sincere in his account of his family history.

Course and outcome. Extensive medical evaluation including SMA-20, thyroid function, VDRL, physical exam, EEG, and an MRI revealed no medical or neurological abnormalities that could explain his mental changes. Mr. A was given a diagnosis of schizophreniform disorder versus schizophrenia, paranoid type, and was treated with low doses of haloperidol, which appeared to reduce substantially his hallucinations and delusional thinking, and prevented him from being hospitalized. At the same time, Mr. A stopped his practice of Qi-gong, because he felt it was not helping him. His ability to concentrate improved, but he still had some residual difficulty. It was unclear if the haloperidol or the cessation of the practice of Qi-gong was responsible for the changes. However, along with these improvements, he also complained of severe akathisia and other side effects, which were not relieved by anticholinergic medication or by the reduction of the dosage of haloperidol from 4 mg to 2 mg per day. After two months of treatment at the clinic, he refused to return for follow-up visits and stopped his medication, despite the fact that he continued to experience the psychotic symptoms that prevented him from returning to work.

Diagnostic Formulation

Axis I:	295.40 Schizophreniform disorder, provisional, with good prognostic features 295.30 R/o Schizophrenia, paranoid type, moderate
Axis II:	Undetermined
Axis III:	Urolithiasis
Axis IV:	Unemployment
Axis V:	Highest past year: GAF = 75 Current: GAF = 35

Cultural Formulation

A. Cultural Identity

Cultural reference group. Mr. A is a first-generation Chinese immigrant from Fukien Province, China. He identifies strongly with his Chinese heritage and also identifies with his adopted country, the United States. He considers himself to be a Chinese-American. Like most members of the first wave of Chinese refugees from the Communist government, Mr. A made a rapid and successful adaptation to Taiwan, suffering only mild difficulties from his dislocation. His migration to the United States was also uneventful. He became a naturalized American citizen and acculturated significantly to his host society. He could be regarded as fully bicultural, exhibiting minimal difficulties interacting with mainstream American society, yet at the same time still maintaining ties with Chinese-American and other Chinese communities. Mr. A often returned to Taiwan to visit his parents until they passed away a few years ago.

Language. His primary language is the Fukien dialect of Chinese, but he also speaks Mandarin. He was able to communicate with his psychiatrist in

English and used Mandarin when he could not express certain aspects of his experiences in English.

Cultural factors in development. Mr. A underwent two distinct migrations during his late adolescence and young adulthood. His move to the United States was prompted by his parents, who felt that he had to leave Taiwan because they believed the Communist government in China posed a constant threat of invasion for the Taiwanese. This second migration involved separating from his family of origin and leaving behind friends and other relatives. His repeated dislocations did delay some important adult milestones, such as marriage, but on the whole Mr. A has been able to adjust very well to his changing situation. He is married, has successful children, and has a good career. At the time of the onset of his psychosis, he was looking forward to continuing his role as chief breadwinner for his family. Losing his ability to work resulted in an unexpected role change into being dependent upon others, and resulted in a loss of self-esteem.

Involvement with culture of origin. He has some school friends from Taiwan who live in the United States with whom he keeps in contact by telephone several times a year or during an occasional visit. He celebrates holidays like the lunar new year. He also occasionally watches Chinese-language television and reads Chinese-language newspapers. Having been raised on the mainland of China, he is familiar with folk healing methods such as acupuncture, herbal medicine, and Qi-gong, but he prefers Western medicine.

Involvement with host culture. He is very involved in the host American culture. He watches American television, reads English-language newspapers, and spends time with American-born people of many ethnicities from work, meeting them for dinner, and attending their parties when invited.

B. Cultural Explanations of the Illness

Predominant idioms of distress and local illness categories. Though diagnosed as kidney stones, Mr. A's backaches could constitute a somatic representation of other difficulties in his life. This hypothesis was not investigated during his presentation or treatment, possibly because his psychiatrist gave almost exclusive priority to the psychotic symptoms. However, since his psychosis emerged rapidly and without previous history in a man in late middle age who was driven to use Qi-gong as treatment of a somatic ailment, it may be interesting to consider the possibility of the backaches as a neurasthenic prodrome to his psychotic break. Many Chinese patients are reluctant to express distress in other than somatic terms, since psychological difficulties may be experienced as potentially stigmatizing. *Shenjing shuairuo*, a form of neurasthenia, is a widespread idiom of distress in Chinese communities;

besides bodily pains such as backaches, dizziness, fatigue, and headaches are common. Somatization may in fact be facultative, allowing the patient access to the health care system, and seen only in the initial evaluation or in other selected settings, such as a physician's office. Provided the somatic nature of the ailment is accepted by the clinician, the person may feel free to explain his/her life difficulties without fear of being stigmatized as a mental patient. Finally, somatization can also be seen as a form of cultural bias. The main Western medical paradigm sees the mind and body as separate, whereas the paradigm for most Chinese patients is holistic—no separation between mind and body. Within this paradigm, it is consistent to present with somatic symptoms as an expression of other life difficulties, especially in a physician's office. It is possible that such a paradigmatic difference underlay the interaction between Mr. A and his Chinese-American psychiatrist, despite Mr. A's obvious biculturality and sharing the same ethnicity as the clinician. If so, that would explain why Mr. A's somatic symptoms were not taken into account during his evaluation and treatment, and may partly explain Mr. A's eventual noncompliance.

Meaning and severity of symptoms in relation to cultural norms. The existence of *Qi* (vital force) and the importance of good circulation of Qi throughout the body via special channels is part of the Chinese health model. These concepts do not correspond with the anatomical or physiological systems described by Western medicine. Used as a method of promoting the healthful circulation of Qi, Qi-gong meditation has enjoyed a resurgence in popularity in recent years as a treatment of various physical ailments and as a general health-enhancing practice. Its popularity is not limited to mainland China (where it has been estimated that 25 percent of the population has made use of it), but has extended to other Chinese communities as well in Taiwan, Hong Kong, and North America.

As a normal effect of its practice, Qi-gong is known in Chinese communities to cause increased sensitivity to outside stimuli (experienced as hearing sounds not ordinarily audible), irritability, tension, altered consciousness, and even hallucinations, but these symptoms are usually transient. However, the Chinese psychiatric literature describes a syndrome called "Qi-gong-induced psychosis" characterized by the appearance of auditory hallucinations and delusions after the initiation of Qi-gong in a practitioner who has never experienced these symptoms before and in whom these symptoms remit soon after the cessation of Qi-gong practice. Patients with Qi-gong-induced psychosis do not show any "negative" symptoms of schizophrenia, such as flattening of affect, paucity of speech, and avolition, but tend to have only "positive" symptoms, such as auditory hallucinations. Cases of Qi-gong-induced psychosis can also display a variety of somatic and psychological symptoms such as dizziness and decreased concentration. Treatment approaches may involve the use of antipsychotic medication, but the illness is by definition self-limiting, and should resolve soon after stopping Qi-gong.

Several distinct types of Qi-gong exist. Mr. A was practicing a variety that is most often implicated in causing psychotic symptoms. This type of Qi-gong aims at inducing a trance state in the practitioner in an effort to attain higher levels of consciousness, where communication with other beings is claimed to occur. This variant of Qi-gong is seen as extreme by many practitioners.

The experience described by Mr. A would be considered floridly psychotic not only according to Western psychiatric criteria, but according to Chinese psychiatric norms as well. Notably, his symptoms did not remit after the cessation of Qi-gong, which raises doubts as to the diagnosis of Qi-gong-induced psychosis in his case. However, a clinician who was not familiar with Qi-gong would have felt that Mr. A was more bizarre than he really was. In particular, the thematic content of his delusions regarding communication with supernatural beings was anticipated by his Qi-gong teachers, and is therefore not individually bizarre; the fact that it is held with delusional intensity and is not amenable to reconsideration, however, makes it of psychotic character.

Perceived causes and explanatory models. Mr. A felt that his backaches were preventing him from working efficiently. Initially, he entertained biological explanations typical of Western medicine, such as kidney stones. When this approach was not able to provide relief, however, he returned to his earlier experiences with folk medicine in China and sought out Qi-gong masters. He began to think that his backaches were caused by his Qi circulating in the "wrong directions" in his body, and that by doing exercises involving synchronized deep breathing and rhythmic movements, he could restore the balance of his Qi, and obtain relief from his backaches. He was vaguely aware of the small possibility of some side effects, but took to his practice intensively. It is unclear whether he or his wife knew that his variant of Qi-gong was associated with an increased rate of psychotic reactions, or whether this information would have had any effect on his practice. Once his psychotic symptoms began, however, Mr. A and his wife felt that Qi-gong had a role in the production and shape of his suffering. He sought help first but without avail from his meditation teachers, and then his wife obtained the assistance of a bicultural Chinese-American psychiatrist.

It is clear that Mr. A and his wife shared a fully bicultural and pragmatically driven explanatory model of his ailments. They appeared to prefer Western models as explanations and treatments of choice, given Mr. A's use of Western medicine both initially and during his most acute stage of illness.

But Mr. A was also willing to commit himself to a folk Chinese healing system after his initial treatment option had failed to produce results. Finally, their bicultural explanatory model is also evidenced by their subsequent choice of a Western-trained Chinese-American psychiatrist, apparently in the hope of encompassing both aspects of their biculturality.

Help-Seeking experiences and plans. As discussed under Explanatory Models, Mr. A and his wife pursued a fully bicultural help-seeking pathway. This pattern of help seeking is common among highly acculturated first-generation Chinese-Americans. It differs from the prototypical pathway seen among many recent Chinese immigrants to the West, that starts with the advice of family and friends, then progresses to Chinese folk healers (such as acupuncturists and herbalists), and finally, and only as a last resort, requests the attention of Western-trained physicians. The fact that Mr. A and his wife had lived in the United States for several decades and were employed in mainstream occupations with high remuneration (engineering, nursing) are surely relevant factors. The fact that it was Mr. A's wife who obtained the eventual psychiatric consultation may be due to Mr. A's cultural reliance on a family member as a health system broker, but also to his relative disability due to the psychosis and to his wife's professional credentials as a nurse.

C. Cultural Factors Related to Psychosocial Environment and Levels of Functioning

Social stressors. Mr. A had suffered from recurrent kidney stones prior to the onset of his behavioral changes. He felt inadequate because he was unable to provide for himself as he had done for over thirty years. In this achievement- and work-oriented family, the illness apparently represented a severe blow to their aspirations and self-identity.

Social supports. Typical of many first-generation immigrants, Mr. A has limited sources of social support. These include his wife, who showed a great deal of concern for him, and some friends from Taiwan that speak his dialect whom he can confide in. Although Mr. A was close to his brother, sisters, and children, they were not told of his difficulties. Mr. A felt that he had to maintain his image as a model eldest brother and father, and could not admit to any weaknesses.

Levels of functioning and disability. Mr. A's level of functioning is lower than we would expect for someone of his educational background and experience. The development of his psychotic symptoms and his subsequent loss of concentration has prevented him from continuing his occupation as an engineer.

D. Cultural Elements of the Clinician-Patient Relationship

Intraethnic transference and countertransference. Mr. A seemed to like his Chinese-American psychiatrist, and superficially the congruence between the clinician, the patient, and his wife in terms of language and culture seemed to facilitate their communication. Even at first, however, when Mr. A was still compliant with medications and appointments, he remained somewhat detached from his treatment. This may have been caused by certain subtle differences between the clinician and the patient and his family that were not explored during their interaction. First, the clinician had little experience with Qi-gong and the diagnosis and management of Qi-gong-induced psychosis. This might have limited his acknowledgment of this explanatory model of the patient's illness as well as the range of the treatment options considered. The psychiatrist was more comfortable with biologically based models of psychiatric disorders and with Western nosological systems. This may have been communicated to the patient in an unconscious manner. The absence of neurasthenia and Qi-gong-induced psychosis among the diagnoses to be ruled out probably also weakened the therapeutic rapport, since this left only diagnoses with relatively higher stigma and poorer prognosis, such as schizophreniform disorder and schizophrenia. Second, the fact of a shared ethnic background may account for the relative lack of detail in the patient's history prior to the onset of his psychosis, probably due to intraethnic countertransference. Since Mr. A's personal background was similar to the clinician's, the psychiatrist may have made assumptions about him and not asked as many questions as he normally would had the patient been from a different ethnicity and background. The lack of background information possibly prevented the discovery of past stressors, which would have informed Mr. A's therapy and possibly clarified his prognosis.

Psychological testing. In this case, psychological testing, such as projective testing, was not ordered, but may have been ordered if the psychiatrist were not aware of the cross-cultural limitations of this modality of assessment. If testing had been ordered, adequate materials would have been available, but the results could be misleading, as is often the case with patients from other cultures speaking languages other than English. In order to have meaningful results, psychological tests should undergo an extensive translation process involving forward and back translation, bilingual committee discussion, and linguistic cultural adaptation. Items must be written with attention to the idioms of distress appropriate to the culture. In addition, psychological tests have to be normed on a similar population to that of the patient to give useful comparisons and results. Thus Mr. A would have had little difficulty with the tests, but they may have missed important data because the testing would be done in English, which is not Mr. A's first language. The treating psychiatrist was appropriate in not ordering psychological testing, which would have added little to the understanding of the case.

E. Overall Cultural Assessment

Diagnosis. According to the DSM-IV system, this patient fulfills criteria for schizophreniform disorder. The presence of good premorbid social and occupational functioning and the absence of a blunted or flat affect qualify him for a specifier of "with good prognostic features." In fact, his overall clinical manifestations (the acuteness of his decompensation, the absence of formal thought disorder and "negative" symptoms, and the retention of insight) augur favorably for the possibility of recovery. On the other hand, the schizophreniform diagnosis must be considered provisional, since if symptoms were to persist for more than six months, he would quality for a full diagnosis of schizophrenia, often with a worse prognosis. Alternatively, we could give Mr. A a diagnosis of Qi-gong-induced psychosis, since his clinical manifestations clearly resemble those described for this condition, and the particular variant of Qi-gong he practiced is known to produce this adverse reaction. Culturally, this diagnosis would have been more easily accepted, and might have improved the patient's and family's participation in treatment. However, Mr. A's symptoms clearly persisted well after his Qi-gong practice stopped, making it difficult to justify this diagnosis. Regarding the DSM-IV psychotic diagnoses, however, we are still left with the unusually late onset of a first experience of psychosis at fifty-seven without clear organic etiology, and we seem to have no clue regarding possible precipitants other than the Qi-gong meditation itself. Does Mr. A suffer from Qi-gong-induced schizophreniform disorder or schizophrenia, or from an abnormally prolonged and morbid form of Qi-gong-induced psychosis? Unfortunately, the patient was lost to follow-up and these questions have remained unresolved. Perhaps it is equivalent to speak of "Qi-gong-induced schizophreniform disorder" as of "prolonged Qi-gong-induced psychosis." In the face of diagnostic uncertainty, however, there may be a pragmatic benefit to the use of the cultural diagnosis (now codified in DSM-IV Appendix 1), since it may have been less stigmatizing than the specified DSM diagnoses and thus more effective in engaging Mr. A and his family in treatment.

Treatment. Mr. A's care would have been improved by the use of a cultural consultant who would have explained the importance of the acknowledgment of Mr. A's practice of Qi-gong, and of the involvement of his family in his treatment, and might have provided some important background information on the practice of Qi-gong and on Qi-gong-induced psychosis. Mr.

A, like most Chinese patients, has strong ties to his family, in this case his wife, that require that they be included in his treatment planning from the outset. A family meeting was held with Mr. A and his wife to explain how medications could help his symptoms, but the practice of Qi-gong was not addressed, nor were their explanatory models, including their notions of his prognosis. The meeting aided in the engagement of the wife, and it was reassuring because it validated her efforts to help her husband, but it could have been more effective. The treating psychiatrist should have shown more respect for the patient's viewpoint and ultimately been an authority figure presenting a strong recommendation for Mr. A's care. Mr. A may not have been lost to follow-up had his explanatory model been engaged and validated.

Finally, this case illustrates that matching the therapist and client's ethnicity, culture, and language is not a risk-free process. The patient had a positive transference toward the therapist; he was going to be cured by a powerful ally. He also was able to communicate easily with his therapist, and trusted a fellow countryman. However, the therapist made assumptions about Mr. A that were not explored, and he did not validate Mr. A's practice of Qi-gong. Thus, a close match between client and therapist in ethnicity is helpful, but not inherently sufficient for effective treatment.

17

Diagnosis and Treatment of *Nervios* and *Ataques* in a Female Puerto Rican Migrant

Roberto Lewis-Fernández

Clinical History

HISTORY OF PRESENT ILLNESS. Forty-nine-year-old widowed Puerto Rican woman with well-managed hypothyroidism who presented to an outpatient Latino Mental Health Clinic in New England after a three-year history of prolonged hospitalizations due to recurrent major depressive disorder with diagnosed psychotic features and chronic impulsive suicidality. Except for partial recoveries lasting less than two weeks, the patient reported several years of chronic sadness; anhedonia; tearfulness; psychomotor retardation; suicidality; guilty ruminations; and decreased sleep, appetite, interests, energy, and concentration. She also suffered from restlessness with pacing, "nervousness," trembling, increased startle, anguish, and severe unmitigated headache.

Patient's "psychotic" diagnosis was due to the occurrence of the following during her affective decompensations: hearing her name called out when alone, glimpsing a darting "shadow" and "feeling" someone behind her. Despite past traumas (physical abuse, husband's murder), she denied intrusive reexperiencing, affective numbing, or stimuli avoidance of post-traumatic stress disorder. There was no history of substance abuse, and her thyroid studies had remained well controlled throughout the course of her psychiatric symptoms.

From *Culture, Medicine, and Psychiatry* 20, no. 2, 155–63 (September 1996) with kind permission from Springer Science and Business Media

Inpatient psychotherapy, antidepressants, and antipsychotics produced a gradual but minor improvement of her depression and suicidality and, no change in her "psychotic" symptoms. Her hospitalization was prolonged by a pattern of increased suicidality each time discharge was contemplated. She was eventually transferred to the Latino Clinic on phenelzine and molindone.

Psychiatric history and previous treatment. Patient was first hospitalized for depression and suicidality at age thirty-two in the context of her youngest son's school truancy. She received a diagnosis of major depressive disorder and was treated with an incomplete trial of tricyclic antidepressants. At thirty-six, she suffered an acute episode of agitation and impulsive suicidality (started to drink bleach) immediately following the murder of her second husband. She required physical and chemical restraints and ER observation for several days but was then discharged and lost to follow-up.

Social and developmental history. Born in rural Puerto Rico, patient dropped out of school during the fifth grade to help raise her siblings and has never worked outside the home. Father was seasonal agricultural migrant, spending several months every year in the United States, where he became an alcoholic. When intoxicated, he was verbally abusive and physically threatening toward patient's mother, but patient denied witnessing overt physical or sexual abuse; she also denied being the object of any abuse during childhood, though she complained of mother's cold distance. At age sixteen, patient married a man eleven years her senior; they had six children, one of whom died at three months of age from pneumonia. Husband's drinking gradually increased until he became very physically and emotionally abusive toward patient. At thirty-one, after he cut her with a razor and broke her arm with his fists, patient ended the marriage by migrating to the eastern United States. She took only the youngest of her five surviving children, leaving the others behind with relatives, a decision that provoked her parents' rejection. After five years in the United States, she returned to Puerto Rico in the wake of the murder of her second husband in a street fight. After her youngest son entered residential drug abuse treatment eleven years later, at age forty-seven, she migrated to a different East Coast city to be near her oldest son from whom she felt estranged.

Family history. Alcohol abuse in father, brother, and two sons. Intravenous heroin and cocaine abuse in one of these sons and a daughter. Depression and anxiety in mother and daughter.

Course and outcome. As part of the Latino Mental Health Clinic outpatient evaluation, the patient's "psychotic" symptoms were reassessed by several Latino clinicians as normative Puerto Rican "spiritual" expressions of demoralization and her treatment with molindone was discontinued. While still on phenelzine during evaluation for family therapy, the patient suffered an *ataque de nervios* ("nervous attack"). In the midst of an argument with her son, she attempted an impulsive overdose with phenelzine after a brief period of brooding and "numbness." She experienced transient dissociative symptoms ("darkness of vision" and "mind going blank") as she took the pills. Minutes later, the patient "came back to herself" and went on her own to the ER. She required ICU treatment and a brief inpatient stay, and was taken off all psychiatric medication. Patient remained intermittently suicidal upon discharge, threatening the stability of outpatient psychotherapy. After several emergency family therapy sessions and as a condition of further therapy, patient's son and daughter-in-law agreed to assume responsibility for her ongoing safety and adherence to treatment.

The patient was then treated with outpatient psychotherapy for a total of five years without need for medication and with no recurrence of major depressive episodes or suicide attempts. After a few months of initially intensive individual, family, and group therapy, patient reduced her participation in psychotherapy. She withdrew from group and family therapy, preferring, individual supportive psychotherapy three to four times a month. Over the five years of follow-up, she had transient but distressing exacerbations of depression, anxiety, dissociation, and somatization that did not meet duration or symptom criteria for dysthymia, generalized anxiety disorder, or a somatoform disorder. Though she continued to perceive "shadows" and hear her name called out, these experiences produced only temporary concern. In contrast, the patient displayed a durable pattern of extreme sensitivity to the possibility of abandonment by significant others, chronic feelings of emptiness, occasional suicidal urges when anxious, recurrent affective instability (sudden depression or irritability), unstable and intense relationships with caregivers alternating between idealization and devaluation, and persistent difficulty in controlling her anger expressed as exquisite susceptibility to perceived slights, meeting criteria for borderline personality disorder.

In 1993, at age fifty-four, patient migrated back to Puerto Rico. Psychiatric evaluation at the time of outpatient discharge revealed reactive anxiety and depression and transient dissociation, usually occurring in response to interpersonal and environmental stressors. These symptoms caused significant distress and impairment (e.g., not eating, isolating self) but only lasted two or three days. Patient then returned to usual baseline state. There was no evidence of formal thought disorder nor loss of generalized reality orientation. There was no suicidality or homicidality.

Diagnostic Formulation

Axis I 300.00 Anxiety disorder NOS
311 Depressive disorder NOS
300.15 Dissociative disorder NOS

Axis II	301.83 Borderline personality disorder
Axis III	Hypothyroidism, controlled
Axis IV	Problems with primary support group (in past: physical abuse, separation from children, and discord with parents and children) Problems related to the social environment (difficulty with acculturation, discrimination) Occupational problems (unemployment), economic problems (poverty)
Axis V	65 (current) 65 (past year)

Cultural Formulation

A. Cultural Identity

1. Cultural reference group(s). Patient is a rural Puerto Rican who migrated twice to the United States since 1969 for a total of thirteen years' residence as part of the "circular" Puerto Rican migration that intensified in the 1960s and 1970s. The "circularity" of this migratory stream consists of recurrent "back-and-forth" moves between Puerto Rico and usually the East Coast of the United States in search of better economic and health care opportunities and in order to reestablish family and cultural links. Like many of these migrants, she was only mildly acculturated despite this extended stay, given the barriers to integration into the United States' mainstream caused by chronic unemployment and limited housing options outside of encapsulated Latino neighborhoods. For the last two years of outpatient treatment, patient spent nearly a quarter of the year in Puerto Rico, signaling her impending return migration.

2. Language. Used Spanish predominantly in daily affairs and doctors' appointments. Poor English fluency and rare use.

3. Cultural factors in development. Patient's childhood contacts were limited to her extended kin group, given the rural isolation of her family compound and her early school termination. This may have intensified the negative impact on her personality development of her father's disruptive and abusive behavior and her mother's affective distance despite the stated absence of witnessed or experienced actual physical or sexual abuse during childhood. These personality patterns were probably reinforced by later adult episodes of physical abuse and traumatic loss. Patient's marriage to a much older man is not atypical for her class and age cohort, and may not have contributed to her symptomatology.

4. Involvement with culture of origin. Predominant. Patient lived in the midst of a Latino neighborhood and traveled frequently to Puerto Rico, where she kept in close contact with several siblings. She had few friends, mostly Latinas, apart from her family.

5. *Involvement with host culture.* Limited, though able to maneuver some aspects of United States urban life well, such as obtaining elderly subsidized housing (though only in her fifties) and disability benefits. She used the public transportation system freely in search of bargains of sundries all over town, from which she made cultural knickknacks (e.g., Puerto Rican flag key chains) for sale to neighbors.

B. Cultural Explanations of the Illness

1. *Predominant idioms of distress and local illness categories.* Patient's illness was described by herself and her community as *nervios* ("nerves") and *ataques de nervios* ("nervous attacks"). Patient's view of her *nervios* was typical of traditional Puerto Ricans, for whom *nervios* is a vulnerability to experiencing symptoms of depression, anxiety, dissociation, somatization, and rarely psychosis of poor impulse control given interpersonal frustrations. The idiom is held together conceptually by the cultural understanding that all its presentations reflect an "alteration" acquired or inherited of the nervous system, and specifically of the anatomical nerves. Patient had suffered from all the symptoms of *nervios* except psychosis. Her acute fitlike exacerbations of *nervios* are known as *ataques de nervios,* and were characterized by paroxysms of anxiety, rage, dissociation, and impulsive suicidality followed by depression and exhaustion in response to acute interpersonal conflicts. *Ataques de nervios* are prevalent expressions of emotional distress and psychopathology among Puerto Ricans; their prevalence in Puerto Rico has recently been established at nearly 14 percent. In patient's case, *nervios and ataques* were associated with her character pathology, but many Puerto Ricans suffer from similar folk syndromes without showing characterological deficits, though the exact relationship between these clinical conditions has not been ascertained. Another aspect of patient's *nervios* was the high frequency and distressing nature of the culturally specific dissociative symptoms: hearing voices, feeling presences, seeing shadows (known as *celajes*). These experiences are very prevalent among Puerto Ricans with and without *nervios,* but sufferers of *ataques* are markedly more distressed by them.

2. *Meaning and severity of symptoms in relation to cultural norms.* Patient's symptoms at the time of presentation were seen by her community to reflect a severe form of *nervios* because they could precipitate rage and dissociation *ataques* with impulsive suicidality and because they had "penetrated deeply," causing her character pathology. Her characterological symptoms were

understood indigenously as a consequence of her *nervios*, rather than as a cause (i.e., a form of bitterness due to her continued suffering), and thus were seen as another sign of severity. Patient was expected to ward against this complication by "controlling" her needs and desires and focusing on the needs of others, such as her children. The community thus validated patient's understanding that reestablishing positive affective links with her family would improve the outcome of her *nervios*. Her achievement of this goal, as well as her coming off psychiatric medications and preventing further *ataques*, were considered signs of improvement.

At first, patient's children rejected the patient's and the community's understanding that her character pathology stemmed from her *nervios* and *ataques*. Her children felt that her symptoms, especially her chronic suicidality, were willful ploys directed at forcing them to put aside their anger at what they perceived as her neglectful parenting. They experienced the patient as manipulative and selfish, uncaring of the effect of her coping mechanisms on them. Family therapy helped patient's son and daughter-in-law to recognize patient's suffering as genuine and to appreciate the limited nature of her past options and current coping skills. In turn, this led them to accept her explanation of the etiological role of *nervios* and *ataques* in her character pathology. Nevertheless, her family continued to be aware that her personality conflicts exceed the norm even for *nervios*, calling her "una persona tremenda" (a difficult, overwhelming person).

3. *Perceived causes and explanatory models.* Her condition was seen fundamentally as a medical problem caused by an "alteration" of her nervous system due to the suffering produced by chronically unresolved family conflicts. Primary among these were the physical abuse by her husband, the parental rejection, and her separation from several of her children during most of their childhood, which led to their ongoing anger toward her. Patient did not feel she was "born with" *nervios*, an alternate cultural etiology, in light of what she considered to have been her "normal childhood." Her dissociative symptoms were attributed to the visitations of deceased relatives, distressing mostly when she was weakened by her *nervios*. Even when improved, however, patient remained leery of these experiences, preferring to pay them minimal attention.

4. *Help-seeking experiences and plans.* Seeing her condition as medical, patient sought help first from internists, who referred her to inpatient psychiatric care. Patient always understood this as being sent to the medical specialists of the nervous system ("the doctors for *nervios*"). Family therapy met patient's need for improving her relationship with her son, but other forms of psychotherapy directed more at intrapsychic change, such as group therapy, were made impossible due to her exquisite sensitivity to offense and her

intense and unstable valuation of the group therapist. Rather than day hospital care, patient sought daily visits with her daughter-in-law. After her family relationships were reestablished, patient left family therapy but suffered only from minor symptoms while her family relationships remained intact. She sought individual supportive psychotherapy with a Latino psychologist and the general "medical supervision" of a Latino psychiatrist. She was also helped by finding a role in the Latino "underground economy" as a seller of homemade cultural artifacts. Patient felt no need to seek help from folk healers for her dissociative symptoms once improved from *nervios*, saying, "I don't believe in any of that."

C. Cultural Factors Related to Psychosocial Environment and Levels of Functioning

1. Social stressors. The main stressor for patient at the time of her presentation was her estrangement from all of her children, which contradicts traditional values regarding an extended and close family centered around a matriarch. Patient felt this was a deserved punishment for abandoning four of her children in childhood. Feelings of rejection by her oldest son precipitated her initial admission and one of her most lethal *ataques*. Once stable, patient tried to increase her contact with her other children but found it too painful since her drug-abusing daughter had lost custody of her own children.

Seen over the course of her lifetime, patient's stressors were severe and included the family disruption caused by her father's alcoholism, her husband's physical abuse, the dispersion of her nuclear family and the consequent discord with her parents and children, difficulties in acculturation to the United States, ethnic discrimination, chronic poverty and unemployment, the murder of her second husband, and her children's substance abuse and subsequent loss of child custody.

2. Social supports. Precarious. As a recent migrant, patient's supports beyond her son, daughter-in-law, and caregivers only consisted of community drop-in centers and a few elderly Latinas. Her lack of supports probably contributed to the length of her hospitalizations, as her fear of going home seemed to worsen her suicidality whenever discharge was discussed. Clinicians' efforts to expand her support system through group therapy membership and psychiatric social clubs were hindered by her character pathology. Most of patient's symptoms, including her suicidal *ataques*, may be understood as attempts to expand her social support network by engaging the attention of family members as well as professional caregivers. The patient always retained the belief that in the face of her overwhelming social limitations and the original recalcitrance of her children, only the full expression of her symptomatology could have produced a positive outcome.

3. Levels of functioning and disability. As a result of her improvement, patient came to see her condition less as a progressive illness without cure than as a permanent vulnerability. However, she attained little insight into her character limitations. Given good family relations and "respect," patient expected to retain her improved state, but she feared decompensation. She felt permanently disabled and expected the government to continue to provide subsidized housing and financial support.

D. Cultural Elements of the Clinician-Patient Relationship

Patient's psychiatric care prior to her referral to the Latino Clinic was hindered by the absence in the diagnostic and treatment process of a culturally normative assessment of patient's character structure as well as of cultural information on *nervios* and *ataques*. Patient's ethnicity was taken into account by assigning her a Latino inpatient caregiver and the use of interpreters, but accurate diagnosis of her character pathology was prevented by the cultural mismatch between the patient and the inpatient unit, which overemphasized her Axis I symptomatology. The joint input of multiple Latino caregivers was able to attain a more comprehensive cultural evaluation and intervention with more successful clinical results.

E. Overall Cultural Assessment

Patient's identity is that of a rural Puerto Rican migrant, speaking Spanish exclusively, who has only lived for limited periods in the United States, resulting in minimal acculturation. Her dysphoria is expressed in the traditional Puerto Rican idioms of *nervios* and *ataques de nervios*. She attributed her relapsing course to unresolved conflicts with her children and did not improve until their affective breach was addressed in family therapy.

Patient's initial treatment proved ineffective partly because of the misattribution of a psychotic label to the patient's dissociative symptoms, which are normative idioms of distress for this population. These experiences were never associated with any loss of reality orientation or formal thought disorder: moreover, they remained, usually with only transient distress, once her overall affective picture improved. They functioned as a kind of diagnostic "red herring." Misdiagnosis exposed patient to the potentially toxic effects of antipsychotic medication and interfered with referral to family psychotherapy. In addition, lack of cultural information also hindered the identification of patient's underlying Axis II pathology and obscured the relationship between her character disorder and her pervasive and persistent Axis I symptoms, including her chronic suicidality and its exacerbations in the form of *ataques*. Pharmacologic treatment of the patient's refractory depression—dangerous anyway, due to other impulsive suicidality—proved unnecessary once intensive family intervention was underway. Her remaining intermittent Axis I symptoms led to periodic distress, warranting NOS diagnoses. But the patient's primary psychopathology proved to be characterological, fulfilling criteria for borderline personality disorder. Like many patients with this disorder, she displayed recurrent dysphoria, though in her case she did not meet strict criteria for dysthymia. Unlike many borderline patients, however, her course was remarkably uneventful once appropriate psychotherapy was instituted, perhaps reflecting cultural variation in the treatment response of borderline personality disorder.

18

Treatment of an Indian Woman with Major Depression by a Latina Therapist

A Cultural Formulation

Maria A. Oquendo and Ruth Graver

PATIENT IDENTIFICATION. S is a twenty-nine-year-old single Christian Punjabi Indian woman living in a large northeastern city of the United States. She is a graduate student at a prestigious business school and lives alone in university housing. She first presented for psychotherapy with the chief complaint: "My mother is driving me crazy."

History of present illness. S had been in her usual state of mental health until approximately six months prior to her presentation, when she first started dating a Hindu southern Indian man. She had been introduced to him by a friend whom they had in common. As the relationship became more serious, S decided to tell her parents about him. They were devastated, particularly her mother. They objected to many things about him. He was Hindu and they were Christians, he was an athlete and not "a professional," and they did not know anything about him or his family. S suspected that her parents assumed that the boyfriend was darker skinned than S, although in fact he was slightly lighter skinned. Her parents refused even to meet him. S was very distressed about their reaction but decided to continue the relationship anyway.

S's mother took every opportunity to discourage S from continuing the relationship. She would tell S that he was only interested in her for "her money" and that she deserved a "better man." S's mother also nagged her

From *Culture, Medicine, and Psychiatry* 21, no. 1, 115–26 (March 1997) with kind permission from Springer Science and Business Media about the difference in their level of education. S was a graduate student at a prestigious business school and her boyfriend had no higher education. S refuted her mother's comments by describing how bright and thoughtful he was, that he made a very good living, and that he owned a house and a car. S tried to persuade her mother to meet him and see for herself, but her mother could not be moved.

S felt that her boyfriend was warm and charming. He made friends easily and worked long hours as a coach. Although he had only lived in the United States for a few years, he had made some close friends, some Indian and some American. S downplayed the differences in religion. Although religion was very important to her family, she was not very religious herself. She also did not emphasize the class differences. She said that she had little knowledge of his family of origin's finances and she did not know his caste, although she could tell from photos of their house that they were comfortable though not wealthy. She was more concerned about their differences in level of education and in the things that they were interested in. For example, S frequently complained that he only liked to eat Indian food rather than experiment and try other cuisines.

As the relationship between S and her boyfriend progressed, S's mother's efforts intensified. S started receiving calls on her beeper at all hours of the day and evening from her mother, who wanted to know where she was and with whom. Rarely, S would become so frustrated she would not answer the page. S started worrying that her mother could indeed track from where she was calling by using caller id. In particular, she was worried that her mother would be further angered to learn that she was occasionally spending the night at her boyfriend's.

As her mother became more persistent, S became more depressed. Although she rarely wavered in her opinion about her boyfriend's motives, she began worrying about her mother's opinion of her and about her ability to tolerate the onslaught of phone calls and pages that she would receive many times a day from her mother. She would cry about her predicament and felt helpless about resolving it. She felt guilty about her parents' disapproval and was upset about disappointing them, but at the same time she felt enraged with them. She felt that her situation was untenable and that she had only two options. She could either disappoint her parents and get married to someone they thought was not worthy of her, or she could risk staying single for the rest of her life. She felt that at age twenty-nine, she was well past her prime.

Gradually, S developed difficulty sleeping and stayed up worrying about what would happen. She was constantly tired and had difficulty concentrating on her studies. Her grades started to drop. Her appetite increased and she gained ten pounds over a two-month period. She frequently thought that she might as well be dead since she could not imagine how she might resolve her quandary.

S had no other psychiatric symptoms, including mania or anxiety. S denied any history of substance abuse. She never used alcohol. She denied ever experimenting with or using street drugs. She agreed to a treatment for major depression, which included medication and twice a week psychodynamically oriented supportive psychotherapy.

Past psychiatric history. Denied.

Social and developmental history. The patient was the eldest of three children born to a Christian couple in the Punjab. Seeking better economic opportunities, when S was five years old, she and her parents and siblings moved to England where a maternal cousin lived. There the patient learned English and started attending school. When the patient was eleven, her parents relocated to a large northeastern city of the United States since many of the maternal relatives had moved to the United States.

Her father worked as a pharmacist and her mother as a physiotherapist. S described her father as a quiet, gentle man and her mother as an energetic, enterprising, domineering woman, who had organized the migrations of the family. The family was extremely involved with their church, attending services regularly and participating in many of the social events sponsored by the church. She had two younger male siblings. S felt that the eldest son, two years her junior, was favored by the mother. He had recently married a woman from the Caribbean whom he had met at church. His wife, who had a lower level of education than he, had been accepted by the family easily. He worked as a banker with a prestigious firm. The younger brother was unmarried and somewhat estranged from the family. He visited rarely. He had a job as a salesman and an excellent income, which he spent on luxury cars and other "extravagances."

S did extremely well in school, earning a scholarship to a private high school. She gained admission to an exclusive, competitive university. In college, she had some difficulties. She tended to feel both isolated and "different." She felt that the other students came from more privileged backgrounds than she and that they did not accept her as an equal.

She graduated from college with good grades and was admitted to business school. Despite her academic success, she perceived herself as someone who had to struggle to effect all of her achievements, unlike others for whom she thought things came more easily.

Family psychiatric history. Denied.

Course and outcome. The therapist recommended both therapy and medication because she felt that the vegetative signs of depression were significant and should be treated.

Although S did not conceptualize her situation as one that could be helped by medicine, she agreed to a course of an SSRI. She was started on Sertraline 100 mg, which she tolerated well. She had some initial headaches, which resolved after the first ten days of treatment with the medication.

Psychologically, S felt trapped in an impossible situation. She wanted to get married and have a family. However, her parents, had encouraged her to pursue education aggressively and had not made any arrangements for her marriage, as is commonly done in India. Yet, her mother felt that she should have a significant influence on S's choice of a husband. S felt her mother was too traditional and remarked that she feared allowing her mother to interfere in her marriage. Previously, S's mother had arranged a disastrous marriage for S's maternal aunt. This aunt, who was living in the United States at the time, married a Christian Punjabi man who was distantly related to S's father. This man would physically abuse S's aunt, who ultimately separated from him and moved to another state with her two children. S complained bitterly that she doubted her mother would make a better choice for her.

S felt that her depression was a consequence of the disruption in the relationship with her mother. Their relationship was an extremely ambivalent one in which S both wished to be close with her mother and also wanted to make a clean break from her. In treatment, S focused on the difficulty of integrating the standards for mother-daughter relationships in India versus in the United States, which she saw as dichotomous and which reinforced her conflict.

In addition, her low self-esteem and her feelings about racism emerged as central issues in her difficulties with relationships. S spoke openly about her feeling of being discriminated against on a daily basis. The therapy attempted to disentangle S's accurate perceptions of racism from her internalized fears of not fitting in and of being rejected. These might have been caused by her early perception of not being as favored as the eldest son and her feeling that being darker than her family members made her less loved.

As S explored her conflict about separating from her mother and her low self-esteem, she became less confused about the decisions she was facing. She became aware of how she contributed to her mother's frequent calling by returning calls and giving her mother detailed answers to her many questions. She realized that her mother's questions regarding her boyfriend's motives for marrying S raised S's anxiety about her self-worth and desirability and clouded S's ability to think clearly about the situation. Ultimately, S decided to marry her boyfriend, and they arranged to finance the wedding on their own.

Much to S's surprise, as soon as she announced the wedding date, S's mother's attitude changed dramatically. S's mother agreed to meet her fiancé and helped S plan some of the details of the wedding. Although she was greatly relieved, S was anxious about whether another change of heart would occur in her mother.

Diagnostic Formulation

Axis I:	296.22 Major depression, single episode, moderate
Axis II:	None
Axis III:	None
Axis IV:	Problems with primary support group (discord with parents) Educational problem (lowering of grades in graduate school)
Axis V:	65 (current) 75 (past year)

Cultural Formulation

A. Cultural Identity

1. *Cultural reference group.* S is a Christian woman born in the Punjab who migrated first to England at age five and later to the United States. She comes from a group that is a very small minority in India. S stated that she felt that the missionaries that had come to convert the Punjabis had been culturally insensitive to the fact that they were placing the new Christians in a difficult position. Now they were "other" in their own country and elsewhere.

Her family had established itself firmly in the middle class in a large northeastern city and were acculturated to a large extent. However, the family kept many Punjabi customs, frequently eating Punjabi food and wearing traditional Punjabi clothes for special occasions such as birthdays, parties, or weddings.

Many of the traditions that were maintained were subtle. For example, the obvious preference given to the male children was something that distressed S, and she frequently complained that it was not "fair." In addition, S's mother's expectation that S maintain very close ties with her and visit weekly made S feel torn. She felt that it was the "right" thing to do and felt guilty if she did not go. She would only reluctantly admit that she in fact enjoyed the time spent at her parents' home. She appeared more comfortable expressing her feeling that it hindered her capacity to do well in school and that she felt that an American mother would be more understanding.

2. *Language.* The patient speaks English fluently with no accent. She spoke

mostly Punjabi and some Urdu at home but was educated in English and spoke English with peers, friends, and boyfriend.

3. *Cultural factors in development.* The patient's early migration to England and later to the United States placed S in a situation where she continued to hold minority status. Her feelings of inferiority may have been reinforced by this and the mother's favor toward the eldest son. In addition, she heard many stories within the family about some lighter-skinned members of the extended family snubbing those who were darker. S considered herself to have dark brown skin. She stated she was darker skinned than her youngest brother but not than her parents.

S's parents encouraged her to pursue higher education. This reflected some level of acculturation on the parents' part since they clearly valued education for their daughter. In addition, they made no provisions for her marriage. A traditional practice in most of India, followed by many migrants to the United States, is for parents to arrange their children's marriages. Frequently the parents will find a suitable mate for their daughter when she is in her late teens or early twenties. There is usually an emphasis on ensuring that the prospective husband have a higher level of education than the bride. Currently, Indian parents in the United States commonly allow the daughter ultimately to decide whether she is happy with the choice, giving her "veto" power.

Not having a marriage arranged for her by the age of twenty-nine left S in a difficult situation. S felt she had been tacitly discouraged from the "distractions" of dating and marriage. Yet this did not gel with her own wishes. S viewed her problem as stemming partly from her previous difficulty in finding a suitable mate. At age twenty-nine, she felt she was in great danger of not getting married at all. She felt that having found an affectionate, hardworking Indian man, she should not pass up what could be her last chance.

4. *Involvement with the culture of origin.* S was involved with the culture of origin in complex and subtle ways. All her dealings with her family of origin led her to be involved with the linguistic, religious, gastronomic, and other aspects of Punjabi culture. Although externally S appeared to be completely acculturated in terms of her understanding of the mainstream culture, unconsciously she was still strongly influenced by her original culture. A central example of this was her ambivalence about how much of a role she wanted her mother to play in her choice of partner.

As S understood it, Punjabi tradition would dictate a mother-daughter relationship in which the mother plays a central role in her daughter's adult life if the daughter is not yet married. This was reflected, to some extent, in S's relationship with her mother. Even when S was busy with schoolwork, S's mother expected to be visited weekly, despite living an hour away. S's mother would spend the day cooking and give S food to take back to her own apartment for the week. S's mother would give opinions about S's clothes, spending habits, and relationships. In addition, S's mother discouraged S from trusting people outside of the family and supported S's close relationships with her maternal aunts.

S felt that this was at odds with what she perceived as the "American" type of mother-daughter relationship. S observed that in many families in the United States, the mother's role changes over time. S viewed the "American" mother as undergoing a transition when the daughter entered young adulthood, from a purely parental one to one in which the daughter is viewed as a more independent adult with whom the mother could be "friends." She imagined that this transformation would set the stage for the daughter to form her own nuclear family, which would be quite independent from the family of origin.

Another example of S's cultural ambivalence revolved around her sexual involvement with her boyfriend. Virginity is heavily emphasized both in traditional Punjabi culture and by her Christian religion. S felt torn about this issue, on the one hand feeling that as a young woman in the United States her behavior was well within the norm, but on the other hand feeling terrible anxiety that her mother would find out.

5. *Involvement with the host culture.* S was extensively involved with the host culture. She attended and succeeded in outstanding American schools. She was quite articulate in English and understood a great deal about cultural expectations in the United States in contrast to India. Her decision to go to business school had been encouraged by her family although they paid neither for college nor for business school. She felt that an MBA would give her the opportunity to have a "respectable" independent career with a comfortable lifestyle. These goals were more consistent with expectations for women in the United States than in the Punjab.

She did, however, feel more comfortable being friends with other "minorities." She explained that most of her significant relationships were with people from the Caribbean or Asian countries. One could see S's situation as typical of the bicultural individual, able to function quite well in both cultures, yet being at risk for conflicts when trying to negotiate the complex and sometimes contradictory demands of each one.

B. Cultural Explanations of the Illness

1. *Predominant idioms of distress and local illness categories.* S's presentation was congruent with the DSM-IV description of major depression. Although some of the behaviors of the patient in the transference could be construed

as being suggestive of dependent personality disorder, the therapist viewed them as typical of the interdependence that is traditionally fostered in Indian women. The tendency to accommodate to others' needs and be interested in finding approval for significant relationships appeared to be dictated by her cultural background and her socialization as a woman. As such, the therapist viewed these behaviors as not pathological but as culturally congruent in this context. Furthermore, S did not exhibit any of the patterns generally seen in a dependent personality. If anything, she was willing to risk losing the affection of her mother in order to choose a mate.

No other illness categories were expressed.

2. Meaning and severity of the symptoms in relation to cultural norms. S's depression and suffering were seen by the family as a direct consequence of her guilt for defying her parent's wishes that she not date her boyfriend. Her mother appeared to attribute little causality to her own perseverance in trying to dissuade S from her choice. The family hid the problem from their community, although S's mother did call her own sisters and instructed them to join in on the attempt to change S's mind. This was especially difficult for S because one of her aunts had been particularly supportive of her and S then felt betrayed by her.

S's distress was also probably exacerbated by a tension between the American (and traditional psychotherapeutic) ideal of independence and autonomy versus the emphasis on accommodating others' needs that is so heavily emphasized in the socialization of women in the Punjab.

3. Perceived causes and explanatory models. Although S clearly identified herself as distressed and needing the help of a psychiatrist, her family did not see her as ill. Rather, they understood her suffering to be self-inflicted because of her "stubbornness" and unwillingness to comply with her parents' wishes.

4. Help-seeking experiences and plans. S identified her problem as psychological and therefore contacted a psychiatrist for help. She did not consider that her problem was one that could be helped by medication since she saw it as being strictly related to a family conflict. Although the therapist asked S to bring her mother for a family meeting, S's mother refused to attend. S's mother's remark to S about this was, "You are suffering from guilt; it is not I who needs to see a psychiatrist." Although S expected treatment with psychotherapy, she came to understand some of her distress as being secondary to major depression. She accepted a trial of an SSRI, to which she responded well. Her acceptance of the medication was influenced by her wish to please the therapist. She was very engaged in the twice-weekly therapy, which early on focused on elucidating the origins of the conflict and the ambivalent nature of the relationship with her mother. Later themes included issues of low self-esteem and self-defeating patterns.

C. Cultural Factors Related to Psychosocial Environment and Levels of Functioning

1. Social stressors. The stressor at time of presentation was S's conflict with her mother, which underlined S's ambivalence about Punjabi ideas regarding the parental role in marriage decisions. The loss of her mother's and aunt's support was severely felt by S because of her feeling that she was "different." S stated that she felt that, ultimately, she only had her family for support because only they could truly understand her. Her difficulty concentrating and consequent lowering of her grades further impinged on her already weakened self-esteem.

2. Social supports. S's social supports were quite inadequate. She was isolated, in part because of her conflict with her mother and other family members. This rift was extremely distressing to both parties. Additionally, S felt that telling others what was happening would be too embarrassing. S thought that the students with whom she was friendly would think her mother's behavior crazy. She felt that the only persons she could talk to about this were her boyfriend and her therapist.

3. Levels of functioning and disability. S continued to function in her relationship with her boyfriend but noticed a decline in her ability to do her schoolwork although she was not, by any measure, failing.

D. Cultural Elements of the Clinician-Patient Relationship

Both S and the therapist were born in countries other than the United States and were "brown" in S's eyes. This had a profound impact on the transference. From the start, the patient had chosen the therapist partly because she was an "ethnic woman" who, S explicitly stated, could better understand the problems that S encountered as a minority professional woman. S saw the similarity in skin color as a shortcut to closeness and sympathy. S felt strongly that only someone of color could understand and tolerate hearing about her experiences with racism. She felt that a white person would regard her distrust as paranoid and her feelings of being discriminated against as defensive. Interestingly, this identification with color seemed more important to S than cultural similarity. Her choosing a Latina therapist highlighted the centrality of her self-perception as a minority woman in an "American" culture.

The patient quickly developed an intense maternal transference that consciously focused on the positive attributes of the therapist and kept negative aspects unconscious. For example, as a way of warding off her anxiety about being rejected by the therapist, as she felt she was being by her mother, and to keep at bay her feelings of inferiority, S would frequently say "I know you are my therapist and not my friend." A year into treatment, as the patient became less anxious about abandonment, she said to the therapist conspiratorially "I can tell you because you are my friend." When asked to explore this, S was able to acknowledge her wish to be close to the therapist in a more personal way and her feeling that the therapist was someone that she could trust.

On a Friday soon thereafter, the patient left her beeper in the therapist's office. She called and asked the therapist if they could meet over the weekend at a restaurant or some "other neutral ground" to retrieve her beeper. The therapist agreed to leave the beeper with the doorman instead. Exploration of this incident the following week revealed the patient's wish to cross the boundary and make the relationship a more personal one in which she might finally gain the favored status she yearned for with her mother. This occurrence underlined S's ambivalence about closeness and distance in relationships, an issue that was the crux of her disagreement with her mother.

For the therapist, treating S meant paying special attention to the patient's fantasy that superficial similarities a priori set the stage for understanding and sympathy. S would frequently make comments such as "you know what that's like" or "don't you agree with me?" which would subtly discourage the therapist from exploring the details of the situation. It was crucial to resist these suggestions especially with regard to racism. S's descriptions of her experience with racism were at times wrenching. For example, S spoke with great resentment about her feeling that whites would keep their distance from her emotionally and frequently literally. She recounted how in the supermarket in the predominantly white neighborhood where she lived, women would literally step away from her in the checkout line. Yet it was difficult to evaluate to what extent these experiences were distorted. S also reported that she had gone to a grocery store in the therapist's office neighborhood and had similar experiences. When the therapist pointed out that the particular neighborhood was quite racially integrated, S seemed surprised. The therapist attempted to maintain neutrality by both validating S's general perception that racism is pervasive and insidious and, at the same time, pointing out when her experience seemed more likely to be due to her own feelings about feeling inferior, undeserving, and not fitting in. Although S usually accepted the therapist's clarifications, the therapist frequently felt trepidation about sounding insensitive, or worse, appearing to deny the corrosive effects of racism.

Overall Cultural Assessment

S is a single Punjabi Christian woman who is extensively acculturated. She had an episode of major depression precipitated by a severe disagreement with her mother which underlined some of the difficulties in integrating opposing cultural expectations regarding love marriages and what qualities make for a good mate. In S's case, the pull from the traditional Punjabi practice of having a mate chosen by the parents was present but confounded by her parents' decision not to arrange a marriage for her. Although she understood this as an attempt on their part to keep her focused on her studies, she also assumed that it implied that she was free to choose a mate on her own, as is the American custom. Her conflict about what is the proper way to proceed drew her attention to heretofore disregarded negative feelings about her mother.

Her preoccupation with racism also had multiple underpinnings. Her mother was in S's own words, "racist against Hindus." Furthermore, the family had expressed strong ideas about the importance of skin color in regard to relationships. These personal experiences with racism within her family made her quite sensitive to racism in general, to which she attributed much personal unhappiness, including her inability to make friends with "nonminorities."

The therapeutic alliance allowed her to examine how she unconsciously reinforced her mother's behavior by answering her multiple pages and phone calls and myriad questions. S came to understand that as much as she detested the torrent of calls, there was something gratifying about the intense attention. As she trusted the therapist more, she was able to decide consciously how to proceed in terms of her relationship with her boyfriend, whom she married a year after the beginning of treatment. Her independence in this decision seems to have been rewarded by her mother, who has now begun to accept her daughter's choice. In this way, the family is perhaps becoming even more "Americanized." As the patient continues to work in therapy, a challenge will be to help her integrate her multiple value systems.

S's therapy integrated psychopharmacologic, psychodynamic, and cultural interventions. The cultural interventions were crucial in the understanding of S, in particular since she presented herself as a completely acculturated individual. Yet unconsciously she clearly had many unresolved questions about the "right" way to make important decisions in her life. Allowing S to understand that she had mixed feelings about being "Americanized," and that her concerns about racism were psychologically rooted in family issues and not purely responses to her environment, contributed to the resolution of many of her conflicts and allowed her to make more lucid decisions for herself.

19

Depression and Back Pain in a Young Male Turkish Immigrant in Basel, Switzerland

A Cultural Formulation

A. Tarik Yilmaz and Mitchell G. Weiss

Clinical History

PATIENT IDENTIFICATION. Mr. Osman is a tall, twenty-two-year-old, single Turkish Muslim man, clean-shaven and casually dressed. He lives with his parents and is unemployed. He immigrated to Switzerland at the age of sixteen to join his family. Two and a half years ago he came to the internal medicine outpatient clinic with symptoms of back pain as well as tiredness in his legs and arms. Because no medical condition was detected that would explain his symptoms, and because he was depressed, he was then referred to psychiatry. The interviews on which this cultural formulation is based were held with him two years after his first presentation; his psychiatrist, a Swiss clinician, was interviewed to understand how he understood the patient's illness, and the patient's father was interviewed in Turkish to identify his understanding of the problem, its meaning, and causes.

History of present illness. When he was referred to psychiatry, Mr. Osman was mainly troubled by feelings of sadness, fatigue, low energy, worthlessness, and back pains. These symptoms had worsened after he came to Switzerland, although many of them had also troubled him since age twelve, but had not caused any major problems in performance at school. The back pains began about six months after he arrived in Switzerland at age sixteen,

From *Culture, Medicine, and Psychiatry* 24, no. 2, 259–72 (June 2000) with kind permission from Springer Science and Business Media

after he took a job as a laborer in a paper factory. Initially the pain came sporadically, then increased slightly and became more constant over the next two or three years. The pain and the fatigue both seemed to increase with exertion.

Examinations conducted by his GP and in the outpatient medicine and neurology clinics could not explain his pain or fatigue. Laboratory tests—including blood count, serum electrolytes, creatinine, liver function tests, thyroid screen, and urinalysis—were all negative, as were serological and other tests to rule out enterovirus, toxoplasmosis, HIV, measles, mumps, syphilis, borrelia, and Herpes Simplex. An EMG, ultrasound, and a skull CT were also unrevealing. Despite treatment with analgesics from the GP, his condition changed very little.

Over the course of two years of psychotherapy, on at least three occasions, he had periods of four to eight weeks when the depressive symptoms were intense, and during such episodes he had suicidal thoughts. During the last depressive episode he was hospitalized for five days in the Psychiatric Crisis Intervention Unit, an inpatient facility of the Psychiatric Outpatient Department of the University of Basel. Psychiatric outpatient treatment consisted of an eclectic psychotherapy—both insight-oriented and supportive—and pharmacotherapy with fluoxetine (20 mg daily). His symptoms persisted throughout the treatment without significant change.

Psychiatric history and previous treatment. Despite long-standing, relatively mild symptoms since age twelve, Mr. Osman had never previously sought medical or psychiatric treatment. His initial visit to a GP before coming to the medical outpatient clinic of the university hospital in Basel was motivated by the increasing back pain, rather than depressive symptoms. He had no history of alcohol or other substance abuse or dependence, and he did not smoke.

Social and developmental history. Mr. Osman was born in a rural village in Central Turkey near the city of Konya and raised in a Muslim religious family. There were no complications at delivery, and developmental milestones and neurological development all proceeded normally. His father left the family in Turkey to come to Switzerland when Mr. Osman was one year old. At the age of four, Mr. Osman, his mother, and his younger brother joined his father in Switzerland, and they returned to Turkey after a year, again leaving his father in Switzerland. At the age of six he came to Switzerland again and stayed about one and a half years before returning to Turkey to attend primary school and, subsequently, a Muslim religious secondary school. His mother stayed in Switzerland. He next attended a higher secondary religious school (Gymnasium), but broke off his studies after a year and returned to Switzerland at age sixteen. Before that, when his mother had already left, he was looked after by his grandmother and two aunts from his father's side of the family. He recalled life at home in Turkey was pleasant for him, in contrast with his stays in Switzerland, which he described as unpleasant, because he felt foreign and socially isolated. In the religious school in Turkey, however, he had also been unhappy, feeling ambivalent about the conservative religious lifestyle; he left the higher secondary school because of that and joined his parents in Switzerland.

A week after he came to Switzerland he started a job as a worker in the paper factory where his father also worked. His job consisted mainly of manual labor, which he viewed as a punishment for having broken off his studies in Turkey. His father and other family members and relatives regarded the patient to be a failure. His father also had health problems at that time and suffered increasingly from insomnia and other symptoms, and Mr. Osman felt it was his fault that his father suffered from these problems. The patient's back pains began within the first six months after he took the job in the factory. He decided to leave the job and attend classes to learn German and begin learning a trade. He sought training to become an electrician, went to school for a year, and then completed a three-year apprenticeship. But after that he could not find a permanent job, and even in the part-time jobs he could find, he was unable to work more than two or three months at a time because of his symptoms.

Family history. Mr. Osman has a healthy brother who is four years younger. His father left the village in central Turkey because of financial problems and immigrated to Switzerland, where he found employment as a laborer in the paper factory when Mr. Osman was one year old. His mother came to Switzerland fourteen years ago, and she also took a job in a factory. Despite their persisting wish to return, financial constraints prevented them from going back to Turkey. Mr. Osman's forty-five-year-old mother has suffered from chronic pain for the past four years, and his forty-six-year-old father has also suffered from symptoms of chronic fatigue, lack of energy, and insomnia for the past seven years.

Course and outcome. After referral by a GP for psychiatric evaluation, Mr. Osman was treated with psychotherapy and fluoxetine (20 mg daily). His first therapist left the clinic, and he was replaced by a second. The therapy addressed feelings of guilt and remorse about his inability to find a job. He had submitted approximately twenty applications in his quest and blamed himself for the poor result, concluding that it was "lack of interest and courage" and speculating that his imperfectly written German in the applications was also a factor explaining his failure. Three notable exacerbations of depressive symptoms occurred in the course of the therapy, each lasting for several weeks, and during these episodes he became increasingly suicidal. In one suicidal crisis he described his experience and feelings as follows:

> Shortly before I broke off my education in Turkey and came to Switzerland, my father had wanted to return to Turkey in the next few months. It was my fault that my father could not return to Turkey and that he had so much difficulty sleeping. Other family members also thought it was my fault. . . . They still think of my problems like that. There are actually three possibilities for me: I could accept everything and not react, or I could resist, or I could kill myself. . . . I have taken the first option so far.

Mr. Osman not only blamed himself harshly for his failure to find a job, he was also ashamed and felt guilty about his depressive symptoms. Overall, the therapy achieved no more than limited success. He symptoms remained for the most part as they were.

Diagnostic Formulation

Axis I	296.32 Major depressive disorder, recurrent
	300.4 Dysthmic disorder
	307.80 Pain disorder associated with psychological factors
Axis II	No diagnosis
Axis III	No diagnosis
Axis IV	Problems with primary support group (meeting family expectations and low status)
	Social and occupational problems (unable to work and earn according to expectations)
Axis V	GAF = 45 (Current)
	GAF = 65 (Highest past year)

Differential diagnosis. Although symptoms of back pain and fatigue were both reported, the latter was mentioned rather than emphasized. Inasmuch as fatigue is also attributable to depression, which was also diagnosed, the diagnosis of pain disorder, rather than undifferentiated somatoform disorder, is preferred.

Cultural Formulation

A. Cultural Identity

Cultural reference group(s). Mr. Osman grew up in a small, rural village in Central Turkey where farming is the major occupation. Although the range of religious practices vary widely in the country, this region is known to be a particularly conservative area. His family owned no land and worked on the farms of landowners. His upbringing was typical of the region in a traditional Turkish Muslim home. They went to the mosque frequently and offered prayers five times daily, and they adhered to dietary restrictions, such as not eating pork. His participation in religious life and practice was encouraged by his family, who enrolled him in an Islamic religious school, called *Imam Hatip Lisesi*, the kind of school that provides training for religious leaders of a mosque (*Imam*). His parents are literate and had a primary school education, but they could be considered representative of people from the low socioeconomic class in the region. Values in their traditional lifestyle emphasized cohesion of the family and extended family group and the importance of meeting parental expectations. Authority within the family is apportioned according to male sex and age. Everyone in the family is required to show respect and deference to others above them in this hierarchy.

Language. Mr. Osman's mother tongue is Turkish; he is now also fluent in German. He can speak, read, and write in German and had no apparent language problems communicating with his German-speaking Swiss psychiatrists.

Cultural factors in development. Mr. Osman was influenced deeply by his traditional and religion-oriented upbringing. Even today, he feels he must not cross his legs or lie down in the presence of his father, which would be considered disrespectful, and he carefully observes these rules. He explained that you cannot argue with your father, and you must accept what older people in the family say. He explained that he had never answered "no" when his father told him to do something. His stays in Switzerland as a child and subsequent experience as an immigrant also had a substantial impact. Here he felt foreign and socially isolated. Because of that, when he was in Switzerland as a child, he longed to return to Turkey, where he had good friends whose company he enjoyed and whom he missed. When he came to Switzerland to find work after leaving school in Turkey, the impact of Swiss culture was even more intense, a force he was required to come to terms with more seriously, since prospects for returning to Turkey were remote. Although he could obtain a job in a factory as a temporary worker within weeks of arrival, manual labor seemed to him degrading, and he also felt disvalued by the indigenous Swiss; he felt they treated him badly as a foreigner. His efforts to learn German and complete an apprenticeship helped to enhance his self-esteem, his position in the family, and his place in the Turkish immigrant society. Ultimately, however, failure to find work in his trade left feelings of humiliation unsoothed. His low status in the family hierarchy was painfully disappointing.

Involvement with the culture of origin. Mr. Osman lives with his parents, and he is ambivalent about the traditional values of his culture of origin. It was because he found the conservatism of his religious school oppressive that he left it, and now he no longer observes required religious practices. He is dissatisfied with the requirements of a traditional lifestyle, especially with his father's authoritarian manner and the family hierarchy. Nevertheless, he accepts his role in the family without expressing his discontent, and he remains entrenched in Turkish culture. Most of his friends are also Turkish immigrants in Switzerland, and he reads mainly Turkish newspapers and watches Turkish TV programs.

Involvement with the host culture. In Basel Mr. Osman lives in a section of the city populated mainly by immigrants from Turkey. He speaks German well, and even though most of his social supports are within the Turkish community and he has few Swiss friends, he tries to make the acquaintance of Swiss people. He accepts the treatment provided by the Swiss GP and psychiatrist, following their directions and attending therapy regularly. He is ambivalent about Swiss culture. He idealizes it but also criticizes it, explaining that he finds the Swiss to be rather distant to foreigners and somewhat rigid. Although he doesn't dwell on this, he explained in one session that "if you want to meet someone here, first you have to make an appointment, and then it takes some time before you can see them. It seems strange." He also feels hurt from his earlier experience working as a laborer in the paper factory, and frustration from his inability to find a job.

B. Cultural Explanations of the Illness

Predominant idioms of distress and local illness categories. Mr. Osman emphasized his pain symptoms, describing them in great detail. He acknowledged that he felt tired, and he mentioned his insomnia without any prompting. In response to further questions about his problem, he explained feeling a lack of interest or taking pleasure in things and low self-worth. He felt he had been a failure since his childhood. He considered himself lazy and blamed himself for not being more active. He felt guilty about this and consequently often withdrew. To a greater or lesser degree he was continually dejected and depressed. When asked to explain what he had learned from all of his contact with medicine, a traditional healer (*hoca*), and psychiatry, he summarized his experience as follows:

> Actually I do not have any illness, it is not really an illness. It is like a simulation; I have these problems as if they were real, but in reality they do not exist; they are like images that have pushed their way into the foreground. The pain is not something that happens through some mechanism in my head, it comes from nerves.

He uses the term *simulasyon*, a borrowed term from English, which is understood, though not common, in Turkish.

In another interview the patient's father was asked how he saw his son's symptoms. He explained that the problems were of two kinds, pain and others, and he focused on the pain. He indicated, however, that there might also be some other problems. Perhaps he was lovesick or had some secret he wouldn't tell his father. He explained that his son had withdrawn socially, and the lack of social contacts was making him more ill. He needed more contact with people like himself, and he was actually suffering from some "character weakness" (*karakter zayifligi*). His use of this term reflects the father's view of the inadequacy of his son's social relations. Establishing key social relationships is extremely important in this community, and a respectable personal identity requires a communal context. Insofar as the father describes the problem in terms of poor socialization and weakness of character, he implies that his son is not really ill, and for him the comments of the Swiss doctors proved that there was actually nothing wrong with his son.

Mr. Osman mentioned that he had no girlfriend and gave no indication of being lovesick. He explained that, being unemployed, he wasn't considering marriage at this point, though he would perhaps consider marriage later. Although his romantic life was not a major topic of consideration in the therapy, the fact that he referred to the question of marriage in the future as something that he might or might not choose reflected an assumption that it was his choice to make. Such an assumption represented an indication of his adaptation and incorporation of Swiss values, since the question of when to marry in the more traditional society of his homeland would have clearly been a matter not for the son on his own, but more for the parents to decide. With that in mind, more attention in his therapy to his relations with women and plans for marriage might have helped to address core conflicts between values acquired in Switzerland and his traditional culture of origin.

Meaning and severity of symptoms in relation to cultural norms. According to Mr. Osman's father, when a youth suffers from loss of interest or pleasure, social withdrawal, and fear of failure, this indicates some problem he cannot tell his parents or close relatives. In a view consistent with the values of a traditional Turkish family, the father considered the depressive symptoms the result of "character weakness." He elaborated, explaining that he thought his son should make more of an effort to overcome his problems. He had not lacked anything; there had always been enough money for his son. Symptoms of pain, on the other hand, were accepted by the father. Mr. Osman had told us that since the pains began, his family—especially his father—had become more understanding and sympathetic; he was no longer treated so harshly. His father confirmed this report. Since his son suffered from pain, he became more tolerant and sympathetic than he would be otherwise, even if the doctors could not find a cause for the pain.

His expression of sympathy was without any indication of self-blame or feeling accountable for his son's problems. In a traditional family, the father is responsible and controls the socialization of his son; migration to Switzerland, however, compromised this father's effectiveness and ability to exercise his control in accordance with traditional values. He showed no indication, however, of any guilt about difficulties fulfilling these obligations, or the possibility of thereby having contributed to the problems, even though he clearly wanted to help his son and relieve his suffering.

Perceived causes and explanatory models. Mr. Osman also distinguished two sets of problems: pain and the rest. As explained above, he considered his depressive symptoms as a "simulation," which he attributed to "nerves" (*sinir*). This is a vague term in colloquial Turkish; it characterizes the nervous system generally and is used to describe the nerves in both the neurological sense and also nervousness as a psychological symptom. In addition, Mr. Osman identified various other factors as the cause of his illness. He thought the poor diet in Switzerland or the change of climate from migration could be responsible, which seemed reasonable to him since he had pain in Switzerland but not in Turkey. He was accustomed to Turkish food. Perhaps he had eaten pork in Switzerland without realizing it. He blamed the arduous working conditions in Switzerland for his pain. In the paper factory his boss had treated him harshly, and the hard manual labor was also a factor. He also explained that perhaps it was his fate to be ill; it could be what God wanted. He considered the possibility that perhaps the evil eye, or magic, as the *hoca* had told him, might also have caused his illness.

In the interview Mr. Osman's father also said that his son was ill because of a poor diet, change of climate, hard working conditions, and social withdrawal. A young man needs friends and social contacts. It was his son's fate to be ill. Unprompted, he told us the evil eye may also account for the problems. His son was well behaved, a good boy, handsome, and very healthy. So it could be that acquaintances out of jealousy did this through "evil eye" (*nazar*). The family, he reported, had also considered magic (*büyü*) but they were not sure about this.

The father's account emphasized traditional ideas and social factors. The variety of causes reported by Mr. Osman reflected a lifestyle striving to come to terms with traditional and Western ways. His various accounts accommodated traditional values and expectations, but the way he described his problem as a "simulation," and his reference to "nerves" conveys both a traditional and a Western meaning. His efforts to integrate aspects of his experience with respect to social, psychological, and somatic Western frameworks, on the one hand, with traditional values and explanations on the other, resulted in a somewhat fragmented account.

Help-seeking experiences and plans. Mr. Osman's explanatory models clearly influenced his approach to seeking help, both the timing and selection among the available options. At the outset he sought no help because he assumed that the pain and fatigue resulted from his work in the paper factory. He thought that when he stopped working, he would no longer suffer from his pains or tiredness. When he left his job, however, and began attending school to begin his apprenticeship, he found that the pain persisted. At school he could not participate in the physical education classes, which also troubled him, and so he went to his GP.

Communicating with the GP was difficult, not just because of difficulty speaking German at that time before he became more proficient, but also because the advice he received from the GP didn't make sense to him. The GP could not diagnose any disease and recommended that he get more exercise, and particularly that he participate in some sport. This seemed peculiar to Mr. Osman, since his difficulty in the physical education class and inability to participate in sports had been an important motivation for coming to the GP. Neither the GP's evaluation nor the workups in the medical and neurology clinics where he was referred revealed any organic basis for his symptoms. The neurologist explained there was nothing wrong with his "nervous system," which Mr. Osman understood with reference to a Turkish concept (*sinir sistemi*). To Mr. Osman the reference to the "nervous system," based on its reference to a technical meaning and its connotation in colloquial Turkish, meant that psychologically he was okay. Consequently, he could not understand why the neurologist suggested that he see a psychiatrist. When he returned to the internal medicine clinic, the internist accepted the advice of the neurologist and made the referral to psychiatry.

In the psychiatry clinic he was treated in psychotherapy and with fluoxetine by a Swiss psychiatrist for about fifteen months; he attended irregularly and found the treatment not to be so useful. When the psychiatrist left the institution, Mr. Osman continued treatment in the clinic with a second Swiss psychiatrist. Discussing his experience in therapy, he explained that he understood that he was supposed to listen and try to understand what he was told, and then put this advice into practice in his life. He indicated the aim of this process as more a matter of following the advice he received, rather than engaging in a process and striving for insight.

His father understood the advice from the medical clinic to mean "you are young and you will get better." It seemed to the father that the doctors had concluded there was no illness. Why, he thought, should he have these pains and feel so tired? It seemed to him that a good-looking young man should be strong, socially active, and motivated. Mr. Osman did not know what to do. When his friends recommended that he see a traditional healer (*hoca*), he did that, returning several times to the *hoca*. The healer performed various rituals to remove the influence of bad magic (*büyü*), and he gave him an amulet to place under his pillow at night. The amulet contained herbs and various other materials, but none of this helped.

C. Cultural Factors Related to Psychosocial Environment and Levels of Functioning

Social stressors. As an immigrant Mr. Osman had a difficult time adjusting to life in Switzerland. He felt disvalued as a foreigner, especially troubled by the low regard he thought his boss at the paper factory had for him. He was very upset by the difficulty of finding work as an electrician after completing his training and apprenticeship. Because of his depressive symptoms and pains, he was no longer socializing as much with friends and younger people with whom he had more in common; he became somewhat isolated. Instead of support at home, it seemed that his family and relatives did not understand these problems; they added to, rather than relieved, the social pressures that troubled him.

Social supports. While he was unemployed, his family provided financial support. This assistance and the support of his Turkish relatives provided a measure of security, both psychological and financial, but not without a price. They were uneasy about his efforts to interact with Swiss culture, and had some concern about this process, fearing it might lead to estrangement from his family and community. Their support, which they felt they were providing as they should, may have interfered with his efforts to integrate into Swiss society.

Levels of functioning and disability. In his everyday life Mr. Osman became increasingly socially isolated. At home he withdrew from family and relatives, and he had little contact with friends. It also became difficult to work on the short-term temporary jobs that were available to him.

D. Cultural Elements of the Clinician-Patient Relationship

Although he was able to speak German well and communicate with colleagues and doctors, he found it difficult to understand the logic of the treatment he was receiving. His language abilities, the way he dressed, and his apparent ease functioning in Swiss culture were misleading. His doctors, particularly his psychiatrists, appear not to have understood the impact of cultural influences on his illness experience, values, and expectations, and they did not understand the impact of their interventions or the way he interpreted them with reference to traditional Turkish values.

The second Swiss psychiatrist, whom Mr. Osman saw for nine months two to four times a month, made a diagnosis of depression and somatoform disorder. The therapist felt that the psychotherapy dealt only with superficial topics, and in his account of the treatment he emphasized Mr. Osman's passive-regressive features. Although the psychiatrist recognized a problem with authority figures, the therapy did not deal with that problem effectively. The therapy did not address the cultural meanings of the symptoms, the traditional attitude toward family relationships, or the particular effects of the illness on the family. The therapist felt frustrated by the difficulties he encountered. "I could not go any further with him," he explained, when asked about the patient. "I just didn't know what I should do."

Efforts to establish common goals and expectations in the therapy that the patient and therapist might agree on were stymied by a failure to consider and address differences in the values that motivated the work of the therapist, on the one hand, and shaped the perceived needs of Mr. Osman, on the other. Consequently, it was never clear to either party what the other expected. This might have been less of a problem for Mr. Osman, whose expectations of therapy were less clear and who was willing to go along with it, just as he was accustomed to following the directives from his father or elders. It was a greater source of frustration for the therapist, however, who was accustomed to establishing a shared agenda in his treatment of Swiss patients.

E. Overall Cultural Assessment

This case illustrates the complexity of illness experience of a young Turkish immigrant man and suggests practical implications and pitfalls in medical and psychiatric treatment. Inattention to and lack of appreciation of cultural values resulted in problems in communication and failure to recognize the coexistence of potentially conflicting traditional and Western cultural explanatory models. An appreciation of cultural values helps to explain the social context, particularly the psychological implications of the distribution of power in traditional Turkish families, like this one, and the socially distinctive responses to particular symptoms. Each of the following four factors significantly influenced the clinical presentation and treatment of Mr. Osman.

Problems in patient-doctor communications caused by ambiguous meaning of "nervous system." When the neurologist to whom Mr. Osman was referred let him know that the evaluation showed the absence of any problem with his nervous system, Mr. Osman understood this to mean that psychologically everything was okay. Even though he did not resist it, referral to a psychiatrist seemed inconsistent with the assessment. He did not question the authority of the referral and continued in treatment for nearly two years without a clear idea of how the treatment would benefit him. It never made much sense to him, and his therapist felt that Mr. Osman was passive, rather than fully engaged, in the therapy.

Coexistence of potentially conflicting traditional and Western cultural explanatory models. Because Mr. Osman had learned a trade and spoke German well, the psychiatrist considered him to be well integrated in Switzerland. He identified the following factors as causes of the illness: negative childhood experiences, separations from parents during childhood, family problems fostering dependency, diminished self-esteem, and narcissistic problems. He also recognized the impact of the difficult working conditions in the paper factory. The psychiatrist was unaware of traditional values that were important to Mr. Osman (such as the importance of not eating pork, even by mistake), difficulty adjusting to the climate, and the importance of fate and possibly magic. Mr. Osman—motivated by worsening depression and consideration of the role of fate and his father's concern about evil eye (*nazar*)—had also sought help from a traditional healer, which was not discussed in the psychotherapy.

Psychological implications of the distribution of power in traditional Turkish families. Mr. Osman was especially concerned about his relationship to his disapproving family. His father considered his emotional problems to be the reflection of a weak character, and perhaps some secret misbehavior. He said his son lacked courage and took no pleasure in life. Experience with rigid power hierarchies in his traditional family influenced the relationship between Mr. Osman and the therapist. The patient expected his own role was merely to listen, learn, and implement the lessons from the therapist, who was there to provide the answers. Although therapists may work with European and American patients with a similar passive style in therapy, the extent to which it is a feature of individual personality, rather than a reflection of cultural values, distinguishes such patients. Failure to appreciate the significance of the elevated status of the patient's father and elders generally in the family hierarchy resulted in insufficient attention in therapy to interpretation of transference, particularly the experience of the authoritarian role of therapist with reference not only to the presumed passive-regressive character structure of Mr. Osman, but also with reference to conflicting social contexts shaped by the influence of Turkish and Swiss cultural values.

Socially distinctive responses to particular symptoms: somatic pain and emotional distress. Mr. Osman distinguished two sets of problems. Those associated with pain symptoms were considered real and explained as the result of harsh working conditions and changes in climate and food. Emotional symptoms, however, such as sadness, fatigue, and weakness, did not really constitute an illness; in his view they were just a "simulation." Although the response to pain symptoms provided some support, because these constituted a "real" problem, his family viewed his other problems as evidence of moral weakness, the kind of problems that should not affect a young, handsome man. These harsh moral judgments of family and relatives contributed to feelings of diminished self-worth, which further exacerbated his depressive symptoms.

Appreciating the influence of these cultural values on what the therapist identified as a regressive, passive-dependent interpersonal style would have helped the therapist recognize the impact on Mr. Osman of his family's judgmental, dismissive view of depression. As a practical matter, this would indicate a potentially useful line of intervention as an alternative to the focus in the therapy on passive-dependence. To the extent that the psychodynamic formulation did not adequately consider the influence of family and culture, it reinforced the father's assessment of "character weakness." Insight-oriented therapy relies on the expectation that personal introspection will lead to adaptation and successful coping with difficult situations and personal problems. The usefulness of these assumptions, however, requires recognition of the role of cultural values and social context in bringing about successful coping and adaptation.

Depression is often associated with feelings of diminished self-worth, for which a social process of validation may be required to bring relief. Psychotherapy that emphasizes the role of individual introspection and insight without due consideration for the importance of these social processes and cultural values may lack credibility, particularly for patients who do not share the assumed values in which Euro-American psychotherapy is rooted. Failure to appreciate implications of conflicting cultural values may exacerbate a key dilemma, making it especially difficult for immigrant patients who are struggling to function in a world that requires them to accommodate traditional values emphasizing social relationships and the Western European values that emphasize the need for individualistic solutions. Therapy needs to be sensitive to this dilemma and address it. The experience of a therapist needs to be calibrated by considering this interaction of culture and individual. Distinguishing the relative influence of each is an ongoing process in the course of therapy, and it is an essential feature of a successful therapy that helps patients negotiate the requirements and constraints of distinctive cultural worlds. The cultural formulation enriched understanding of various aspects of clinical problems and indicated approaches to core issues that otherwise remain obscure and neglected.

20

Sakit Jiwa, *Ng(amuk)*, and Schizoaffective Disorder in a Javanese Woman

A Cultural Formulation

Kevin O. Browne

Clinical History

PATIENT IDENTIFICATION. Anik is a twenty-nine-year-old Javanese woman (interviews occurred during 1996; "Anik" is a pseudonym). She was born in a rural area about twenty kilometers east of the south-central Javanese city of Yogyakarta, and had lived in the city for four years. She had been married about a year and a half, but was very unhappy with her husband and family obligations. Because of her illness, Anik was unable to care for their eight-month-old daughter. She had hoped her mother would do so, but was told her mother was too old to care for a baby, so her daughter was being taken care of at the time by Anik's aunt in Jakarta. I first met Anik in the inpatient ward of a public mental hospital in Yogyakarta. She agreed to be interviewed after I explained my research into cultural aspects of mental illness experience and treatment in Java. I met with her sister-in-law six months later, and twice I met again with Anik herself, once seven months after the initial interview, and then a month after that. While Anik's first language is Javanese, she is also fluent in Indonesian. The interviews were conducted in Indonesian.

History of present illness. Anik said her current illness resulted from the stress of her marriage, the enormity of her family obligations, as well as being

From *Culture, Medicine, and Psychiatry* 25, no. 4, 411–25 (December 2001) with kind permission from Springer Science and Business Media

"startled" (*kaget*) by a harsh encounter with her landlady. Hospital intake notes also describe that her baby became ill after drinking an oil commonly used for household cleaning, which also served as a major stressor. Anik said the illness began six months after the birth of her daughter, that is, about two months before she was hospitalized. Anik described in some detail her situation and the events that precipitated her current symptoms, though the timeline she provided was vague. She was having marital conflict, describing a "lack of openness" and "compassion" from her husband, and she was very jealous and suspicious that he was having an extramarital affair. She said he was disappointed about her inability for a period of time to produce breast milk for their daughter. This, along with the stress of having to work at her job and take care of an extended household, caused her to become quiet and ruminative (*melamun*). She said she also became easily angered, such as when her house was messy and noisy, was quick to take offense, and sometimes slammed doors (*ngamuk*). She also reported feeling persistently sad, crying easily, feeling guilty, and having suicidal thoughts. Another precipitant was an incident when her landlady spoke harshly to her, which scared and startled her. She also described a distressing incident when she was six months pregnant, and a strange man entered her room at home and startled and disturbed her.

Anik said that at the beginning she considered it a "small" illness. She said it began when she became quiet and ruminative and then began to not sleep or eat. She also developed hallucinations (seemingly both auditory and visual), though the exact time frame in which these symptoms emerged was difficult to determine. My sense in talking with Anik and reviewing hospital accounts is that the hallucinations probably coincided with her social withdrawal and ruminative behavior, that is before the sleeplessness, loss of appetite, and other depressive symptoms, though how long before I could not determine. In general the voices Anik heard were accusatory toward her husband, his family, and their landlady, though they seemed to keep up a running commentary during our first interview as well.

It also appeared that Anik suffered from jealous delusions regarding her husband's supposed infidelity. While I have no evidence whether or not he was having an affair, both the hospital intake notes and Anik's sister-in-law report jealousy and suspicion of delusional intensity.

Anik claimed that these startle episodes frightened her and also caused her to remember her acute childhood fear when her mother was mentally ill. As a result of these stressors, she said she became fearful and irritable. Her sister-in-law reported that Anik had long been a quiet person who tended to be open about her problems, though sometimes sought attention through "overacting" her feelings. She said that recently, however, Anik got "angry without reason" nearly every day.

Anik was brought to the mental hospital by her brother, and had been there four days before I met her. Her clinical symptoms recorded on admission included *mondar-mandir* ("wandering without purpose"), *ngamuk*, being easily offended and suspicious, talking to herself, crying, insomnia, and *melamun* ("daydreaming"). Her affect was noted as "labile," and both visual and auditory hallucinations were noted. On admission her diagnosis was recorded as schizophrenia, paranoid type.

While in the hospital Anik was treated with antipsychotic medication, specifically chlorpromazine (100 mg three times a day) and haloperidol (1 mg three times a day). It is common, at least in the hospitals I am familiar with in this area of Java, for these two antipsychotic medications to be prescribed simultaneously. In addition, she was prescribed the antidepressant moclobomide (100 mg three times a day).

Anik also received a course of electroconvulsive therapy (ECT) (six treatments). Though there is some variation, in my observation of psychiatric practice in this and several other hospitals both in Yogyakarta and neighboring Central Java Provinces, ECT is routinely used to treat severely depressed, aggressive, as well as psychotic patients. A typical protocol was described to me by one psychiatrist as one or two treatments per day (up to three for depressed patients), usually three to six times total, with twenty-five to thirty being the maximum. In social and economic terms, ECT was seen by psychiatrists and often by families as desirable, as it tended to reduce symptoms more quickly and allow the patient to return home. At the time of this first interview, Anik had already received three treatments. Two days later (and after a fourth treatment) her status was noted as "improved." It is probable that her symptoms were more acute on admission than by the time I interviewed her. She did show some dullness during the interview, which may have been a side effect of the ECT treatments.

Depressive symptoms were prominent throughout her hospital stay, though there was no evidence of a manic or mixed state. Anik was discharged from the hospital after two weeks, with a designation of *sembuh sosial* ("socially recovered"), although there were continuing symptoms including poor insight, anxious speech, and "mimicry." Since it appeared she was no longer psychotic, I interpret this symptom of "mimicry" as indicative of Anik's ruminative anxiety, that is repeating words to herself, rather than as a sign of echolalia or echopraxia, as I had detected no signs of such catatonic symptoms. The discharge prognosis was stated as mixed. Her tendency toward introversion, along with the early onset and type of illness, pointed toward a poor prognosis, while her socioeconomic and family status, and the presence of psychosocial stressors, were considered better prognostic signs.

Psychiatric history and previous treatment. Anik had reportedly been experiencing significant distress since about age thirteen. During our last interview she admitted that she had "relapsed" four times since she first became ill. Her sister-in-law confirmed that Anik had experienced emotional stress and had been "apprehensive" since she was a teenager. Anik had been in the hospital on two previous occasions. The first time was in 1992, when, according to hospital records, she was admitted because of being *ngamuk* and "wandering without purpose." She was hospitalized for two weeks at that time, and discharged as *sembuh* ("recovered"). The second time was in 1994, when her symptoms included anxiety and jealousy. She was in the hospital for three weeks and again discharged as *sembuh.* From what I could learn of her clinical history, Anik had typically responded well to antipsychotic medication, and her psychotic symptoms seemed to be in full remission between these episodes.

In my experience with mental hospitals in Yogyakarta, the designations of *membaik* ("improved"), *sembuh*, and *sembuh sosial* can have a range of meanings, including that the family wants the person home or that finances have run out. This often means there has been a reduction in affective and psychotic symptoms, though there may still be significant impairment in cognitive and social functioning.

Social and developmental history. Anik is the sixth of seven children. She was born in an economically poor, mountainous rural area of Yogyakarta Province, some twenty kilometers east of the city. Both her parents are Javanese. Her father died when she was just out of high school, though he was living in Jakarta at that time. She does not know what caused his death. Her mother continued to live in the family home. Anik completed high school, and worked as a civil servant in one of the government administration offices in the city. She, along with her husband, daughter, nephew, and mother-in-law, rented a room in a neighborhood not far from her office. She said she did not have close friends. When asked, she could only name her husband, her brother, and the office supervisor as people with whom she felt close.

Family history. When Anik was a child (sixth grade of primary school), her mother was *gila* ("crazy") for a period of about three months. During this period her mother was often *ngamuk.* Anik described her mother's behavior as being "like a tiger," screaming, scratching, and striking people, including the children. Anik remembered being very frightened. She said her mother's illness occurred because of poverty and having to care for seven children. Her mother was first given traditional herbal remedies, and when they did not work was taken to the mental hospital, where she "recovered." Anik did not provide further details about the course of her mother's illness.

Mental state exam. Anik is a thin woman with a fragile-looking appearance. Her conversation style was quiet and shy at first, though she seemed to grow more comfortable as the interview progressed. Her speech was coherent though sometimes tangential. During the initial interview she was agitated and cried at several points, and expressed guilty thoughts. At subsequent meetings she was more calm but her composure seemed fragile, with a great deal of sadness beneath this calm exterior. During our interviews she did not express much anger, though one of the primary reasons she was brought to the hospital on this occasion was the expression of aggression and suspicion.

At our first meeting she seemed to be suffering from auditory hallucinations of an accusatory nature toward her husband, his family, and their landlady. Her attention sometimes wandered and she appeared to be "blocking," as if listening to other voices. She had some looseness of associations, at one point blurting out that my research assistant was an "angel," because her Muslim-style clothing was white and "radiant." Another time she began crying and said that I looked like her dead father. She did not express suicidal ideation at the initial interview, but both prior to and subsequent to this time did express such thoughts.

Anik's memory was mildly impaired at the initial interview, perhaps related to her lapses in concentration and auditory hallucinations, or perhaps because of the several ECT treatments she had just received. She offered contradictory information when recalling events, dates, and hospitalizations. Questions often needed to be repeated or rephrased. At subsequent meetings her memory improved.

Anik is of average intelligence. She had significant insight into the relationship between her mother's illness and her own, and into the conflict between cultural pressures to restrain her emotions and behavior and the strength of her personal feelings. Her insight into her current illness episode and her marital and personal situation was rather poor. She was able to develop good rapport.

Course and outcome. Six weeks after her discharge, Anik suffered a relapse and was again hospitalized. She was expressing suicidal thoughts, was talking and ruminating to herself, crying frequently, and had not slept for three days. In addition it was reported she was *ngamuk* (banging doors). Her sister-in-law added that Anik was so frequently performing Muslim prayers (*sholat*) that it was a cause of concern, and had asked to be taken to a Muslim boarding house (*pesantren*). She was suspicious and jealous, and her affect depressed. The admission lasted two weeks. Her discharge status was noted as "improved."

During each of my subsequent interviews with Anik she appeared emotionally fragile and admitted that she was easily upset, angered, and offended. Her speech, however, was coherent and logical, and I detected no evidence of thought blocking or other symptoms of psychosis. Her sister-in-law, however, said that since her discharge she looked pale and talked "randomly." On the occasion of our second interview she called me from the hospital where she had been waiting four hours already to have her prescription refilled. She said that she came once a month for a refill (she called it "*kontrol*"), and that her taking medication (chlorpromazine 100 mg three, times a day and haloperidol 1 mg twice a day) was now "routine," though her sister-in-law said this was not completely clear. Anik denied that she had relapsed since our first meeting, which was contradicted by hospital records and by her sister-in-law's account. Whether she was confused, forgot, or wanted to appear as "better" I cannot say. She reported that when offended she became quiet, and often went to the mosque to pray. She was now separated from her husband and living with her mother. She maintained that her husband did not understand her and that she wanted a divorce. She described her condition as "improved."

Our third meeting occurred at Anik's office. While she appeared sad and fragile, she seemed more composed. She said that what she needed was "compassion." At this time she was still living with her mother.

Diagnostic Formulation

Axis I:	295.70 RIO schizoaffective disorder, depressive type
Axis II:	None
Axis III:	None
Axis IV:	Birth of child
	Illness of child
	Marital stress
Axis V:	GAF = 30 (Current)
	GAF = 48 (Highest past year)

Differential Diagnosis. The past history I could obtain, along with my clinical impressions during the interview, suggest that a diagnosis of schizoaffective disorder, depressive type is most consistent with Anik's current symptoms. While it seems likely that her auditory and visual hallucinations emerged before her major depressive episode, this is not completely clear, nor is it clear that the time frame was at least two weeks prior. If the depressive symptoms in fact emerged first, then a diagnosis of major depressive disorder with psychotic features would be more appropriate.

Some of Anik's symptoms, such as irritability and increased religious activity, suggest the presence of a mixed episode, but she did not report sufficient manic symptoms to confirm this diagnosis. More detailed information about her past episodes is necessary to completely rule out by history a bipolar I or II disorder with recurrent psychotic features, presenting in a predominantly depressed state during the current episode.

It is also possible that she suffered from post-traumatic stress disorder (PTSD) with psychotic features. She reported strong fear and a threat to self during her mother's mental illness, as well as irritability relating to her recall of this stressor. She described that when she heard her landlady's harsh voice, she imagined her mother's screaming, but it is not clear whether such experiences constituted dissociative flashbacks. Nor is it clear how serious was the actual threat of harm during her mother's illness. She did not seem to have a sense of a foreshortened future, emotional numbing, nor detachment from others. Moreover, her startle response is a common occurrence in Javanese culture, where being surprised or startled is a frequent explanation of illness.

I also considered the possibility of a brief reactive psychosis. Given that the psychotic symptoms had apparently persisted for at least two months, however, this diagnosis must be rejected. Finally, it seems unlikely that her illness had a postpartum onset, given that the episode reportedly emerged about six months after the birth of her daughter, and that she claimed it was precipitated by factors other than this birth event. Given the uncertainty of the actual time frame involved, however, this possibility must also be considered.

Cultural Formulation

A. Cultural Identity

1. Cultural reference group. Anik is ethnically Javanese. The people of the Yogyakarta region of south-central Java pride themselves on being especially refined (*halus*) with regard to emotional expression and outward demeanor. This ideal of presenting a smooth and tranquil affect to the world has been noted by many ethnographers, such as Clifford Geertz, and is said to reflect inner calmness and spiritual attainment. Many of Anik's symptoms, such as anger, suspicion, and sadness, are likely to be viewed as pathological both in the community at large and by clinical personnel.

2. Language. Anik speaks Javanese as her first language. She is also fluent in the national language, Indonesian.

3. Cultural factors in development. Anik's perception of Javanese cultural ideals has influenced her illness, especially regarding emotion, aggression, and social connection. Her high emotionality, hostility, and "daydreaming" are considered symptoms of illness by Anik and others alike. When offended or angry, Anik tried to cope by becoming quiet. Though social withdrawal is also socially disapproved of, it is less stigmatized than anger and violence. Her desire to deal with her distress by being an "obedient" Muslim, praying regularly, and even requesting to live in a *pesantren*, reflect the strong influence of Islam in her perception of self, mental health, and sense of community.

4. Involvement with culture of origin. Anik and her family, like many Javanese both rural and urban, perceive a wide range of causes of mental illness. These include sorcery, spirit possession, stress, and the idea that it runs in families. Anik said she did not believe that evil spirits caused her mental illness, though she did link both her vulnerability to such illness and her recovery to the idea of religious piety. Like many others dealing with the exigencies of mental illness in the Yogyakarta area, however, Anik also sought alternative treatments, along with her religious efforts and psychiatric treatment, that often would not fit with the stated ideals of "modernist" Islam. Such alternative treatments for mental illness range from herbal preparations to prayer to the retrieval of lost souls, among other methods.

B. Cultural Explanations of the Illness

1. Predominant idioms of distress and local illness categories. Anik's description of her illness as *sakit jiwa* denotes a disturbance of mental and especially spiritual balance. While *sakit jiwa* can also refer to a range of anxiety or mood disturbances, it is very often applied to experiences that involve psychotic symptoms. While Anik's lament about her husband's lack of compassion and communication, and the enormity of her family obligations, are common complaints among Javanese women, her extreme reaction to her situation, in particular her hallucinations, delusional jealousy, and her *ngamuk* and *melamun* behavior, was considered evidence of psychosis.

Ngamuk is strongly associated with *sakit jiwa*, and is a dominant cultural marker of mental illness in Yogyakarta. It is a Javanese verb that can designate any form of loud, violent, or disruptive behavior. While such aggressive behavior is viewed by both clinicians and laypersons as a primary symptom of an emotional/spiritual self "not in order," the term is applied to persons in both psychotic and nonpsychotic states. While her family focused on this loud and threatening behavior, Anik identified more with her feelings of disappointment and loneliness.

In its application, which frequently includes women as well as men, *ngamuk* stands in contrast to the more restrictive clinical term *amuk*. *Amuk* is a noun and psychiatric term that references rare cases of extreme violence, which, according to the DSM-IV and many previous researchers, are said to be almost exclusively limited to men. In the global circulation of psychiatric knowledge, *amuk* has developed into a potent symbol of homicidal rage. Lucas and Barrett argue that as such a symbol of extreme violence, *amuk* in effect collapses categories of culture, person, and mental illness into a reductive icon of Malay/Javanese culture. Unlike *ngamuk*, it is a term that is rarely encountered in psychiatric hospitals or in everyday usage in Yogyakarta.

In Anik's situation her *ngamuk* behavior, apparently confined to slamming doors and loudly expressing resentment and suspicion, can be linked to her other depressive symptoms. Given the cultural premium on the suppression of both angry and sad affect in the service of a "smooth" presentation, when people experience overwhelming emotions the range of acceptable behaviors is very narrow. Many people, like Anik, seek to cope and to achieve smoothness through piety or social withdrawal, though they may experience serious symptoms of depression. In some instances, at moments of vulnerability these suppressed feelings may emerge in angry and/or threatening ways, and immediately be labeled as *ngamuk*. While in part, then, *ngamuk* can be seen as a response to cultural constraints on emotion and behavior, it is not reducible to that. As a discursive practice *ngamuk* also highlights pervasive social preoccupations and vulnerabilities with regard to emotional expression and social harmony.

An idiom that describes these feelings of anger, resentment, and depression is *sakit hati* (literally "liver sickness"). Anik used this term to describe the feeling she had when her landlady spoke harshly to her. *Sakit hati* may arise after feeling mistreated, being scorned by a lover, or from feelings of powerlessness. The experience of *sakit hati* is often accompanied by feelings of sadness, hopelessness, and social withdrawal, and sometimes substance abuse and suicidality.

Anik also admitted to frequently "daydreaming" (*melamun* or *merenung*), a term that refers to concentration lapses, whether in the sense of pleasant distracting thoughts, anxious ruminating, or dissociative states. *Melamun* is also strongly related to conceptions of mental illness in Yogyakarta. It is often said to make one have "empty thoughts," and renders one vulnerable to excessive emotionality or to being entered and possessed by evil spirits. I frequently heard people warned not to daydream, or they might become possessed. The admonition references Javanese preoccupations with always remaining conscious and aware, both as a means of spiritual attainment and to control one's emotions. Anik's tendency to withdraw and ruminate is seen by both clinicians and family members as a symptom of her continued vulnerability and illness.

Anik said *melamun* leads to a lack of concentration and then to confusion.

She said she began to *melamun* at the beginning of this episode, wondering "how things got this way," which caused her to feel sad. She engaged further in *melamun* in order to try to solve her problems, to try to become more quiet and pious.

2. *Meaning and severity of symptoms in relation to cultural norms.* The type of psychotic *sakit jiwa* such as Anik experienced is considered a very serious illness in Javanese society. With the importance of emotional and spiritual control in the delineation of social status, *sakit jiwa* is constitutive of a self that is "not in order," and psychosis is considered to be perhaps the greatest such disturbance. The stress placed on her marriage and other social relations is one indication of the seriousness of her illness. While *sakit jiwa* carries significant social stigma, there is also often community sympathy and tolerance of symptoms provided the behavior is not dangerous. The accommodation made by Anik's supervisor and coworkers reflects such acceptance of *sakit jiwa.* I encountered such occupational tolerance on many occasions during my research in Java. This ability to provide meaningful work conveys some cultural buffer for many suffering from such illnesses.

Anik's strong expression of sadness and resentment does not conform to the cultural ideal of a "smooth" affect. Her *ngamuk* behavior is viewed as one of the most prominent symptoms of *sakit jiwa* in the Yogyakarta area. In a community survey I conducted in two different neighborhoods, for example, *ngamuk* was the most prevalent characteristic of *sakit jiwa* mentioned, and a major reason why families would bring an ill family member to the hospital.

Anik lamented that communication with her husband had been lost, which caused her to feel lonely. Loneliness or social isolation is a deep concern to many Javanese, who see such isolation as a cause for pity and concern. Anik's desire to enter a *pesantren* may be interpreted as a means to express her piety, and a place to find compassion and the feeling of emotional and spiritual *kontrol* that she sought.

3. *Perceived causes and explanatory models.* Anik's explanatory model is that her *sakit jiwa* is attributable to her vulnerability, which derives from the stress of her mother's illness, her unhappy marriage, her baby becoming sick, and to the shock (*goncangan*) from her harsh encounter with her landlady. Being shocked or startled (*kaget*) is an idiom that is strongly associated in Javanese culture with illnesses such as soul loss or the condition of *latah.* It goes beyond this, however, reflecting the widespread experience of the self as vulnerable to harsh disturbances of the ideal calm, leading to a variety of illnesses, including psychosis. Anik mentioned that she was also *kaget* when her brother brought her to the mental hospital. The idea of being influenced by the stress from unexpected or harsh events or encounters reflects a com-

mon Javanese idea that some people are by nature weaker and more easily distressed by such events and therefore susceptible to mental affliction. Shock is thought to lead to disorganized thinking, lack of concentration, and to a general disturbance of self.

Anik admitted she was vulnerable to stress and to *kaget*. She said that this susceptibility derived from her exposure to the "stress," "panic," and "uproar" (*gara-gara*) of her mother's *sakit jiwa*. Anik said she too became ill, was influenced by that experience, and was fearful she would become as sick as her mother had been.

Anik said there was a lack of openness in her household and wished her husband was more straightforward. That is, she was frustrated about his lack of communication and wanted him to be more understanding of her needs. She said she had been disappointed in her marriage and wanted a divorce.

Anik saw herself as a strong Muslim, and said that she did not believe that evil spirits had anything to do with her illness. Anik's husband, however, believed her illness was caused by spirit influence, which is typically seen as a primary cause of *sakit jiwa*. She said her brother brought her to the hospital so that she "would not become possessed." Her symptoms, including hearing voices, *ngamuk*, *melamun*, and social withdrawal, are frequently associated with spirit possession or sorcery. Anik's overall assessment was that her "*kontrol jiwa*" ("mental/spiritual control") was "not in order." She said those who become *sakit jiwa* are people who don't want to follow their religion, and who "daydream" and lack concentration.

4. Help-seeking experiences and plans. Sakit jiwa is considered by most people in Yogyakarta to be primarily a spiritual illness, and the first treatment choice of families there is usually to seek some type of "alternative" or spiritual treatment. While Anik denied that evil spirits were involved in her illness, she did strongly embrace the idea that her illness was spiritual in origin, and on several occasions she sought alternative treatments for her illness apart from the psychiatric.

Between our first and second meetings Anik sought the help of three alternative healers. The first was a thirty-five-year-old Muslim woman, whose treatment consisted of saying prayers over water, which was then given to Anik to drink. She said there was no change as a result. The second healer was an older Muslim man. He gave Anik a piece of coconut tied with paper, to be carried with her. She was then told to bite the coconut and then throw it away. She had this treatment three times but felt no change.

The third healer was a forty-year-old Christian man, and this time Anik fell the treatment was more effective. She was again given blessed water along with paper on which were written prayers in an Arabic-like script locally known as *bintang rajah*, a kind of mystical writing used by some healers in the area. The water was to be taken to her house for two weeks. She was then instructed to drink the water, and her hands and scalp were also massaged. On another visit she was told to cook and eat a rooster in order to find out the kind of evil spirit that was bothering her. Finally, she was instructed to perform *sholat tahajud* (to pray at midnight) for seven nights in a row while reading Koranic verses. After these treatments Anik said she felt calm and had not been *ngamuk* or easily angered since then. She held to her belief that spirits were not the cause of her illness, and thought perhaps part of this improvement derived from a suggestion from within herself to feel calm, that is, to consider the blessed water to be like medicine.

Anik also continued to take anti-psychotic medication. She described her visits to get this medication at the hospital pharmacy as *kontrol*. This idiom is pervasive among patients and families seeking follow-up psychiatric care. It refers not only to visits to obtain medication, but also a state of being "in control" of oneself, that is, not overly emotional or psychotic. For Anik, *kontrol* was seen both as a relief from symptoms and hope for spiritual health. As an emblem of psychiatric knowledge and practice, *kontrol* also exacts a conformity of standards and discourse, and a measure of compliance, producing an ideal of mental health and a routinization of medication visits.

C. Cultural Factors Related to Psychosocial Environment and Levels of Functioning

1. Social stressors. Anik's illness, along with her jealousy and suspicion of her husband, was a matter of considerable social embarrassment. While divorce is fairly common in Javanese society, the apparent dissolution of her marriage led Anik to return to her mother's rural home to live. As a result, she had to take a public bus two and one-half hours each way to work.

2. Social support. Both Anik and her sister-in-law report that Anik had a good relationship with her mother. While she said she missed her husband, her insistence on a divorce would mean further social isolation and lack of support. She did derive social and financial support from her job, where she was given wide leeway to work (or not) as she was able. She had a good relationship with her sister-in-law as well. Otherwise she was not able to name any good friends, and appeared to be fairly socially isolated.

3. Levels of functioning and disability. Anik was generally able to work, unless she was ill. She was able to continue to work at her job despite her illness because her supervisor and coworkers understood her difficulties and allowed her to miss work when needed, and did not require more of her than she could do. Although she had had several relapses in the last few years, she was apparently not in danger of losing her job. In between these periods she seemed to function reasonably well. At the time of our second and third interviews she appeared fragile though personable and coherent. Her psychosis and suspiciousness appeared to signal the end of her marriage, and she felt a certain hopelessness about the future. She described her hope for the future as to be able to care for her daughter again and to be *iman* ("pious").

4. Cultural elements of the clinician-patient relationship. Given the cultural premium on affective and social "smoothness," strong emotional expressions, *ngamuk* behavior, and social withdrawal tend to be pathologized by Javanese psychiatrists and other clinical staff. Anik's crying on the hospital ward and expressions of resentment elicited nervous reactions from the nursing staff.

According to her hospital chart, clinical staff also conducted at least one outpatient psychotherapy session with Anik to address aspects of her depression and marital problems, which suggests that her prognosis was considered better than that of many patients. When I observed it, such psychotherapy was usually brief and seemed to reinforce Javanese cultural norms, often taking the form of advice about acceptance of one's difficult situation and the importance of ongoing medication use.

My relationship with Anik was affected both by my status as a foreign researcher, as well as by my appearance that reminded her of her dead father. My sense is that she felt a mixture of hope, sadness, and vulnerability through our association. My interest in hearing her story was clearly unusual compared to the hospital staff, who focused on reducing her symptoms. Her crying and confusion during the initial interview made clarifying her history and situation more difficult. She called me from the hospital to arrange our second interview, however, and at these subsequent meetings she seemed more clear and eager to talk with me, perhaps feeling some benefit or anxiety reduction through our conversations.

5. Overall cultural assessment. Anik presented many of the symptoms of a recurrent psychotic illness that responded well to medication, as well as those of a current major depressive episode. Her experience of *sakit jiwa* and the relationships in which it occurred highlight not only the cultural elements that shape her illness but also some of the dilemmas of constructing a psychiatric diagnosis in Yogyakarta. This cultural influence in the development of her symptoms can be seen most strongly in the conflicting pressures she felt to express her personal feelings—anger, sadness, and disappointment—on the one hand, and cultural preoccupations with emotional restraint and behavioral control, and the presentation of a "smooth" affect, on the other. Anik herself is acutely aware of these contradictions, expressing guilt about her illness while also partly blaming Javanese social and gendered constraints, such as her family burdens and her husband's lack of compassion, for her illness.

In Javanese society there are very few viable options to express and resolve such strong emotions. There is pressure to accept her fate with regard to social and family obligations, that is, to uphold gender and other cultural norms. Anik's tactic for dealing with these burdens was to become quiet and withdrawn, but these behaviors are also seen culturally as problems. Her psychotic behavior, suspiciousness, and depression have also led to significant stigma, marital problems, social isolation, and loneliness.

Anik's story centers around several key Javanese idioms of mental health and illness. Her *ngamuk* behavior practically guarantees a designation of *gila* or *sakit jiwa* and a family intervention. Her experience of *melamun* is taken both as a sign of her weakness and vulnerability to illness or spirit attack, as well as a continuing symptom. And her invocation of *kaget* as a causative factor is utilized to explain the illness and evoke sympathy, but is also seen as a sign of personal weakness.

This cultural premium on affective smoothness, broadly shared by clinical staff, patients, and family members, affects the treatment and diagnosis of patients. Economic limitations, along with a desire to reduce affective symptoms rapidly, results in most patients receiving ECT. Symptoms such as Anik experienced could also shape a number of diagnoses. *Ngamuk* and *melamum* are noted as serious symptoms on many hospital charts as well as invoked by families, but as broad markers of a social preoccupation they do not translate into precise diagnostic categories, and may indicate a range of psychotic and mood disorders. Moreover, an overemphasis on *ngamuk*, for instance, may obscure other symptoms or facets of a patient's history or social situation. In Anik's case, for example, a lack of attention to her sense of personal and social vulnerability and history of trauma make a consideration of PTSD very difficult.

Acknowledgments

I would like to thank the Indonesian Institute of Sciences (LIPI) for granting permission for this research, and the Center for Southeast Asian Studies at the University of Wisconsin–Madison for a Research Travel Grant. I also wish to thank Rita Eka Izzaty and Esthi Damayati for their invaluable assistance with this research, and the hospital staff who made these interviews possible. Special gratitude goes to "Anik" for her indulgence and patience with my questions. I would also like to thank Roberto Lewis-Fernández and the anonymous reviewers of this article for their very helpful comments.

Index